PRAISE FOR DETOX NOURISH ACTIVATE

In these volatile and difficult times many are looking to complementary healing modalities to assist in achieving optimum physical, emotional, mental and spiritual well being. *Detox Nourish Activate* explores healing dis-ease at the root level. Packed with information, meditations, and plant based formulas, this book should be on the bookshelves of every lightworker.

Steve Nobel, Author, Spiritual Coach and Founder of the Soul Matrix Healing System.

Healing is a process without a direct trajectory or a one-size fits all solution. Luckily, *Detox Nourish Activate* serves as a playbook and in depth workbook that will help each person who reads it discover their own unique nature and heal the core blockages to wellness and freedom. No book I've come across encmopasses such an eclectic approach to healing and self actualization.

Blake Myers, ND, Physician, Teacher, Author of *The Natural Apothecary*.

Detox Nourish Activate is an impressive and exciting book of information as well as experientials to guide one on a deep and profound journey of healing at all the levels of our being: physical, mental – emotional and spiritual. For those who want to work on healing themselves outside of or complementary to the allopathic paradigm, this is the book to accompany you on that journey. This is also a great book for those who just want more out of life and want to live life to their fullest capacity.

Lisa VanOstrand, President Barbara Brennan School of Healing.

Adora Winquist is a plant whisperer who teaches us how to understand plant languages for our own specific health issues. Her new book, *Detox Nourish Activate* is a treasure trove and a wonderful guide for authentic self-care.

Mary Bemis, Founder, Insider's Guide to Spas.

Detox Nourish Activate is a groundbreaking book that inspires the reader to take charge of their physical, emotional, mental, and spiritual well-being with a powerful integrative approach for sustainable health and vitality. LuLu Shimek, ND and Adora Winquist masterfully interweave years of wisdom, expertise and experience, while offering the reader a guide for self-empowerment to overcome the health challenges of today.

Donna Evans Strauss, Author, Senior Faculty, Barbara Brennan School of Healing.

The authors of *Detox Nourish Activate* aims to empower readers to "unlock the unlimited healing powers" held within us. This book is a great self help tool for everyone interested in seeing and acting beyond the ordinary.

Nasrin Safai, Author, Mindfulness Coach, and Spiritual Teacher.

The information contained in this book is for the reader to make life altering changes by not continuing to repeat the same patterns. A passage from the book "everything you need to live the life of your dreams is within you." The answers are contained in the words from the authors. Making these life altering changes requires a person to heal at the subconscious level. Learning to connect with your authentic self and grow into your truth as a divine being of light is the challenge. This book gives you the answers you need. Happy Reading.

Robert Allen Walls, President of Inner Search Foundation, Author, Publisher, Teacher, Healer.

Detox Nourish Activate speaks of the infinite possibilities of health, peace, and joy that is attainable to all seekers. Adora and Dr. LuLu are undoubtedly long practicing experts in their fields, with vast knowledge beyond what we learn in the everyday world. This book is anything but ordinary and deserves to be picked up, explored and implemented. It takes you to a comprehensive depth with the invitation to take back the power of your health, your life and your ultimate freedom.

Kristin Rocco, Yoga Teacher, Author of *50 Days of Grace*, Owner of Breathing Web Farms.

Whether you're just beginning to tap into the wisdom of vibrational medicine or are an avid practitioner, this book offers a wholesome, practical step-by-step process to identify key areas for healing the emotional, spiritual, and physical aspects of dis-ease. Adora and Dr. LuLu offer compassionate, integral, and resourceful guidance that is beautifully reinforced with illustrations, diagrams, and meditations that welcome you to connect and receive the botanical, the crystal, and the animal kingdoms as your silent benefactors on your path of self-healing and transformation. This book will become your ally for each new layer of your evolution.

Patsy Balacchi, Feng Shui Consultant & Energy Healer, Creator of Zenotica.

This book couldn't be better timed, as we now know that our DNA does not solely determine the health we will experience. The *Detox, Nourish, Activate* book shares how we can empower and optimize our DNA through powerful tools, techniques and lifestyle changes, many of which are all shared. This book invites you to take a whole person approach to clearing away that which no longer serves your health in your mind, body, heart and spirit. Thanks to this book you have the tools to enable you to effectively nourish and replenish your energy in order to activate your optimal health. The time to begin transforming your health and wellbeing is now, happy reading!

Dr. Rachel Dew, Doctor of Natural & Integrative Medicine, Author of *Healing the Total Self* and CEO of ModiHealth.

DETOX NOURISH ACTIVATE

DETOX NOURISH ACTIVATE
Plant & Vibrational Medicine for Energy, Mood & Love

LuLu Shimek, ND and Adora Winquist

AEON

First published in 2021 by
Aeon Books
PO Box 76401
London W5 9RG

Cover Design and Illustrations by Patsy Balacchi, USA

British Library Cataloguing in Publication Data

A C.I.P. for this book is available from the British Library

ISBN-13: 978-1-91280-796-3

Typeset by Medlar Publishing Solutions Pvt Ltd, India

www.aeonbooks.co.uk

Loving Disclaimer: The formula and treatment information contained in this book is not meant to take the place of direct medical advice, but rather, as an educational and informational resource on your personal healing journey Although the dosages and recommendations through-out the book are generally safe adult doses, readers should always con-sult with a medical professional regarding their current health. This will ensure that any health decisions you make are not only in your best interests but also are safe with medications or supplements you make currently. Readers who fail to consult any appropriate health providers do so at their own risk of injury or harm. The authors and publisher bear no responsibility for errors or omissions.

DEDICATION

We offer this book to all seekers on the path of health, wholeness, and freedom. May these pages of wisdom offer a guide to deepen self understanding and the ability to transform your life into one of love, happiness and infinite energy.

It is with great gratitude that we offer a blessing to both of the lineages seeded within our DNA, to bring this divine knowledge forward for the benevolence of human evolution.

We pledge our devotion and mission to the activation of the ancient wisdom of the plant, animal and mineral kingdoms that has been forgotten. May this book ignite the deep knowledge innate within all of humanity for the healing and renewal of our sacred planet.

"Dare to declare who you are. It is not far from the shores of silence to the boundaries of speech. The path is not long, but the way is deep. You must not only walk there; you must be prepared to leap."

– Hildegard of Bingen

"You stand with one foot in the physically based reality, and the other in the spiritually based reality. What is in between, is the solid ground of your core."

– Barbara Brennan (Heyoan)

TABLE OF CONTENTS

FOREWORD

From the moment I started reading this book I recognized that it is much more than what I imagined it to be. The authors have gone far beyond what one could imagine on a topic that is already vast. The focus is clearly to interact with the book through integrated healing and a personalized journey of taking back your life through multiple modalities relating to health and wellbeing. It begs you to ask what is next and how do I get there to reset the clock and unlock the power within knowing that you are much more than your thoughts, memories, pain and suffering and beyond living in survival mode.

The book starts off with some poignant questions we do not often like to ask since we may not want to know the answers. There is always a fear that we may find out that our whole existence may not reflect who we really are. This confronts the reader to look within and then to continue onward. It invites you to see yourself exactly where you are, knowing that everything you have done has brought you to this moment. This is a reassuring start and a sign that you are in the right place with thoughts of a life of unlimited possibilities; seeing who you really are is not always who you have become. You are taken through a journey of your own evolving self.

To achieve this the premise is simple: detox, nourish, activate, and heal yourself from your past, present and future through a clearing and reversing of the cellular damage in your genetic DNA. After all, DNA stores the memory imprints of physical, emotional, mental, and spiritual trauma. In some respects, it involves reverse engineering your life backwards and forwards to a place where trauma is cleared to regain your life force in order to align with your destiny. Detoxing, not just of the body, but in the letting go of everything that is no longer needed or desired.

When I first met Adora, over twenty years ago, I felt that I had known her well before I knew her and like a labyrinth heading towards the center, we collided while on an aromatic tour of southern India. In one moment of opening myself to nature, in its purest form, I was met with an equal force of love from my divine opposite. In our twenty-year journey as friends and colleagues I have witnessed firsthand her evolving, self-rising and falling only to reappear in a new version of herself, integrated through incredible hardship and loss. Like a plant, she has grown, learned, distilled, and re-emerged from the ashes in a new form and where each time more of her greatness has been revealed. She is clearly one of the world's authorities in vibrational medicine and she clearly practices what she teaches.

I met Dr. Lulu for dinner in a cozy French restaurant in the heart of London. From the first moment I sensed her extensive wisdom and playfulness in a way that she sees the world in its beauty and magic. I was immediately captured by her brightness, quick wit and her core passion for health and physical well-being. Her masterful approach to healing encompasses leading edge genetic medicine, intertwined with the versatility of herbal therapeutics to offer a unique insight to restoring vitality. Dr. Lulu's passion and dedication in the world of healing shines brightly through her work. Her path of healing is recognized through her commitment to DNA level healing.

Adora and Dr. Lulu clearly want you to be active participants as part of their journey. They weave their own personal healing stories of recovery into the mix, a process that gets you to see them as real and authentic teachers who clearly walk the same path as they teach. On the one side, the book is very logical, specific, instructional, and informative and on the other it is energetic, alchemical, and magical. The path is to resolve trauma and to claim back what is rightfully yours—your health and well-being, in a playful and interactive format. It is easy to read and comprehend and nudges the reader to dive deep and absorb a lifetime of information in one sitting. It is a recovery manual where I clearly learned something about myself in the process. The result, being a journey within of listening and rediscovering my own passion and life purpose through the silence of connecting my heart to the unknown parts of me found in my DNA.

In almost 40 years of my commitment to healing and vibrational medicine, I have concluded that the topic is far too great a subject to understand in a lifetime. Truth be told, I have understood more than I have integrated. It is my conclusion that it is not what we know that transcends us to greatness, but how we live our life based on the direct action that we take. What I have discovered is that we are far greater than anything we know or have learned. From our genetic past and need to connect with a higher power is a desire to be heart awakened and not so mentally driven. I recognize that without change everything around us, including ourselves, withers on the vine and what is ignored will undoubtedly come back to haunt us. What we think is the truth is often the opposite and when we are still, everything is revealed on a need-to-know basis when the time is right. From the unconscious to the conscious, from DNA to life well beyond the physical; from the need to know everything to being in the moment; we often do not have any answers to the questions that confront our very existence. From quantum physics to quantum mechanics there is nothing that is off limits when it comes to the mysteries of the universe. Yet, life is clearly passing us by, and we are often none the wiser.

And then there is plant-based healing and vibrational medicine where all the questions have answers that can be found in the life of plants: from their physical chemistry, color, odor, aroma shape, location, extraction, and vibration that cannot always be seen but can surely be felt. Plants have existed from the very beginning of time to the present and they hold the answer to where we have come from and where we are heading. They have adapted, transmuted, distilled themselves, evolved and hold the answers to life's biggest mysteries of why we are here, what we need to know and how to change. However, plants do not speak our language and instead communicate through their entire being made up of matter and a complex chemistry containing thousands of constituents. All one needs to do is to observe everything a plant is by recognizing that like humans, plants are an expression of the natural world for us to use in diluted or concentrated form. To pay attention to what we see and what cannot be seen that can only be felt when we feel the vibrations within our hearts. Like us, plants are whole, and every part of their existence has meaning.

This book connects to the reader not just in words but through directions, empowering diagrams, exercises, making of aromatic blends, light wheels, and continues to connect beyond the pages into online meditations. What is described is clearly more than just the physical and involves the emotional and spiritual as well as a necessary change in our internal chemistry through a connection to the heart, the body, the earth and to higher states of consciousness. This is beyond esoteric beliefs and the focus is clearly on what it takes to detox, nourish, and activate the heart, adrenals, and the brain. These three organs are vital to how we feel regarding our vitality, moods, how we see the world and the need to reboot and recharge. Solutions are offered to these organs through aromatherapy, botanical medicine, light wheels, crystals, stones, energetic and vibrational techniques, flower and gem essences, alchemy, recipes, intentions, meditation mudras, sacred spaces, rituals, sacred geometry, and nutrition. In short, the merging with the plants, minerals, medicine, magic, and aromatic interventions. All represent love and how it interweaves into all aspects of our lives through what can be found in nature and beyond.

Michael Scholes
Botanical Formulator and Owner of the Laboratory of Flowers

ACKNOWLEDGEMENTS

At first glance, it is impossible to fully decipher the myriad of possibilities contained within an idea. When we first discussed the writing of this book, our original concept appeared much more simplistic. The further we immersed ourselves into the writing journey the more voluminous and expansive it became. What first began as a synergy of aromatherapy and botanical medicine quickly evolved to intertwine other interventions of divine knowledge and medicine from the animal and mineral kingdoms. There was and is so much more to be shared.

We thank the spirit kingdoms of the plants, minerals and animals for their wisdom and transmission. To spend time in stillness was incredibly potent and allowed us to hear their stories filled with universal truth and healing energy.

We express our gratitude for healing and teachings that came through our own DNA and our family blood lines seeded from our parents and many previous generations. We thank all of the teachers past, present and future for their higher knowledge, patience, love, and spiritual growth. We are eternally grateful as it has brought us here, now.

We thank our creative director, Patsy Balacchi, for the brilliance of the cover and illustrations, especially the Freedom Photon Wheel. She is a true visionary and master of intuitive design and evolved the vision for the book cover and exceeded our expectations tenfold.

Thank you to Oliver Rathbone and the Aeon Team. Meeting you in London was incredibly auspicious. We appreciate your guidance and patience with co-authoring this book. Your dedication to bringing new works to the field of natural and alternative medicine is beautiful to witness.

We offer gratitude to each other as colleagues and writing partners, as we have lived the journey that is written upon these pages. It has been a fulfilling journey and the work is even more magnificent than we envisioned.

I, Adora, would like to thank first my parents Richard and Patricia for all their love, care and life lessons. I would also like to express my gratitude for the Infinity Team and specifically the brilliant members of my design team that work on the illustrations: Ahliyah Gavin, Lila Beavers, Wiralpach Nawabutsitthirat, and N'Dia Allen. Your passion and creativity is inspirational. I am deeply grateful to Dr. Dava Michelson for her curation of the acupressure points based on Five Element Acupuncture in our Essential Oil Based Tapping protocols to Detox, Nourish and Activate each bodily system. Her vast breadth of work and practice spanning three decades lends a tremendous depth of wisdom and knowledge for this unique intervention. Thank you to all of my friends that supported me and my children during the writing of the manuscript. It consumed me in ways I could not have anticipated, and I was often in a reverie that seemed to place me between time, space and dimensions. Love and gratitude to my daughters, Lillyan and Violet. You are both my gems and beautiful teachers of wisdom and truth. I know that as I continue along my own healing journey, you will also shift and heal deeply. To my beloved John, your love, support and deep understanding of me is one of the greatest gifts and healings of my life.

I, Dr. LuLu, first in deep gratitude, thank my dear parents, Sarah and Brent, for bringing my soul into this world, loving me unconditionally and nurturing my unending desires for individuality and determination to make a difference on this beautiful planet. Second, I thank my dear husband, Dave, the journey through writing this book was an adventure of my own self discovery and you lovingly supported me every step of the way. I am forever grateful for you, making me laugh and find the joy in every moment. I thank all of my friends, teachers, guides, mentors, and universities for igniting the path within me of a healer and physician. I lastly honor my plant allies for reconnecting with me in this lifetime and for providing the profound healing wisdom within this book.

WE WELCOME ALL OF YOU AND THE ALL OF ALL OF YOU

If you have picked up this book, we are thrilled that YOU have taken the initiative and realized that your whole health is the key to unlocking the door to your freedom. Have you been feeling like you have been traveling down a road and now you have reached a dead end? Or maybe you lay in bed and think life must be better than this. What if I could just get out of bed today feeling energized, not wanting to crawl back under the covers and just give up! Perhaps you hear a voice within hinting that there is some other and greater purpose for you.? Well, you are not alone, phew! We have helped countless patients and clients find their freedom and rewrite their health story by healing and unlocking or activating their DNA.

We would like to offer this book to you as an invitation to see beyond the limitation of your current sight, to open yourself to fully feel the exquisiteness of being completely alive, loved, and whole. We invite you to allow the rich abundance that is your birthright to flood every cell, molecule, and particle within your body and to experience the satiation of what is possible in living life beyond limitations. We beckon you to break free of the constraints and constriction of this third dimensional reality of pain, struggle, and negativity, sometimes referred to as the "matrix," to the multidimensional creative nature of your being that exists here and now and in every moment.

The truth is that YOU and every person on the face of this beautiful planet have a unique light and gift, and every moment of your life thus far has prepared you perfectly for this moment. It is often what seems like breakdown, which ultimately becomes *breakthrough*. Often, our deepest physical or emotional and spiritual challenges and pain lead us to our greatest strength and talents. It is this process that lends itself to the inner alchemy of distilling our own "quintessence."

Now take a moment, close your eyes, and take a deep breath. If you had a "secret power" to unlock your unlimited healing potential, what would it be? Who would you be? We are asking you to DREAM BIG! There is nothing holding you back from expressing your biggest self. So, put on those tights and cape because it's time to embrace your inner superhero! Follow your passion, invite in your greatest purpose and open your mind, heart, and soul to find and follow your inner voice. What you can create is truly a life beyond your wildest dreams.

In this book, you will discover how to unlock or activate the power in your DNA, to heal and transform the places in your being that are calling to you, with simple yet profound tools. We are the ones we have been waiting for! The cycle of staying and playing small, shrinking and diffusing your light is complete. Bless it, open and RISE!

Your Infinite Health Is Your Freedom

As we write this introduction, we stand at an unprecedented time on Mother Earth. The entire planet and all kingdoms of life, including the human race are experiencing a pause and a reset – an invitation to seek the "Temple of the Beloved" within, the source of divine consciousness that exists above and below and infinitely around us. We stand at this threshold to query the depths of our being: Who am I? Why am I here? Where have I been? What is my high path, my true path? What truth is begging to come to the surface of my consciousness? What is next – for me personally? In my relationships? My communities? The human race?

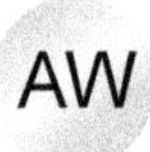

Through the writing of this manuscript, I was guided to go through the journals I have been keeping from the past two plus decades as a healer, teacher, student, formulator, and seeker. I was struck by the common theme or message through my writing and the subsequent sessions and programs created during these years: the quest for freedom. Through my personal journey of healing, I was paving the pathway for my own sovereignty to emerge. Through all the levels of pain and suffering, there was a place of driving certainty and a fervent commitment to the quest. Who was I really, after all the layers of family dynamics were peeled away? How could I fully express who I was without the need for approval or acceptance? What would it be like to live in abundance versus lack? What if my decisions were no longer based on base survival? Ultimately, what does it mean to truly be free?

We are collectively in the void; everything we thought as being certain, no longer is. Nothing is finite and everything is in flux. The beauty of this void, or as you will see it written throughout these pages as the zero-point field, is that all creative potential is possible here, it is limitless. Anything and everything can be transformed, recreated, and born anew.

We invite you to ponder these questions wholeheartedly and to breathe into the places where you feel fully free so that they may expand. To the places within that are bumpy or sharp as you ask these questions, may all the breath gently move through you so that new awareness and shift may unfold with ease and grace.

Do I feel free to fully express myself and move unhindered by the limitation and constriction of the third dimensional matrix?

Do I feel free to live, love, and love myself completely without guilt, shame, self judgement, or uncertainty?

Am I living free from survival mode of not having enough money, love, or fulfillment?

Do I feel free to live the life of my dreams? Not my mother's or father's dream for me or for themselves. Not my spouse's or society's dream for me. Am I living the dream that comes from deep in my soul?

Do I feel free to rest, relax, to settle and "be" without doing, working, or justifying my worth in some way?

Do I feel light, joyous, invigorated with the spark of youthful innocence and life force?

Do I feel free to believe in myself no matter what, regardless of what others think of me?

Yes, these are some rather BIG questions, AND this is the perfect time to dream as BIG as YOU CAN.

We developed a three-step process called *Detox. Nourish. Activate*© to heal the DNA on a physical, emotional, and spiritual level to ignite the healing power within every cell. Our cells experience dysfunction or mutation from many factors including but not limited to: environment, heritage, emotions, conception, trauma, stress, and many, many more. These cellular changes affect every aspect of our life and when not addressed continue to cause deeper damage. If you think of the inside of your cell, it's filled with many, many organelles or aspects for cleaning, energy, and providing nutrients to the body. Did you know that you have trillions and trillions of cells in that miracle of a body you walk around with every day? That is the real deal we will come back to and expound upon shortly.

Your cells represent your life force or stream of energy running through the body, and when the cells are toxic or malfunctioning the whole system starts to fail. Mayday, Mayday – the system is failing, are you listening? Sometimes you might not notice the body's messages to you, "system error," but then finally your body sends a louder message which you finally hear and take notice of.

The *Detox. Nourish. Activate* system is designed to not only address areas of distress in the body but to heal damage and trauma that has been in your body and energy field in this lifetime and many generations back. You are the microcosm for the macrocosm of your DNA and genetic heritage. When you bring healing and transformation to yourself, you bring it past, present, and future to your genetic line and every person you are in a relationship with. From a planetary and cosmic perspective, when we heal at the DNA level, this clearing gets posted on the grid for our entire species for planet Earth, the web of life, one person at a time. As this shifts the planetary grid it lifts vibration for every member of that species.

Have you ever heard of the hundredth monkey phenomenon? Essentially, when approximately the hundredth monkey of a species learns a new habit, what could be considered critical mass, then the entire species makes this leap of consciousness. What a powerful reminder to our connectivity in the web of life. We can similarly view this opportunity from the human perspective, that when we receive a certain level of critical mass in our awakening, we also quantum leap our collective consciousness. The micro perpetuates the macro and vice versa.

HOW TO USE THIS BOOK AS YOUR TRANSFORMATIONAL GUIDE

Throughout this book you will discover diagrams within each chapter to empower YOU and give you the tools to heal and obtain optimum health and well-being. This book is divided into three systems: heart, adrenals, and brain, which we discovered were at the seat or root of all core dysfunction. These physical aspects of the body also correspond to three primary energy systems or chakras: heart, root, and crown.

Your heart represents your connection to each other, to humanity and holds all your relational experiences and beliefs. It is only with an open heart that we may experience the true richness of life and love. The adrenal system is connected to the root chakra which represents your connection to the Earth, your sense of belonging on the planet, in your family of origin and your physical body. This healthy connection is paramount to be able to receive the nourishment and abundance of Mother Earth. Your brain represents your relationship to the Divine and your ability to connect with higher states of consciousness and knowing. It is one of the greatest gifts of humanity as it allows us to receive high level concepts and execute them to form (with the assistance of course of our Earth and other primary connections). The balance of our brain chemistry is instrumental to how we think, feel, act, react and a myriad of other brilliant aspects to thriving in this earthly realm. These three organs correspond to our primary energy vortexes that we perceive and navigate life through.

At the beginning of each system, there is a *Freedom Photon Wheel* for using all the sacred alchemical interventions for each system including aromatherapy, herbs, and crystals, and much more. You will discover within the system the power to heal areas of distortion, dysfunction, and trauma. At the end of each system, there will be another *Freedom Photon Wheel Ritual* for you to activate and assimilate the healing paradigm shifts you have excavated within that system.

Each organ system then has two diagrams. The first diagram shows the location and physiology of the organ system as well as the connection to disease states. The second diagram shows the energetic components of the organ system and the psycho-spiritual connections to trauma contributing to mental (thoughtform), emotional (feelings), and spiritual (belief system) distortion or misalignment.

Discovery Dives are in each section of the book to guide you deeper into awareness, healing, and transformation. Also, within each section there are links to guided meditations online for complete integrated healing.

As you navigate through the coming chapters to completion of this manuscript, keep an eye peeled for signs, symbols, your dream states, the people that appear in your life, miracles that find expression in your day to day, and how your health and happiness evolves in greater ways. This is more than a book; it is a revolutionary journey of your rebirth into a life of self-mastery.

The Journey of a Superhero – You Have to Go Through It to Get to It

We often have unrealistic expectations, of ourselves and others. This creates resistance and enforces old patterns of struggle, disappointment, and failure. Have you ever wanted, or strived for something greater in your life, and dove towards it falling short? You are not alone. We all have this place within. It's OK, together we can learn how to fail forward, learn from the past, and soar freely towards the future. You cannot bypass your pain, whether physical, emotional, or spiritual.

The only way out is through. AW This was an often-repeated phrase at the Brennan School when I attended. It was a gentle reminder that the process of healing and transformation requires a certain level of emotional acknowledgement for sustainable change. It is not solely a decision we choose at the level of the mind, and with that decision we are free from our pain and suffering. Nor is it a process of getting stuck in the trauma emotionally and continuing to re-wound ourselves. We have come here to learn how to use our entire beings: our mind as well as our emotions, our physicality, strength, and determination, AND our vast spiritual connection, our vision for a greater life, healthier relationships and dreams as big as the stars. Moving through the heaviness of the emotional debris connected to our pain allows us to create a new path. This is not an invitation to get stuck there, to continue to feel the pain over and over again, no. It is an invitation to garner the wisdom, to polish the edges of the DIAMOND, distinct from the coal. You are the diamond in the rough, waiting and ready to shine in all your glorious luster with facets that can beam only your light in greater ways.

"YOU are the greatest gift, the greatest treasure you can ever give yourself."

Together, we shall explore some of the pyscho-dynamics crucial to initiating new levels of understanding within you. These may be new concepts to you. GREAT!

Throughout this book we will reference the magical and transformational Discovery Dives, and now's the time to start with the first one. Yippee, the transformation journey is beginning! OK, we got super excited for you!

DISCOVERY DIVE – EMBRACING YOUR SECRET POWER, AKA SUPERHERO

A superhero … me? Yes, you! Are you wondering what could you possibly have as a secret power? A playful approach to this process is paramount. Just as the subconscious mind holds all past experiences and trauma it also receives inner knowledge from your soul. It is a reminder that "everything you need to live the life of your dreams is within you."

To open to this state of limitless potential, we recommend immersing yourself in your favorite setting, preferably in nature, to sink into the Earth, activate all your senses. Inhaling your favorite essential oil synergy, playing a beautiful piece of music, and so on. By relaxing the mind in this manner, we open to the alpha brainwave frequency and open the communications to the subconscious.

Tapping into this key information further opens the subconscious mind and allows for your innate inner knowledge to flourish. Our feelings are one of the most significant indicators of our thoughts and beliefs. Our feelings also fuel our intentions, conscious or not. Have you ever heard the phrase, "Where our intentions go, our energy flows"?

Thinking back to your early childhood, we will talk more about this "treasure map" in the coming pages. It is rich with clues. What secret messages are held within your youth?

What inspired you when you were young? Nature, culture, or music?

What type, art, or literature?

What was your favorite subject?

What did you love to imagine yourself as? A doctor, lawyer, fashion designer, artist, musician? What did you dream about? Travel to far-off lands?

What are the elements of desire you have carried into your adult life that have not yet been made manifest?

Authentic desire mirrors the longings your soul has come into this lifetime to create and your unique superpower acts to propel you for this unfoldment.

Consider the previous questions and sit with your journal as you start to trace out your own treasure map. Open yourself to any answers that come forth without considering them to be foolish or impossible. This book is an ally and guide to your biggest and best life.

For example, I AW spent countless hours in nature as a child. I felt as though I could hear the flowers sing and see them dance with each other in the most exquisite harmony. I found more comfort with the flowers, trees, and soil than I did with children my own age and most often, my family of origin. Their colors, aromas, and shapes made sense to me. There was no conflict in their interaction, and I could see how they exchanged energy with each other in the most natural of manners. These moments offered the greatest amount of peace and calm. Fast forward a few years. I habitually escaped the dinner cleanup with an excuse to use the restroom. Little did anyone know, until about twenty years later, I would sit and mix "potions" from all my mother's expensive creams, perfumes, and powders with the meticulous concern of a chemist. Who would have thought that several years later, I would create a nationally and internationally recognized brand from this desire.

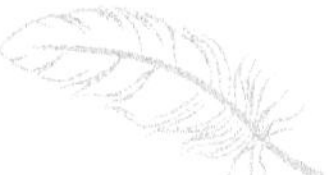

Congratulations! You have now activated your secret power to help ignite and accelerate your healing journey in this book and as we like to say, "*To Infinity and Beyond*." Did you see the golden feather at the bottom of the page of your Discovery Dive? You will see this golden feather throughout the book to assist you in activating your DNA with extra love and guidance as a crucial element to true transformation: self-care! Stand by for more of a download on this vital ally along your journey.

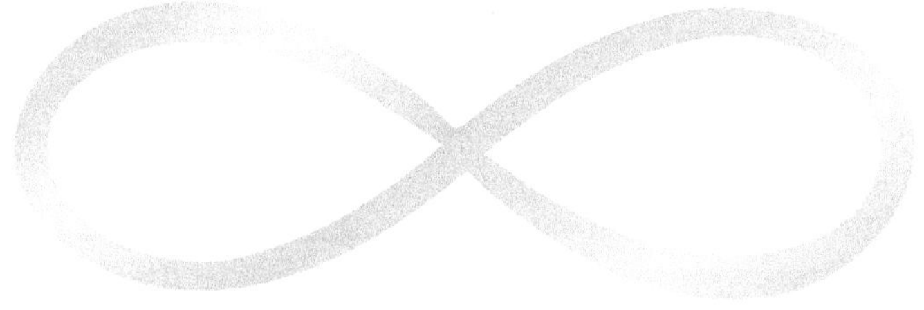

You will also notice a golden infinity symbol throughout this book. This form of sacred geometry is a potent actuator of shift. It invites multiple paradigms of intelligence and opportunity from all time continuums into the present moment. From one angle, we see the microcosm and the macrocosm; for sustainable healing, we must activate both pathways from the external using vibrational healing elements like aromatherapy, sacred geometry, and crystals, to internal pathways, like botanical medicine and whole foods, then both circuits meet in the middle, intermingling and creating a synergistic harmonic to change. All pathways of the infinity symbol come back to the center.

The infinity also represents both bloodlines, from the mother and father that run through our genetic heritage, meeting at the concentric point of cellular consciousness in the zero-point field of limitlessness, where quantum shifts take place. This holographic healing is then communicated through the trillions of cells and the DNA, and we connect in with INFINITE consciousness, expanding our awareness and understanding of ourselves, and what it means to have "the world as your oyster."

SELF CARE – FREEDOM FORMULA DISCOVERY DIVE

Self-listening is a skill to cultivate. It is a vital ally in our daily intentional practice of self-care. All the alchemical elements in the Freedom Photon Wheel coming up in the next chapters will work as deeply and sustainably as your practice of self-care and self-love allows them to. Be curious about your intention when configuring your synergy of alchemy for your Freedom Photon Wheel Ritual. From a multidimensional perspective, the Freedom Photon Wheel morphs in its own superhero way into a deeper journey of your own healing spiral. Imagine a nautilus shell and how its sacred geometric form depicts a journey into the center. The treasure at the center of your journey is filled with the golden divine light of your "quintessence" and the unique offering that only you can bring to the world and the greater healing and evolution of humanity.

Your love is the light that opens, illumines, enlivens, and connects your spiral of healing and transformation with that of humanity. In order to fully embody this teaching, we must look at the ways we love, honor, and take care of ourselves. What voices, images, beliefs come forward when you want and need to rest, relax, read, just "Be," instead of the popular decree of "Do." When we say listening is a skill to cultivate, we are offering the invitation to learn to listen to your body, and other perhaps new aspects of yourself, before all other senses.

At this moment, are you breathing? Is it full or shallow? Did you know we cannot experience anxiety or fear when deeply breathing? In the fullness and silence of our breath, we can learn to listen to our body. Start here, your body speaks volumes. As it starts to open and communicate with you, be curious about what you need to come back to balance. Is it rest, water, a bath, herbal tea, exercise, contact and touch with another, a good cry, music? Your life and health will transform radically as you deepen your contact, communication, and true listening to yourself.

AW I have personally experienced a great dichotomy of self-care, my old patterns of caretaking, over giving and over doing stemming from places within, where I didn't feel worthy enough. This dictated actions and outcomes that would leave me feeling depleted and betrayed, pushing myself past the point of exhaustion to work harder and harder to collapse. It was not until my forties that I could see the belief system in my father's lineage or bloodline that the only way to succeed or have anything without guilt was to work hard. I had glimpses of this my whole life, but it did not become crystal clear, or a light filled with readiness to shift until I was ready to let it go. Still, there are moments when the choice to go down that old path arises, as they may in certain areas of your journey. This is a great time to explore the ways in which you work hard to acknowledge yourself, find approval, and value or devalue yourself.

The way we love ourselves benevolently changes EVERYTHING around us.

Within each of us is a "wise one" or higher self, cultivating a clear and consistent connection with this aspect of us who always knows the truth. This is now the time to tune in! It will serve you in the greatest of ways.

As you begin to explore your relationship with self-care, have an open compassionate listening ear and heart. Feel free to journal your answers and carve out time for rest afterward. Enjoy a cup of tea, light a candle, have a picture of yourself nearby.

Do I rest when I am tired?

How is my hygiene? Do I bathe regularly and groom my hair, skin, nails in ways that honor my health and vitality?

Do I overwork? What is my definition of work?

How do I nourish my body? Do I eat food that I know is good for me?

What is my relationship with alcohol and drugs? Do I use them to numb or escape myself?

Is my self-talk loving and compassionate or am I verbally abusive and over critical?

Do I exercise consistently in a way that is healthy for my body?

After exploring your answers offer a prayer of gratitude:

"In my sacred human heart, I give and receive my love."

Remember that throughout the book the golden feather tips help you nourish yourself with deep self-care.

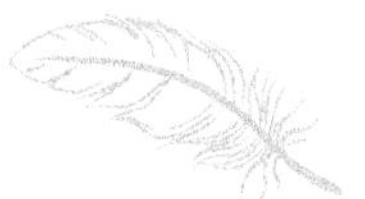

CHAPTER 1

Grounding Down – Getting to the Root

In this day of advancing artificial intelligence, you may have heard the term holographic or hologram. No, this is not an intro for a stellar science fiction read. A bit of a cliché but stick with us for a moment. When your DNA was seeded cellularly at the point of conception, it was imprinted with intelligence. Filled with the genetic coding of every physical, emotional, psychological, and spiritual experience that your parents have encountered throughout their lifetime, as well as their parents and down the line of family heritage. Studies are now showing that our DNA links back to over six generations. This DNA link can be life changing for how the DNA of our body functions. For example, if your great, great, great grandfather worked in a mine, lung

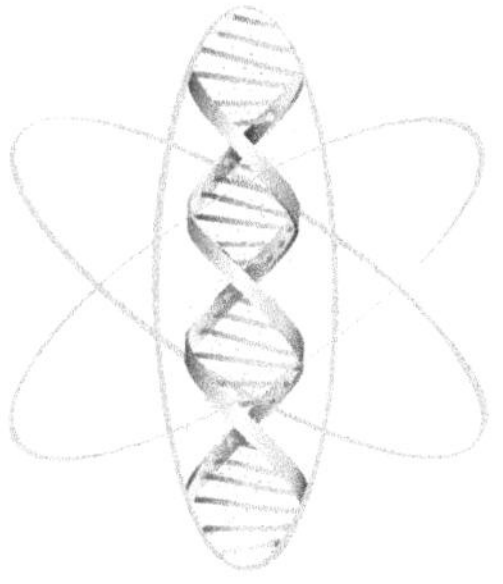

disorders or trauma connected to grief could be the core of your genetic illness or cellular dysfunction.

Each one of the trillions and trillions of cells in your body, which are the smallest unit of life, contain quantum information about you and your entire family lineage. Think of the complexity of experience and intelligence that you hold within you, that you are. Let's go a step further down the rabbit hole: these trillions of cells in your body communicate through LIGHT. Known in quantum physics as biophotons, these emissions of light, which travel at the speed of light, are filled with this intelligence. Our auric body, or energy body, is also filled with information and intelligence, that which we know about ourselves as well as what has yet to be discovered in our past and what is still unfolding in our future. In this regard, the healing interventions that we apply to our cellular, DNA level affect our subtle energy bodies and vice versa. The holographic connection makes more sense now, yes? This will become even more clear as we explore different plant and vibrational medicines and techniques for sustainable holographic healing.

Another term we will introduce to you is alchemy. Traditionally, alchemy is spoken of to transform base metals into gold. However, the true path of alchemy is the path of the seeker. We are all seekers on a journey of exploration and excavation in this life. We have the grand opportunity to explore ourselves authentically, inviting in greater self-awareness Then to excavate and transmutate the places of pain, struggle, and suffering, transforming them into places of empowerment, passion, and purpose.

We all have a unique light, a gift, and every moment of your life thus far has prepared you perfectly for this timely opportunity to heal and grow into the full expression of your soul or life purpose. The true alchemy is the distillation of your quintessence, golden light or soul purpose. Getting to the root of it and releasing the limitations you carry, and we all have them, is paramount to this quintessence surfacing and shifting from a life of "surviving" to a new life of "thriving."

PERSONAL EVOLUTION: SOUL HIGHER PURPOSE TRIAD

Alchemy in this regard invites you to move beyond all third dimensional thoughts and beliefs of what is and what is not possible. Let's consider the nature of every human on the planet Earth right now.

HORIZONTAL INFINITY SACRED GEOMETRY

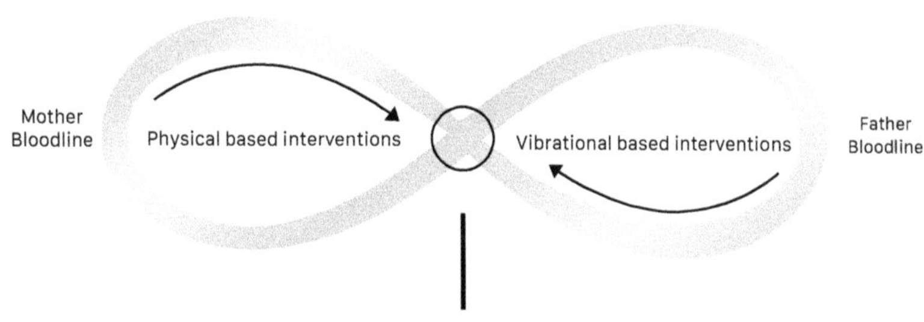

ZERO POINT FIELD OF
LIMITLESS POTENTIAL

HOLOGRAPHIC & INFINITE HEALING OF THE DNA (MICROCOSM TO THE MACROCOSM)

We live in a planetary construct based on the Law of Three, or the Triad. We can see this manifestation in the holistic concept of body, mind, and spirit, of the triple goddess, Maiden, Mother, and Crone, and the Holy Trinity, "Father, Son, Holy Spirit," and the sacred geometry of the great pyramid.

We are each configurations of the pyramid or triad. The three aspects of our own trinity are alive, engaged and although often vying for separate and singular expression, they are longing for unity.

In one corner, we have our "mother" aspect, representing our relationship with our mothers, all information and intelligence held within our family lineage on the female side, and then from a higher spiritual perspective our views and relationship with the Divine in female form. Our feminine principle is yin in nature, receptive – reflecting our power

SOUL HIGHER PURPOSE TRIAD

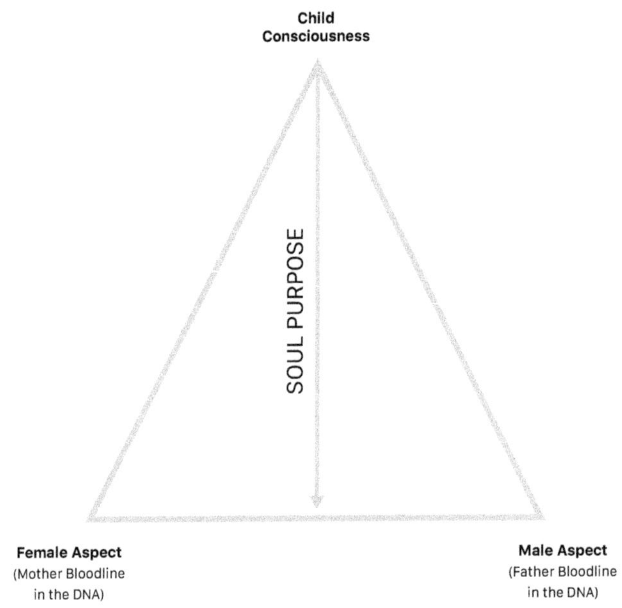

The Triad or pyramid represents our three aspects of personality to heal and unify so that our soul purpose may enter our consciousness and actualize on the physical level.

inward; it is intuitive, wise, and sensual. Our feminine nature represents the creatrix of all things, infinite wells of creativity and nurturance.

In the next corner, we have the "male" aspect, representing our relationship with our fathers, all information and intelligence held within our family lineage on the male side, and then from a higher spiritual perspective our views and relationship with the Divine in male form. Our masculine is yang in nature, and represents courage, strength, confidence, leadership, and power outward. This is not to be confused with a masculine nature out of balance demonstrating power over another.

The third points to our "child" aspect, representing the "child consciousness" and all core wounding and trauma that took place in our early stages of development. The child is always looking for "perfect love" and for someone outside of themselves to fill the void. Confusion is often present when the child's consciousness is engaged.

In this parent-child triangle, an alliance is formed with one parent over another. The child begins to view the opposite parent through the eyes of the ally. That view and all the perceptions held therein begin to mold the belief system and vantage point of the child. For example, if the child allies with his or her mother, she begins to absorb the mother's beliefs, images, and viewpoints of men, positive and negative, as truth. The wounding we experience through trauma from the point of conception through the developmental stages of youth holds all the information we require to sift through the lessons required to actualize our life purpose on a personal and planetary perspective.

In the very center of the pyramid lies our life or soul purpose. When we have reached a critical mass within our own healing trinity, our soul purpose emerges with greater clarity and the path of self-mastery. It is then we can anchor and actualize our soul purpose for incarnating in life and achieve quintessential fulfillment. Every purpose is unique, based on the lessons your soul has come into incarnation to experience, assimilate, and evolve from.

CHILDHOOD MAPPING

We touched upon the "treasure map" of our youth. Our family heritage core dynamics form a guiding map to source our divine quintessence and life purpose. From the point of conception through the developmental stages of our youth, experiences imprint on our cells through physical, emotional, and spiritual events. Those that shock our system with pain, whether perceived or actual, are traumatic to our physical and nonphysical bodies and are stored and repeated through similar patterns and dynamics until the core pain is released and our beings assimilate the wisdom of the experience for our soul's growth. The more awareness, healing, and light that we bring to these parts of ourselves, the closer we come to actualizing our soul or life purpose on a personal and planetary level. Even unresolved past life experiences are held in this "map" as well as the genetic and auric field. Our child aspects hold all unresolved or traumatic experiences, even if based on perception versus actuality. Even irresolute past life "time capsules" are held in this map and therefore the auric field and the cells and DNA. As we experience a physical pain, disease process, or an emotional feeling or memory, we can access the energy points to move along our own timelines to find the "roots" to clear and allow full spectrum healing to transform our past, present, and future selves.

AW My early childhood environment was chaotic. My parents' disagreements and alcohol use created volatile emotional peaks and valleys. This perceived lack of safety and love imprinted on my cellular consciousness. As I grew into my adolescent and more formative years, this distortion arose in feelings of depression, anxiety, grief, and rage. My anger was toxic, and I can recall taking pleasure in making teachers, waitresses, and often strangers cry with a sense of distorted power. The rage I felt towards my family situation was overwhelming. Underneath the rage was a deep sense of grief, dis appointment and betrayal.

My child consciousness had gotten stuck in the pain of an abusive and angry mother. For the sake of survival and search for love, I had allied with my father and took on much of his energy, pain, and belief systems. In doing so, I deeply rejected the feminine within me and learned how to operate from my masculine. I became excellent at doing, working hard, focused on the outer vs. the inner. I learned how to push through and create from my will. I learned to bury my emotions, temporarily of course, and I paid a heavy price. In my late teens, I began to experience great pain in my abdominal area.

I was not diagnosed with endometriosis until I was twenty-one. The years in-between were difficult. I made such frequent trips to the doctor's office with severe, debilitating pain. My doctor was quick to dispense pain medication and I could feel his uncertainty in treating my symptoms. I lost a great deal of work to the pain and other symptoms including adhesions to my stomach wall, which resulted in chronic nausea and vomiting. I ended up hooked on the pain medication. It became the only sense of support I felt I had. After examining me and doing an ultrasound, my doctor said the only problem I had was in my head because I had not accepted the fact that I was a woman, and women were born to suffer. This infuriated me, and yet it also confirmed the belief system I picked up from my father. Women were somehow weaker and more emotional than men.

Healing didn't happen overnight. The descent into the underworld of our subconscious is cavernous terrain to navigate. After numerous surgeries, tests, and medications, and with no end in sight, I hit a wall.

I can remember it as clearly as yesterday. I was driving to work, getting on the ramp for the highway. I was in another morning of pain pill fugue and I almost hit another car. It was at that moment I decided to take control of what was happening to my body and ditch the medicines, over testing, and the expectation that someone was going to "fix" me. This crucial point in my journey drew me deeper into the study of two passions: plants and vibrational healing. I also worked with acupuncture, chiropractic, and started therapy. The deeper I began to excavate myself within my healing spiral, it became clear that an enormous part of the transformation was reconnecting with my own feminine and healing the split therein.

It took time, and I am grateful to the part of me that said no to the hysterectomy that was proposed by my physician at the age of twenty-one with what was diagnosed as stage four endometriosis. Even with the pain, and the inability to function at my normal pace, there was a voice, deeply feminine, that assured me I would be alright and that I would heal. That aspect of my being also knew I was to give birth to two children. I did so in my mid to late thirties, and they are the most incredible individuals I have come to know. We all have a voice of truth and wisdom inside. It is always present and accessible with cultivation. You have a voice within your being, within your cells that knows things your mind cannot fully understand, and this voice will always steer you in the right direction.

The wounding and trauma that each of us brings to this Earth to heal is voluminous. It is specific to the journey of our souls and yet we are not alone along the way. Oftentimes we need a reminder, so we can unite in healing and live in a compassionate way with ourselves and each other.

For me, it took many years and personal process work to release the negative emotion I felt towards my parents. What I could not see or understand in those early years was the deep pain that both my mother and father had experienced in their lifetime. The layers continue to rise, as they represent so much more than the two individuals that consecrated our spirits and souls into matter. There were guides along my journey to greater self-understanding, healing, and evolution.

Now that we have explored some of the psycho-spiritual aspects of healing, let's move along the continuum of the infinity symbol, the macrocosm down to the microcosm, back to the physical body.

HOW THE BODY RELEASES TOXINS

THE ROUTES OF ELIMINATION

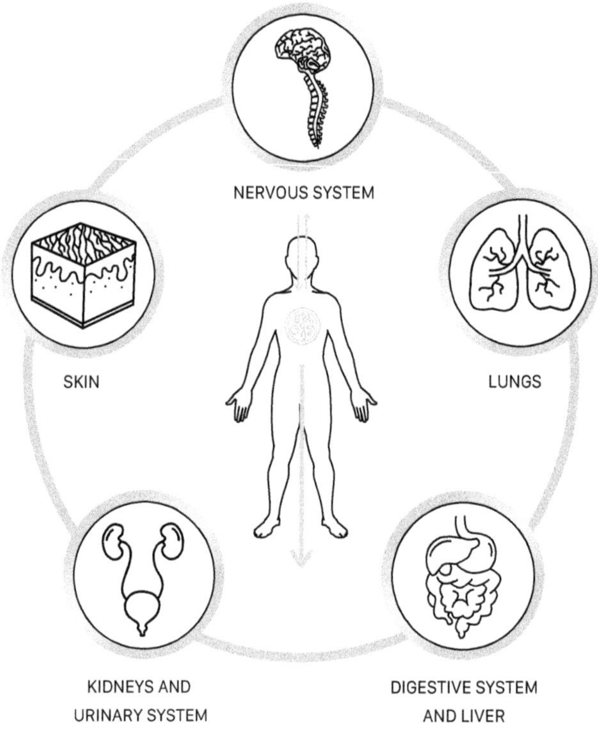

HOW THE BODY RELEASES TOXINS

How does the body release the cellular toxicity or cellular imprint of a physical impairment? Well, physically the body has routes of elimination, called emunctories, which are organs or areas of the body that assist us in eliminating. When these emunctories become blocked the body is not able to release and then the toxins build up layer upon layer. Let's take a super magnified view of a cell for a moment. Our cells have little gateways where nutrients as well as toxins enter and leave the cell. When the cell is filled up with "debris," it becomes very challenging for the cell to function optimally, leading to congestion or a clogging of the system. Well, what happens when this toxic cell or poorly functioning cell replicates? The body becomes burdened or overloaded with toxicity and systems in the body begin to fail and shut down. This is when your body is sending you warning signals which we commonly ignore.

What about pharmaceuticals and drugs? Yes! These also leave a cellular imprint especially when they have been used for many years for a chronic health condition or an addiction such as opiates. Even after discontinuing the use of pharmaceuticals and drugs, cells still have the memory and to remove this imprint proper Detoxing, Nourishing, and Activating the cells is necessary for complete clearance and healing. (Note: Throughout sections in this book there will be links to meditations you can listen to online to enhance your healing process.)

Your DNA also stores the imprint or memory of emotional and mental and spiritual trauma. The requirement of healing is the removal of any toxin. This is great, but how do we do this? By using the Freedom Photon Wheel interventions in this book!

So, let's talk about toxins. What is a toxin? A toxin is a natural form of cellular metabolism coming from inside the body, endogenous, or outside the body, xenobiotic. The body is sometimes able to recognize the toxin and discharge it from the system, but other times the toxin will build up in the body and cause disturbance in the terrain. An example of this is a heavy metal or pesticide. The body can also experience emotional toxins: over stimulus, bad jobs, fear, loss of free will, or loss of self-expression. Disease can happen in the body on any level when there is an imbalance physically, spiritually, emotionally, or mentally.

How do the cells play a role in detox? If we understand how our system and cells work in the body, we can understand much more about how our body ends up in a chronic disease state or dysfunction. Chronic disease starts with multiple organ system imbalance, but It really starts with conception! As you have learned in the previous section, the genetic impact is greatly affected by your heritage.

So how do you remove cellular toxins? Your first step is to recognize where the toxin is in the body on a systemic and physiological level. The body can't get rid of the toxin until it sees the toxin as a foreign substance. You then open the systems in the body and neutralize the toxin. This is a crucial step! If you don't do this step you will get sicker. Then you can safely eliminate the toxins from the system without a backfire.

What are the requirements for cellular healing? First you need physical rest: this allows your muscles a period for recovery to assist in the removal of toxins. Second, you need physiological rest with enhanced techniques to increase elimination. Fasting from eight to twelve hours is an easy way to give your body a much-needed break. Third, you need mental rest. The brain and central nervous system (CNS) require sleep for recovery, a minimum of seven to eight hours per night.

What aspects damage the cells?
∞ Poor diet ∞ Insufficient sleep ∞ Sleep at the wrong time of the day ∞ Lack of exercise and movement ∞ Toxic water ∞ Overwork and stress

All of these create free radical damage and lead to chronic inflammation.

DNA & CELLULAR DAMAGE

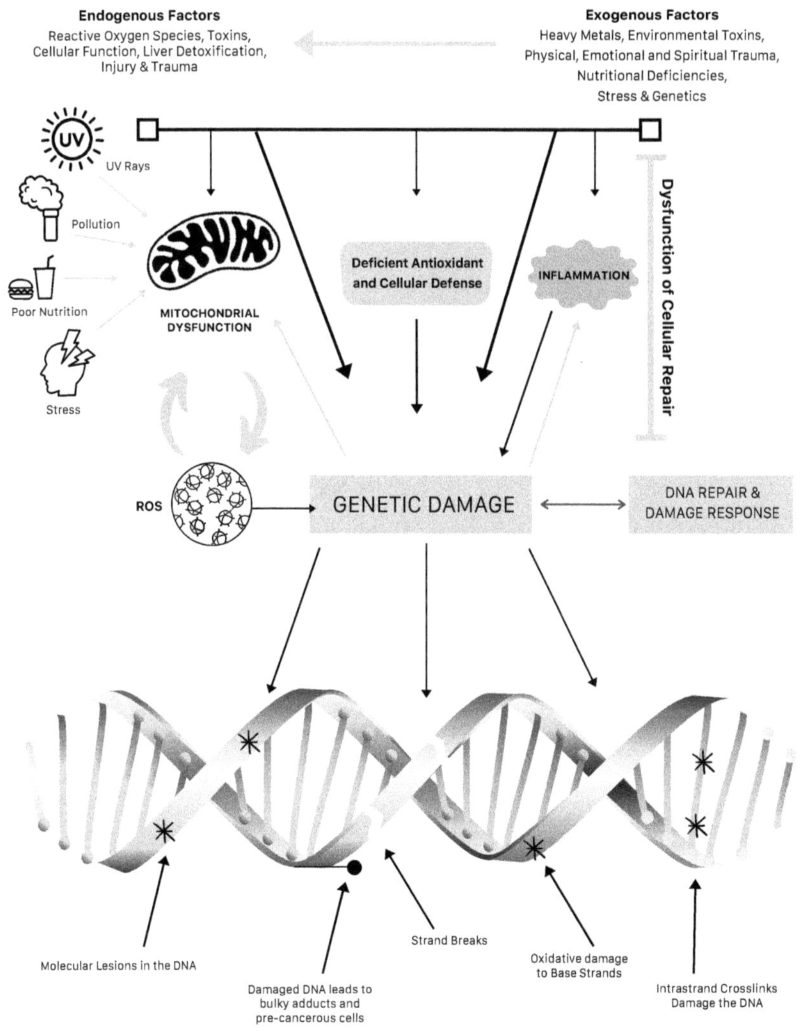

YOUR DNA IS INFINITE

LEVELS OF THE AURIC (ENERGY) FIELD

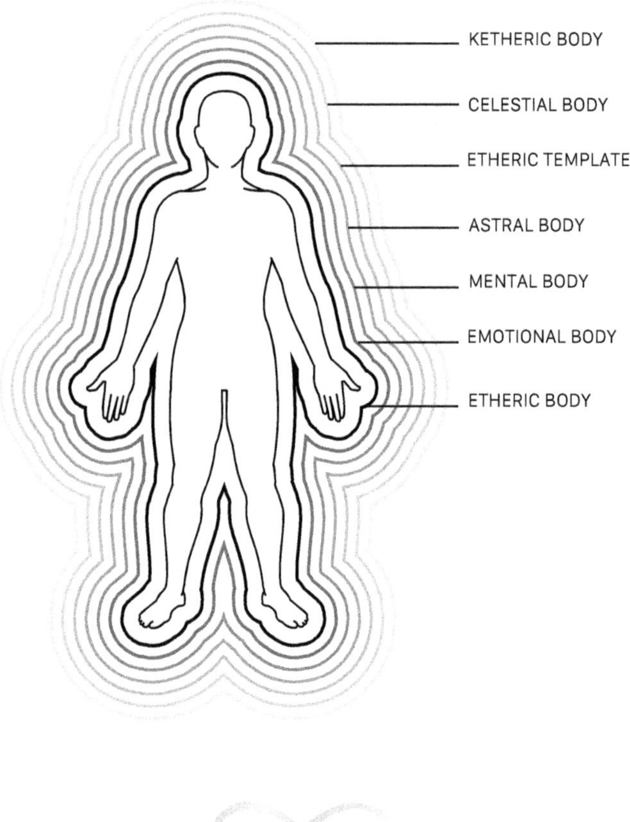

∞ To access the DNA Activation meditation please go to www.zenergy-medicinals.com

When we look at each system of the body, it is imperative to view it from a holographic perspective. The physical body is the perfect tool for that. Our bodies are the guides that can illuminate the pathways of where to direct our innate healing energy through intention and action. Although physical disease begins on the outer layers of the auric field, from the spiritual levels down to the mental and emotional bodies, all points of connectivity meet in the physical. Past trauma is rooted in the energy and physical bodies and compounds that energy through repeated experience that proves the pain and dysfunction we perceive to be true.

One client, Mary, experienced a chronic autoimmune illness that limited her physical and sexual quality of life. Upon deeper explorations of her past, we discovered that Mary had a long history of feeling as if she did not belong or want to be present in her body. She chronically experienced negative patterns of self-talk that she was worthless and unable to succeed in her proven field, despite great brilliance in creativity. Further discussion of her past spoke of suicide ideation in her mother from a very young age. This distortion was energetically imprinted on Mary's cellular consciousness and she felt trapped to its beliefs.

Whether the trauma we experience is real or perceived, it imprints throughout our multidimensional nature, from our energy bodies to our physical cellular consciousness. When we approach sustainable change and healing in our lives, it is crucial to address from a multifaceted perspective that can co-mingle and merge, as shown in the horizontal infinity symbol, through communication with our physical as well as psycho-spiritual natures.

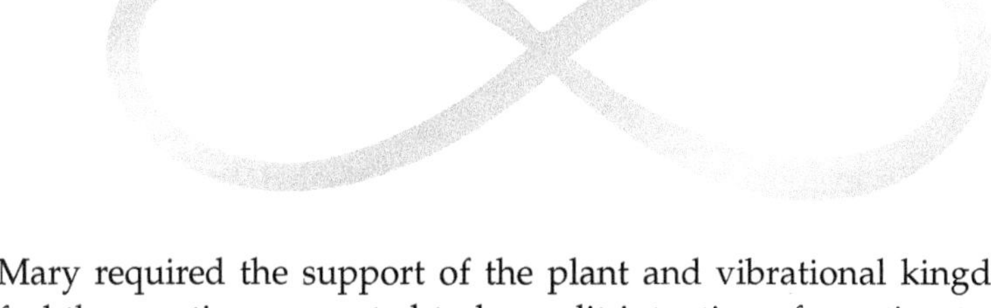

Mary required the support of the plant and vibrational kingdoms to feel the emotion connected to her split intention of wanting to have a healthy, successful life juxtaposed with her genetic coding and current life belief system of not wanting to be physically here. Ultimately, Mary was able to make a quantum leap in her relationship and career fields into the unknown and create new healthier experiences. Although there was tremendous terror attached to taking these steps, the alchemy of the plants and energetic techniques created a bridge for Mary's transformation.

Trauma holds limiting beliefs, unhealthy and toxic patterns, and trapped energy, creating experiences we intrinsically know do not serve us. These patterns and beliefs are passed down through our genetic code or bloodline. It is critical to fully explore these areas in ourselves, still in shadow, to find the roots, clear them, and begin the healing process, layer by layer. Once we can make the connections from a mental perspective, we can then move through the emotions to free the life force held as trapped energy consciousness and then nourish the physical body to allow sustainable health to proliferate.

The more we clear the unresolved places within our past and the DNA, the closer we become to fully actualizing and expressing our life and soul purpose. Every being on this planet has come to create, experience, and grow at the soul and personality levels and contribute to the greater good in a specific way.

Our choices are typically based on our perceived reality of past experiences, either positive or negative. For every choice we make, there are consequences and then based on those consequences, lessons. The lessons then impart further intelligence for us to continue to choose from. What happens when we get stuck in the patterns of distortion and dysfunction and our emotions run rampant? How often do we react from a place of defense versus presence in the now moment?

Here are a few ways that subconscious trauma expresses itself in our pyscho-spiritual dynamics:

∞ Resistance
∞ Projection
∞ Emotional reaction
∞ Cycles of struggle

This offers us insight to the importance of personal process work to clear the traumas and patterns of limitation. Our emotions offer us the clay that can be sculpted to our deepest desires and soul's longings.

HIGHER SELF, LOWER SELF, AND THE GREAT MASK

The human experience offers many perspectives competing to be expressed in each moment. We all have a higher self, lower self, and a masked way of being in the world. The more deeply we navigate our

VICIOUS CYCLE OF AN EMOTIONAL REACTION

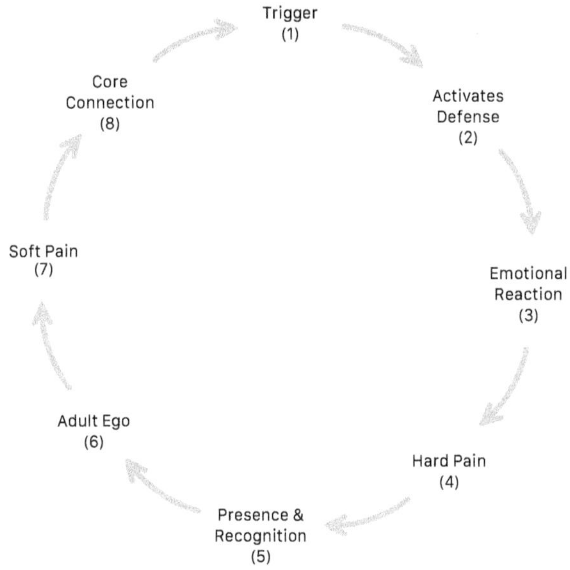

"What we demand from another is what we are called to give to ourselves."

1. A trigger is activated through internal or external means: related to a past trauma.
2. Defense mechanism is activated.
3. Irrational blame and demand is projected onto another.
4. Feelings of hopelessness and helplessness are experienced. Resistance to feeling the original pain (trauma) re-creates distorted patterning.
5. Presence in the moment recognizes child consciousness is engaged.
6. Alignment with positive intention engages healing.
7. Allow the soft pain of the child to be felt and released with self love.
8. Deeper connection to core releases held "quintessence" and lifeforce to flood the body and aura with radiance.

healing spiral, the more awareness we bring to each aspect, allowing for an "in the moment" appraisal of who is "running our show" and how to pivot accordingly. Here are a few characteristics of each aspect of self that can help to identify which perspective we are relating from.

Our higher self has a positive intention to align with divine will. When we approach life from this perspective, we are clear, spontaneous, creative, and undefended. When we are aligned with our higher self, we accept ourselves, we create from effortless intention and energy flow, communion, pleasure and fearlessness. We have the intention to beautify and express our own Divine nature.

When we're in our lower selves our intention is to separate, to be selfish or willful, defended, prideful, closed to feeling pain, impatient, and resistant to union. The lower self-perspective is that of self will, pride, self-importance and superiority ... Anything that separates us from the other. Our lower self loves to judge another. Judgement of the other damages the self in far greater ways, ultimately diminishing the parts of us that deeply and innately long for unity.

Consider the possibility that there are many more ways than one to:

∞ Live ∞ Grow ∞ Feel ∞ Expand ∞ Pray ∞ Eat ∞ Move ∞ Create ∞ Heal ∞ Journey

When we wear the great mask, we're in our idealized self-image – pretending, fake, inauthentic, denying fear. When masked, we are disconnected from ourselves and lack the ability to be in contact with another. We're in denial of our own negativity, our own pain and brokenness.

PAST LIFE CONNECTIONS

Although our childhood mapping contains the roots of any unresolved past life experiences, it is oftentimes beneficial to revisit lifetimes where unresolved issues may be contributing negatively or of course positively on the current one. This can expedite healing and understanding from the soul to the personality aspects.

Do you recall any past life experiences? If so, do they share a common theme, pattern, or traumatic event? Our past lives are not all places of pharaohs, queens, and royalty. Each time your soul comes into embodiment, it chooses a comprehensive path of lessons and experiences designed for you to receive greater understanding about yourself, your relationships, and creative principles, all with the ultimate design for self-mastery and enlightenment. For this to occur, all perspectives and vantage points of life and the masculine and feminine principles within must be assimilated and balanced.

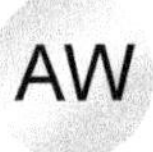

My first trip to India shook me to the core; it rearranged me at the molecular level, and I was forever changed. I had wanted to travel there since I was a small child and in my very early

twenties that dream became a reality. I was green in the world of aromatherapy, healing, and business and had the privilege of traveling with pioneers and leaders in all three fields of study and practice. There was a magical rose farm in the South that seemed to exist both on Heaven and Earth. I met a young boy there, maybe about five years of age. I was struck immediately when I looked into his eyes. He began to follow me and my new friends through the fields of rich color and heady scent. As we walked near each other, I felt a profound connection to this young child I had just met. At one moment, I could have sworn he said to me, "So, what do you want to talk about?" which was of course impossible as he didn't speak any English whatsoever. When it was time to board the bus and leave the farm, I was overwrought with a deep sadness. I wept for the next hour on the bus. At that point in my life, I had no children of my own, but I was certain that this boy had been my child in the past. He stood staring at me through the windows in the bus until we left, also with some sort of recognition. I was not sure then, and even now, what those tears washed away, yet I am certain something deep inside of me healed, opened, and paved the way for my children to be able to come many years later.

CREATING SACRED SPACE AND AN ALTAR

As you use this book and the Freedom Photon Wheel sections, we give instructions on how to create or add to your sacred space and altar for enhanced DNA healing. After you create your altar, use these suggested rituals for your meditations, Discovery Dives and Freedom Photon Wheel experiences. This will energize your sacred space and create greater ease and flow in your intentional practices.

Gather these items:

∞ Mirror
∞ Two white candles

Instructions: Add one item to each of the areas listed below

Air element – East on your altar: a feather, incense, a bell, or photo of winged creatures (butterfly, bird)

Fire element – South on your altar: a candle, incense, or an image of a dragon or phoenix

Water element – West on your altar: a bowl of water, seashell, or a chalice

Earth element – North on your altar: a crystal, salt, a bowl of soil or coins

Akasha element – Center on your altar: an image of sacred geometry, the cosmos, or a pyramid crystal

5 ELEMENTS ALTAR PLACEMENT DIAGRAM

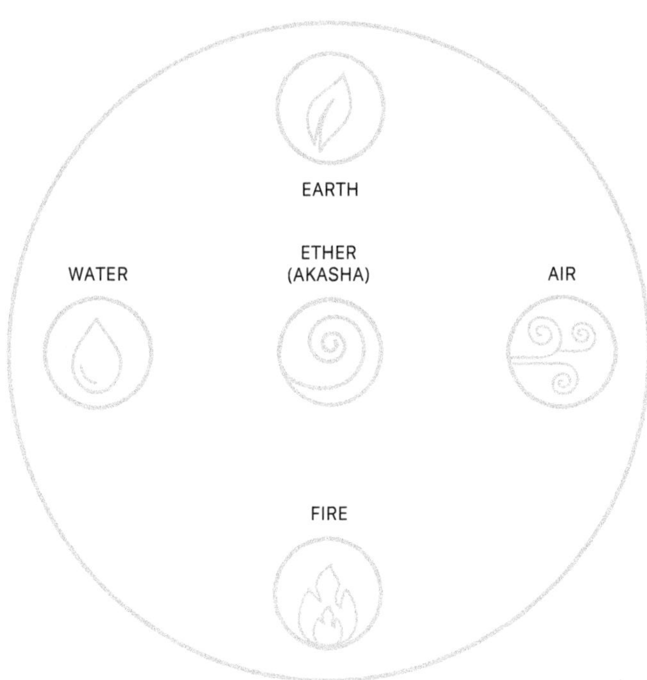

∞ Any other items you wish. There are some other suggestions in the Freedom Photon Wheel section.

Ritual:
Set up a mirror with two white candles, one to the left and one to the right. If you have not already set your sacred space and altar, do so now with the invocation, journal, and pen.

INVOCATION OF THE DIRECTIONS

- ∞ To access the invocation of the directions please go to www.zenergy-medicinals.com

Take a deep breath in as we invoke the directions and the elements.

- ∞ In the direction of East: We call forth the element of air. Sacred sound and thought of all the winged creatures. The eagle, we welcome thee now to come in a good way. Thank you.
- ∞ In the direction of South: we invoke the element of fire. Sacred transformation and transfiguration. The energy of the phoenix, we invite thee to come in a good way. Thank you.
- ∞ In the direction of West: we call for the element of water. The sacred fluid bodies upon mother Gaia. Deep emotional cleansing, purification, and healing. The energy of the dolphin and the whale, we welcome thee to come in a good way. Thank you.
- ∞ In the direction of North: we call forth the element of earth. The sacred ground beneath our feet. Of structure, strength, nourishment, abundance, healing. Guardians of the north, we welcome and honor thee to come in a good way now. Thank you.
- ∞ We invoke the elements of Akasha of all that is seen and unseen; past, present, future, still unfolding. The essence of alchemy. We welcome thee now to come in a good way. Thank you.
- ∞ We activate the memory deep within our DNA of communing with these elements and working with them in great respect and honor as powerful forces for healing, manifestation, and illumination.

PAST LIFE DISCOVERY DIVE

Practice this Discovery Dive within three days of the full moon.

Dream Tea and Detox the Heart – Spikenard Medicine to Connect with Ancestry Wisdom (page 107) recommended for the ceremony.

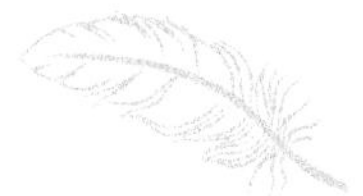

Dream Tea

Ingredients:

15 g Chamomile – *Matricaria recutita*
15 g Lemon balm – *Melissa officinalis*
15 g Kava kava – *Piper methysticum*
15 g Valerian – *Valeriana officinalis*
7 g Catnip – *Nepeta cataria*
7 g Rose – *Rosa centifolia*
5 g Lavender – *Lavandula angustifolia*
5 g Lemongrass – *Cymbopogon citratus*

Combine all ingredients.

Infuse 17 g in 236 ml of water for 4 minutes and drink 30 minutes before bed.

Now that your sacred space is set, you can refresh it as often as you feel is right. At least every thirty days, it is good to cleanse the space and your elemental representations with incense, sage, or palo santo. This will allow you to reinvigorate the energy and lift the vibration consistently. This process is also a great reminder that we are constantly changing, healing, and growing. That you are not the same person you were last week or last month. Every day is a new opportunity to harness the higher vibration of the elements and draw into your cellular consciousness and mental, emotional, and spiritual bodies for greater healing and personal growth.

We recommended taking a bath in Epsom or sea salts prior to this ritual to cleanse your energy field. You may add the Spikenard Medicine to Connect with Ancestry Wisdom and sip your tea while bathing. When you are ready, sit in your sacred space. Inhale your essential oil blend for 30 seconds and invite in this intention:

- ∞ In the name of the Holy of Holies and all that is of sacred light, I invoke communion with the Divine Consciousness, my I AM presence and highest self, and all my spiritual teachers, guardians, and guides. I ask to be shown which incarnations are currently affecting this one and allow for the most benevolent outcome of information and understanding to come forth for my best and highest good.
- ∞ As you continue to breathe in, soften your gaze into the mirror. After some time, you may notice your face shape-shift into that of another. Be patient. As your visage changes, invite in an intention for any

information you require to assimilate the lessons of this life to come forward. You may see an image, or color, a sound. You may feel emotions that arise and find a connection in your current life. Allow this to happen organically and jot down anything you see, hear, feel, or imagine.

∞ When this feels complete, offer a prayer of gratitude to yourself and the Divine Consciousness for its guidance. Sometimes, this unfolds with practice as you learn how to open your channel to HSP (high sensory perception). For everyone it is a little different. You may be highly visual, seeing colors or imagery. You may be more clairaudient, able to hear. You may have more kinesthetic HSP, and a feeling of empathy, or you could experience direct knowing, where you "just know." Everyone can cultivate this skill set, with practice. It is the pathway to finding your inner authentic voice. Have fun with it!

THE VICTIM STORY – NO ONE WINS IN THE BLAME GAME

The victim story is one of the biggest pitfalls that the collective consciousness of humanity holds. It consistently attempts to engage us through the voice of the lower self and unconscious negativity.

In its syrup sweet voice, the inner victim will softly tell you that what you are experiencing is not your fault. It will make excuses for you for everything from why your relationship ended, why you overslept, forgot to pay the utility bill, got fired, missed that deadline, why you overate, over drank, or some way checked out of your life. It will blame outcomes and experiences on your past, your parents, your spouse, kids, boss, or neighbor. It will justify your emotional reactions, self-abuse, misconduct, and every way you have not and do not take care of yourself in a "good way."

Here is the good news: We have all been there and are still invited to return, but we don't have to. The more parts of ourselves that we heal, bring new light and consciousness to the victim's voice within, the more it will continue to become smaller and smaller with your positive intention and deep commitment to your journey of self-mastery.

The voices of unconscious negativity never completely take their leave; however, you can come to a place within yourself where they don't control you. Instead, you can become a witness to that aspect of your humanity, have compassion for it, and apply one or a combination of skills you will find through this book. You will re-pattern your pathways and expectations for your life. This takes a consistent commitment to self-responsibility. Consider the possibility that you are the creative generator for your life experience.

In order to shift the victim story, you must get honest with yourself. Your LIFE depends on it, the quality of joy, health, abundance, love, relationships, and so on. Whether you are reading this thinking you have healed every part of your blame game, or if you are really pissed off right now because we have offered a completely new life concept that is making you squirm, stick with us. The victim story is insidious; its roots delve further into the soil than you would like to admit or believe. Until we can decipher its voice and excavate its roots, we can never fully be free or accept our superpower and "quintessence." It's part of the rub AND the opportunity of the human experience.

Your superhero journey and transformation requires self-responsibility and truth, accountability and compassion TO and FOR yourself. The only way out is through, and you aren't going alone. You are held, supported, encouraged, and respected for all the pathways that it took to get here, now. The plants, minerals, animal spirits, essences, and other interventions within these pages offer their medicine, magic wisdom, and vibration for you to return home to the truth of who you are as a divine being of light.

DISCOVERY DIVE – YOUR VICTIM STORY

Everyone has a victim story or a victim recovery story! Anytime we give away our power to someone else and we engage in the blame game we are delving in the victim rabbit hole. Breaking apart these patterns allows us to break through the limitations of our victim story and remove our blinders. It is only when we can see beyond our own confines that we can create a new story of empowerment.

How do you project blame? Is it a quiet voice within that is hidden on some level? Is it vociferous and blatant? Is it self-blame and belligerence?

What do you blame your parents for? Do you hold them responsible for limiting your life in any way? How is this blame limiting you in your current family dynamic?

Do you blame your children for not achieving your goals? Financially? Career or relationship wise?

Do you view your boss as an authority figure that somehow limits your success?

Do you blame God for your not having the love, money, or happiness you deserve?

Sometimes our victim pattern is more insidious. Perhaps you find yourself more often in the role of the rescuer. Either speaking up and out to a potential perpetrator or saving the perceived victim only to find a pattern of over giving and feeling drained and ultimately resentful. Right around the corner of the resentment lies the victim in its masked nature.

GROUNDING MEDITATION

To access the meditation please go to www.zenergymedicinals.com

Grounding Synergy Oil

∞ 2 drops Vetiver essential oil (*Vetiveria zizanioides*)
∞ 3 drops of Patchouli essential oil (*Pogostemon cablin*)
∞ 1 drop of Sandalwood essential oil (*Santalum autrocaledonicum*)

Blend into 1 tablespoon organic jojoba. Note that Sandalwood is endangered and should be used in reverence and moderation; the New Caledonian species is our preferred Sandalwood for this sacred healing work.

∞ Be seated comfortably either on the ground or in a chair, making sure that your arms and legs are uncrossed unless you are sitting Indian style or in the lotus position. If you have created the Grounding Synergy Oil listed above, please have it handy.
∞ Apply a drop of your synergy oil in the palm of your hands … dropping into the left hand. The left palm receives higher frequencies. Rub your hands together and take a deep breath in for about 30 seconds. You may also rub this oil onto the heart, the dantian area below the navel and at the soles of the feet. Set the intention to connect with your body and Mother Earth in a new and deeper way.

Take a deep breath in, exhaling slowly, feeling your entire body relax, open.

∞ Hold your focus on the dantian point which is about an inch and a half below the navel. This can be viewed as a ball of light and the single note or frequency that holds you in physical form. It's the point that's referred to often in martial arts as a center of power.

∞ See, feel, allow, imagine yourself sinking into the warm mossy deep green earth. This moss feels so inviting, nourishing, safe, protective, imagine it circulating your entire energy field. The utter delight of sinking into profound contact and connection more deeply into our bodies and into our earth mother.

∞ Release all the stress of the day, of the year, of your life, and back to the universe to be transmuted into light. Bring your awareness back to that golden line of light connecting with the Earth. Allowing that to come back up, you can envision this as an amber light, this magnificent representation of life force coming up from the Earth encoded with the frequency for deep healing and nourishment from the mother of all mothers. Allow energy of great abundance, physical safety, protection to charge your physical structure, lifting your vibration.

∞ This is your safe haven, your personal connection to the core of the Earth. A guiding force of light, love, life force, vitality, and vibrancy that is yours in every moment, and deepens every moment that you intend to make contact to open yourself.

CHAPTER 2

You are the Ancient Tree of Life

We invite you to envision yourself as a beautiful ancient tree, the tree of life. Starting with the analogy that like a tree, our body holds trauma to its core roots and then creates offshoots or branches of compounded, compacted energy and emotions held in the body. The emotions left unresolved create physical disease as a messenger to the pathway of healing. Healing core trauma unlocks the life force from our Earth connection to nurture, strengthen, and stabilize our physical, emotional, and spiritual bodies. When trauma stays unresolved, it continues to project its distortion around us, just as a movie projector does. This is not a punishment; it is a way to bring our attention to its continued existence. When we continue to see the same patterns in our life surfacing, and similar outcomes because of that, we can more easily focus our intention for healing.

Transformation at this core level becomes the gateway to allow the compounded energy and emotion to heal, opening our hearts and our being to the work of our soul, or life purpose. When we tend to our own tree, or body, we not only feel a deeper connection to our own healing but the healing of the community around us.

THE TERRAIN OF YOUR TREE AND DNA

Let's first examine the soil, or terrain, of your tree. The terrain contains all the energy and nutrients feeding your tree. But go a little deeper here at a tiny, microscopic level and think about all the DNA filled cells living in your terrain. The terrain is fed with nutrients from your environment: sun, air, water, food, and emotions. This DNA in your terrain has two main hereditary lines, from both your father and mother, tracing back through many, many generations. Your terrain can become imprinted during conception with trauma that has been held within your family's DNA. Let's look at an example here to help further your understanding of this concept.

Amelia, a forty-five-year-old woman, came for a consultation suffering with chronic bronchitis, allergies, and eczema. When we dived deep into her trauma tree, we learned several things about her terrain. First, her great grandfather worked in a coal mine for several years and died of black lung disease. Second, growing up her family lived very close to a paper mill which released toxic pollutants into the air. Last, she experienced a great emotional loss three years ago, when her twin brother passed away in a tragic car accident. When we examine these three on her trauma timeline, we can see how not only the history of physical respiratory ailments contributed to her current lung dysfunction but also from an emotional level we can see that grief is deeply ingrained in her DNA life story. When this toxicity level reaches a "danger level" and the body is not able to eliminate it, your internal life force or internal battery becomes depleted, and disease sets in at a deeper cellular level.

TREE OF LIFE

Trunk of the Tree

The trunk of your tree has many layers from the inner core, through the rings, to the outer bark layers.

As we experience different life experiences these form the rings of the tree and when we have deep traumatic experiences these form not only throughout the rings but more deeply on the outer bark. You can think of these layers as a protective defense mechanism to create a shell around the tree. This shell or shielding layer protects us from further

TRAUMA TREE

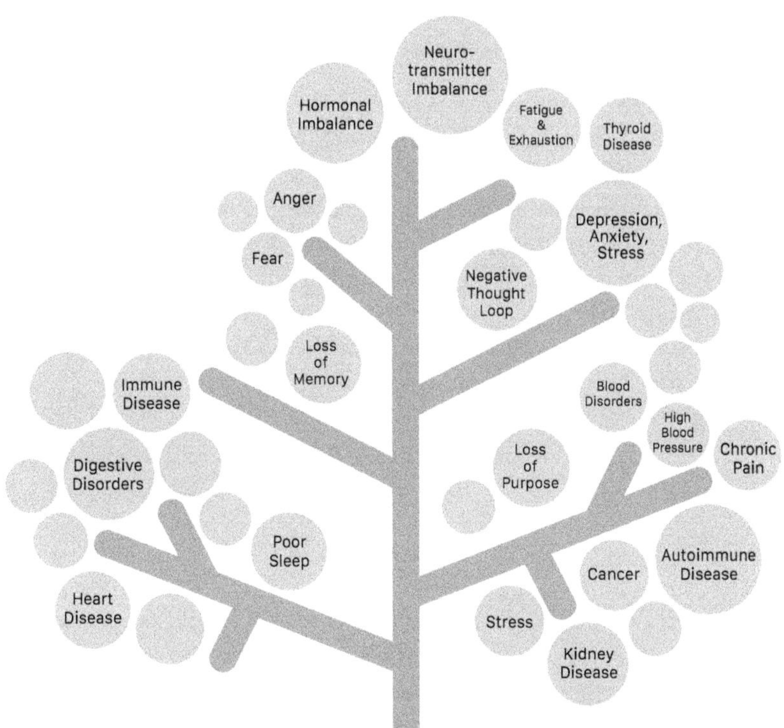

CELLULAR DYSFUNCTION & DIS-EASE

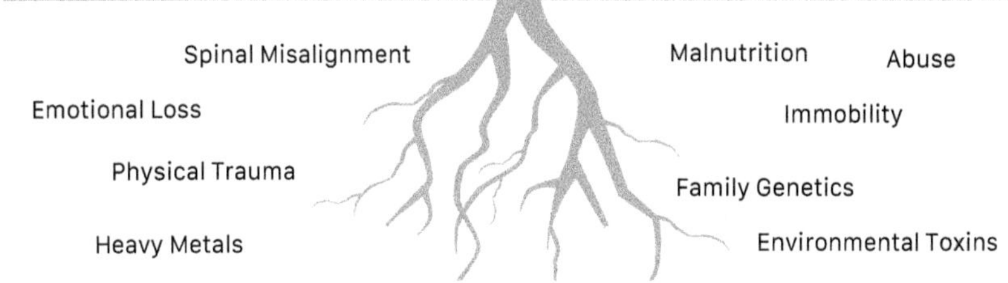

ROOT CAUSE OF TRAUMA

traumatic damage but at the same time can backfire and prevent us from releasing the trauma.

Branches of the Tree

As the branches of the tree move further and further out from the trunk, the disease and discomfort become more and more compounded, and the dysfunction intensifies. Imagine layer upon layer of trauma intertwining, much like an ancient tree filled with knots: these twists and turns of pain and trauma must be unwound for true healing to begin.

So, you have deep layered trauma, great – now what? Time to experience healing to the deep core of your tree. Are you ready? See the meditation below as well as the link for the audio meditation to really get to the root of it! OK, cheesy tree analogy.

TRAUMA TREE CROSS SECTION

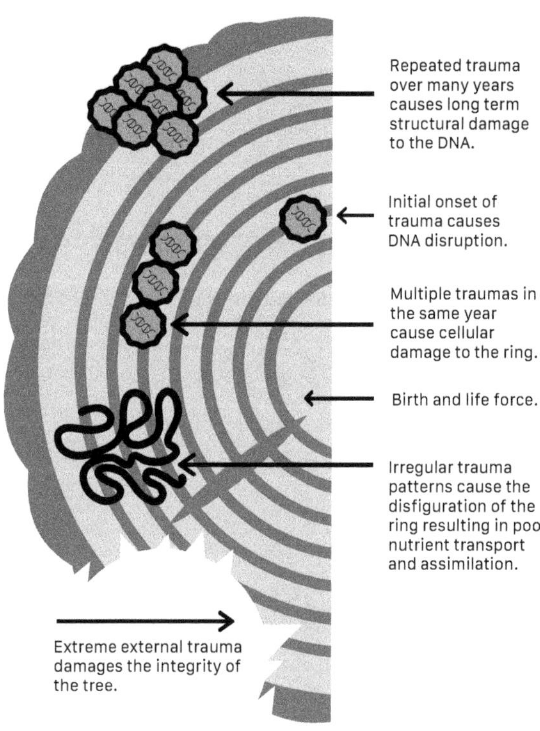

MEDITATION – VISUALIZING YOUR TREE

∞ To access the meditation please go to www.zenergymedicinals.com

Cistus Trauma Release Synergy

∞ 1 drop Cistus essential oil (*Cistus ladaniferus*)
∞ 1 drop Immortelle essential oil (*Helichrysum italicum*)
∞ 1 drop Rose Otto essential oil (*Rosa damascena*)
∞ 1 drop Sandalwood essential oil (*Santalum austrocaledonicum*)
∞ 3 drops Lavender essential oil (*Lavendula angustifolia*)

Blend into 1 tablespoon of coconut oil to create your own alchemical medicine. Anoint your body reverently and sparingly over any places that hold trauma, especially your heart.

All trauma is stored in the physical body and rooted in emotion. This lends with precision the focal points to which we need to bring our attention and awareness for healing. Pain can be a clear indicator to where disease and trauma are stored. Yet pain is not always present, and it often arises when we have not been hearing our body's more subtle messages. The visualization below will help you to identify where there is trauma stored in your body and then to follow the thread further to identify where the roots are connected. Remember to be gentle and loving with yourself. The healing journey is a spiral within to source greater knowledge of the self as a Divine Being of Light and greater expression of the quintessence that you embody, that light unique to you represented through your distinct gifts.

∞ Take a deep breath in through your nose, inhaling your synergy, exhaling slowly, allowing your intention to form. Calling in the support of your spiritual teachers and guides, guardian angel and highest self, begin to see, feel, allow yourself to experience yourself sinking down into the safety, support, and nourishment of Mother Earth, Goddess Gaia. Begin to breathe in through the soles of your feet, imagining deep roots pouring through them deep down into the core of the Earth. As the energy comes back up from the Earth you are filled with a sense of protection and calm.

- ∞ On your next inhalation begin to see, feel, allow, imagine yourself as a tree. Notice the elongation of your trunk as the energy reaches up to your main limbs, and then forms more and more branches. Allowing the energy to flow down through your leaves and branches, limbs to trunk and roots into the ground, notice the areas where the energy seems to get stuck, where it is heavier or seems nonexistent. Are the leaves and branches full and green or sparse and faded? Is your tree in a grove or does it stand alone? Visualize your tree now superimposed onto your physical body, and notice where the energy is blocked, inflamed, where it is lacking. Does it have color, sound, an image, word, or any other communication?
- ∞ Take a few minutes and continue to collect information and if you feel comfortable, open a dialogue asking more specific questions about how you can bring back flow, balance, and healing to those places within. When this feels complete go ahead and jot any notes down on the "Your Tree of Life" worksheet. It may seem like you will never forget the information you have given, but because we are often in an elevated form of consciousness during meditation it is sometimes easy to forget the full context of guidance.

Finish with an intention of gratitude. This will forge greater connection and communication with your wise self.

YOUR TRAUMA TREE

Using the Trauma Tree as your guide, fill in the tree with your personal dysfunctions or illnesses.

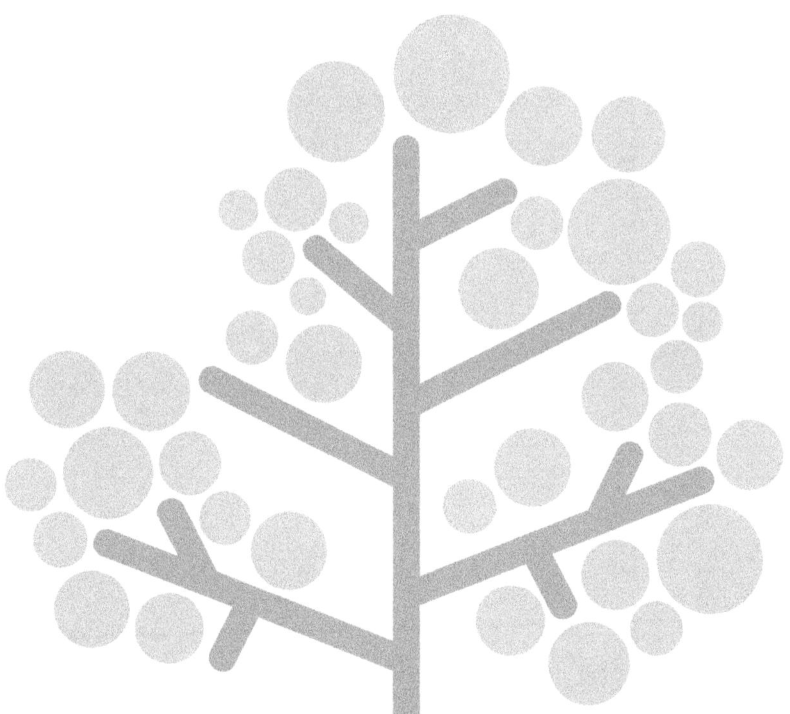

CHAPTER 3

Trauma – Your Portal to Freedom

TRAUMA IS YOUR PORTAL TO FREEDOM – AND THE KEY TO UNLOCKING IT!

Let's go back to the "treasure map" concept. As we bring awareness to physical pain, disease, or an emotional feeling we can access the points along our own timelines to find the "roots" to clear and allow full spectrum healing to transform our past, present, and future selves. Yes, we did just say your future self! The journey is not just about bringing healing into the past and present but projecting and visualizing healing to and from your future self. Sometimes working on the healing of your future self can bring an easier sense of ease and release of trauma because it allows us to disassociate from the current level of trauma.

It's important to note that everyone's journey is unique. We all have come into this life to experience different lessons for soul growth, and we are all at different points along our individual healing spiral. As unique beings, we each have a specific formula for our optimum healing and personal growth. In the coming chapters we will offer you numerous tools and interventions, both tangible and intangible for you to masterfully create your map to freedom.

TRAUMA

Trauma can take many forms, and we want to stress the point here that trauma is not always a "bad" aspect of your life. Did you hear that? NOT ALL TRAUMA IS BAD! In fact, trauma can be beneficial. It is what shapes us and our life into who we are. We would like you instead to think of trauma as a point on the road of your life, or the *Trauma Tree* we discussed in Chapter Two, where you have gotten derailed, stuck, or lost. You might be saying, well, I don't have any trauma, how did my life get all F*$*# up? Often when our body experiences a traumatic experience or life changing event, it's deeply ingrained in the brain or neural pathways (don't worry, we will discuss this in more detail in Chapter Eight). Think about it this way, you are traveling down a beautifully wooded trail and a majestic moose crosses your path, so you take note of all your surroundings, the smell of the pine trees, your accelerated heart rate and breathing, the cool mountain air on your cheek; maybe you can even see the glistening sweat on the moose's back. These heightened senses create a stronger "groove" in your memory where similar circumstances can bring up these same feelings of the encounter all over again. These memories are held throughout the body and respond through various "triggers" that we shall explore in the coming pages.

LIMBIC CENTER – BRAIN AND EMOTIONS

The limbic system is a combination of the mental and emotional layers into one system forming memories. When you experience trauma, it affects the hormonal and chemical regulation of the limbic center. You then begin to assign a label or multiple labels to the experience and we then store it in multiple parts of the brain – this is called the Genetic Blueprint. This genetic blueprint can be activated by a song or smell of a particular food that draws up memory from within the brain.

When damage is done to one part of the brain, you may still have a memory stimulated by an event from another part of the brain because you store information according to the input of sensations. You can have multiple events and triggers from which to pull these memories.

After so much of this "stress" or overstimulation the limbic system begins to disassociate. The brain will disengage during a traumatic event, numbing, avoiding, and having restricted affects. In this post-traumatic or traumatic state, the pain "numbing" and "shunting" occurs because the brain has released its natural opiates and hormones to place the body back into the parasympathetic mode of resting and digesting. These responses then become a part of the Genetic Blueprint and can result in a much longer state of disengagement.

These changes create a toxic chemical environment which causes cell death and structural alteration of the DNA and the brain. On an actual MRI you can see the changes of the traumatized brain: functional, structural, chemical, and biological. These reduce your future coping skills and ability to adapt and respond to stress.

THE LIMBIC SYSTEM AND AROMA ENERGY HEALING TECHNIQUES FOR RELEASING TRAUMA

∞ To access the meditation please go to www.zenergymedicinals.com

Where our intention goes, our energy flows. Sound familiar? Essential oils follow suit. Where the blood goes, the essential oils go; deep into the cellular consciousness, crossing the blood brain barrier because of their lipophilic nature of fat solubility.

This allows access to the limbic system and central nervous system, our bridges to our cellular consciousness and auric fields, and therefore holographic healing. Essential oils support the release of deeply set emotions and trauma, with the lock and key mechanism of the limbic system allowing us to re-pattern our neural pathways to higher levels of light and new expectations for a better and healthier life on all fronts.

Associated with primitive functions, the limbic system was originally identified as the smell brain. This is a key concept pointing to the significant benefits of using essential oils. Complex in nature is a multitude of structures for me equated to the New York City subway system with pathways that are numerous and far reaching. The limbic system is closely linked with the hippocampus and the hypothalamus. The former connects and coordinates all sensory applications, including emotional drives and instincts and the latter institutes physiological reactions, including neurochemical and hormonal responses and regulation such as the mood enhancer serotonin and endorphins. The connection between the limbic system and the nervous system allows the essential oils to have a powerful effect on supporting, balancing, and strengthening this primary bodily command center.

The limbic system is likened to a lock and key concept. When you first inhale an aroma, you are creating the lock. And then again, when you inhale the same scent it becomes the key to unlock the memories and psychophysiological responses associated with that memory. The more you utilize your oil and recognize it as a potent intervention for transformation, the more quickly you can accelerate your path of healing and ultimately self-actualization.

Creating deeper contact with ourselves creates increased awareness of our emotional trigger points. Refer to the emotional reaction diagram. How do you get triggered and what is your emotional response? Aromatherapy offers us potent alchemy to shift the trajectory of our emotional response in the moment because of the limbic connection. When an unwanted emotion or pattern arises, try gently inhaling a blend of the following oils for a minute or two, focusing on the positive affirmation to dissolve the emotional imprint in the cells and to create and solidify new healthier memory cells in the limbic brain. Then, continue to use that blend whenever you want to access the new positive connection.

Be sure to pay attention to your dreams and guidance after working with your oils this way because you've created a pathway for your soul and personality to communicate with you far more easily. Here are a few for you to start with; feel free to create your own combinations.

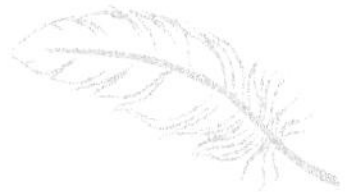

Take a moment to imagine on this trail of your fabulous life, that each trauma or life event is marked by a golden feather. These golden feathers create sparks in your memory that you are easily triggered by either in a positive way or a negative way.

- ∞ Anxiety: Breathe in patchouli and frankincense and affirm – "I am calm and capable."
- ∞ Depression: Breathe in orange and ylang ylang – "I choose health and joy in body, mind and spirit."

YOUR PORTAL TO FREEDOM

Sounds pretty sci-fi! Well, we are not talking about a portal to another galaxy but rather a doorway to unlimited creative potential, optimal health, and the fullness of self-expression. OK, so, let's go back to the golden feather concept we discussed above. When you start to use the tools in this book, botanicals, essential oils, crystals, and meditations, you begin to access this portal and the golden feathers act as keys. As you access each key, the door(s) unlock, and new discoveries of your health unfold. The trauma begins to lift, you feel lighter, and you move forward into freedom. This is one of the reasons the limbic connection is such an integral aspect to healing. You become the key-master and the gatekeeper of your journey. Magical healing bonus – don't forget the meditations on trauma to accelerate your healing.

How can trauma be the key to unlocking your freedom to health? You are most likely asking yourself right now, do I have to go through trauma to achieve health and freedom, to live a joyous life. Absolutely not! But what we found is that when you are stuck in a pattern or merry-go-round of illness and disease that you just can't seem to get off of, the key to getting back on track is addressing the trauma.

Trauma is Your Portal to Freedom. In the web of life, everything is connected. We are deeply connected to each other and to the earth. In your community of friends and family, the medicine of healing is held. Our human nature is designed to heal through relationships. It is through this presence of love, compassion and greater understanding we can shift collectively. On some level, we empathically experience everyone's trauma, and to fully heal ourselves we must address the healing each other and of the Earth's DNA. Then we can let go of not only our trauma but of those around us. This can be a simple process by using the tools in your Freedom Photon Wheels you will be learning and creating throughout this book.

TRAUMA TIMELINE DISCOVERY DIVE

Trauma takes on many, many forms. In fact, there are so many that we created an easy worksheet for you to recognize your own trauma and

NAME it. Use this trauma worksheet and start answering the questions as you continue along through the chapters in the book. When we experience trauma, it can affect us on a physical, emotional, or spiritual level – and we know you are asking this – so yes, you can have trauma on multiple layers of the body at the same time and many of us do. We are amazing but complicated humans!

A great deal of trauma is held at the subconscious level and, with the innate wisdom within you, surfaces when the time is ready. Be patient and gentle with yourself as each layer rises to the surface to heal and transform. It will set you free!

YOUR TRAUMA TIMELINE

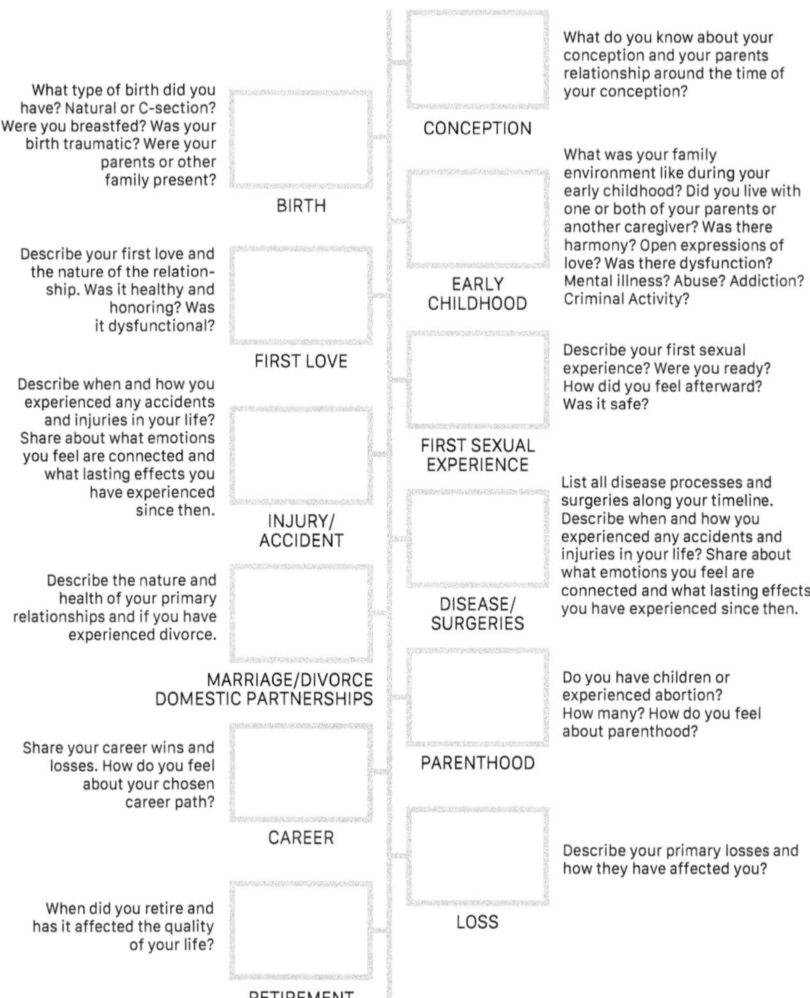

Instructions:

The explorative process of self discovery for the trauma timeline offers the opportunity to document and witness, with loving compassion, your core experiences that have imprinted on your DNA and physical and non physical bodies. They hold unlimited potential for exploration, transformation and a deeper understanding of yourself and human nature. Be gentle with yourself as you fill in your timeline. You can create your own ceremony to honor your journey of life experience.

Suggestion – make a copy of the worksheet so you can use it to work through different layers of trauma.

TRAUMA DISCOVERY DIVE

Please only use this worksheet after reading the above section and completing your Trauma Timeline. This will ensure you are prepared to start releasing your inner trauma – but let's face it, this can be intense!

How to use this worksheet:
This worksheet is for your eyes only, so HONESTY IS KEY. Healing is all about YOU so why shield yourself from freedom??

Dig deep, folks – to the deepest darkest place of your soul where you just want to let out the biggest scream of frustration, anger, hurt, or abuse. If you don't remember anything or can't think of anything, that's OK! Your Freedom Photon Wheel interventions will help with the connection and release of your inner trauma!

Step 1
List and name your traumas – you can be general until you are ready to be more specific.

Examples:

- ∞ I experienced a childhood trauma
- ∞ I was in a life changing car accident
- ∞ I have a debilitating chronic disease

Now you give it a try.

Step 2
Take each of the traumas listed above and describe how it is affecting your life emotionally.

Example: I have a debilitating disease and I am emotionally and physically exhausted.

Step 3
Take each of the traumas listed above and describe how it is affecting your life physically.

Example: I was in a life changing car accident and I have chronic pain.

Step 4
Take each of the traumas above and describe how it is affecting you mentally.

Example: I have chronic fatigue syndrome and it is hard to focus, remember, and even think about the simple tasks and responsibilities in life.

Step 5
Do you notice any connections between the traumas you listed above?

Example: After I experienced the car accident in 2003, I began to feel more and more tired and lost my sense of passion and joy for life. The chronic fatigue symptoms then began to manifest over the following two years.

Step 6
What emotions came up for you when listing these traumas?

Example: I began to have a tightness in my chest and tears came into my eyes – I also felt angry: Why me!

Step 7
What actions are you ready to take to step into your freedom?

Example: I am ready to do whatever it takes – I can't live like this anymore.

HEALING TRAUMA

∞ To access the meditation for releasing trauma please go to www.zenergymedicinals.com

Healing trauma is a layered process, like the peeling of an onion. As we bring the light of awareness into a specific layer with our focused intention for healing, applying the interventions included here we begin to clear the pathways of stuck energy, disease process, and limited thinking to allow for the next layer to surface. This process of peeling is not finite: layers surface to be cleared. This release allows greater levels of love and light to nourish the fullness of our being as we elevate our consciousness to greater points of self-mastery free to live the lives we have always dreamt of.

A cautionary note. Sustainably shifting deep levels of trauma requires the support of qualified, seasoned practitioners to assist and support the healing process as it unfolds. Be sure to vet your support team from education to experience. With that said, innately you are the MVP of your healing journey. Invite the intention of those practitioners who hold the most benevolent medicine for your awakening and healing to be clearly brought to your path.

CONCEPTS FOR CONTEMPLATION – THE LIFE PULSE AND SELF AWARENESS

THE LIFE PULSE

Everything has a life pulse. Aligning with greater understanding of your relationship within the principles of and phases of the life pulse increases self-awareness and your ability to balance the aspects of expansion, contraction, and stasis.

Let's look at common aspects of each stage. In a state of expansion, we are moving outward. We are active and searching as if on a quest propelled by an inner calling. We're creative, building, growing, learning and experiencing oftentimes outside our norm or comfort zone.

When we are in a place of contraction, we bring the experiences and interactions of expansion inward for deeper introspection. We search to understand and find balance through a new level of equilibrium.

It is important to note that both the expansion and contraction phases have a negative potential as well as positive, based on our intention. Negative expansion can appear aggressive, dominating and willful. Negative contraction can show as regression, withholding, seeking safety through isolation, or separation motivated by fear or mistrust.

In the stasis phase, we assimilate the wisdom of experiences garnered in the expansion and contraction phases. This aspect is imperative for full integration at the physical and soul level. Stasis allows for rest, renewal and ability to move forward holistically. When our relationship to these phases is out of balance there is no movement, no growth. We can become stagnant and stuck. If we believe that contraction is negative, then that surfaces in our negative intentionality. Are we resisting our natural flow of life to move to be inward or outward, or to be quiet, silent, or resting? Questions to ask in contradiction: Am I moving backward rather than inward. Am I afraid? Of what? Do I feel a sense of distrust? The inability to give? Do I feel the need to protect myself or to separate myself from others? The antidote for a contraction is: What am I afraid of that I might find inside of me? What within me do I mistrust? What within me do I think is so bad that I protect myself from it?

As we explore our trauma, we begin to understand ourselves at a deeper level. Our trauma can be connected to not feeling worthy: of love, money, health in our bodies and in our relationships. It can be connected to not feeling safe, not trusting, feeling alone, feeling shame around sexuality and sensuality. We can push away our feminine or our masculine. We can push away God, our loved ones, pretend we are fine, bury ourselves in addictions of all sorts. OR, we can invite the light of truth deep within and pivot. We can align with our heart and positive intention, to deepen the connection with ourselves. We can move through our trauma, bring light there, healing and opening to our essence, our gifts, our "quintessence."

AW There was a time in my life where I felt lost. Truthfully, there have been many times I have felt this way, but I am defining one moment here. I had this repetitive feeling, "I just do not know what to do with myself." I've been thinking about this phrase often. It brought me to a new level of realization, a new way of looking at myself. I don't know how to be in stasis … stillness, quiet without it being a collapse, a loss, numbing, numbing pain. I don't know how to just sit with myself and not do it in a way that is outwardly put upon me. Where I get so stuck in overwhelm to the point of being incapacitated.

I love the stream of life expansion, I love it. I'm great with that. It is my zone. I am most comfortable being expanded. Contraction is also highly familiar. This deep, dark place of retreat where I won't let anything come close. It touches on such a young place of safety, the only place I could go to feel safe when I was young … a small, dark closet.

But stasis, stillness, this is the place I judge myself the most, not acting, not doing. How do I find a place of self-resolve, of loving self-care?

Where I can just be and allow what is happening to occur without needing to label it. How can I let go of the demand for expansion or contraction, avoiding the collapse and the booming voice of the great self-judge within? This represents an enormous aspect of my own healing journey.

Where is your comfort zone in the continuum of the life pulse? Where is your discomfort?

What phase frightens or seems elusive to you? What fears are held deep with you? Where do you feel unworthy of love?

Mental illness runs rampant on both of my bloodlines. Depression, alcoholism, addiction, chronic anxiety, suicidal ideations and the act itself, mood disorders, and many, many gradations in between. I understand the fear of getting stuck in the mire of feeling unwell on multiple levels, becoming trapped in the stillness and enveloped by the darkness. I know these places, I have felt them, explored them, been immersed there, felt stuck there, and also risen up out of them. That does not mean perfection, but it is a great shift and healing.

When we move through and heal our trauma, we find that the other side is filled with light, ripe with possibilities, miracles. This is where compassion is born and the ability to open our hearts with greater understanding to others who have walked similar paths.

Healing is the path to freedom; it takes courage and commitment and a tremendous amount of support and it absolutely frees us to be the most amazing versions of ourselves. You've got this! You have everything you need within you to heal at the core level, on every level.

Clearing trauma opens a path to fulfill our biggest dreams in ways that in the past have seemed impossible. All the life force, or energy encapsulated in the layers of trauma, sometimes referred to as "blocks," is filled with our "golden quintessence," our greatest gifts and unique talents. As we heal, we break open these places within, and the calcified energy consciousness held in the trauma blocks breaks apart becoming nutrients for our soul growth. This allows filaments of bright light, our "essence," which is filled with the remembrance of our own divinity. The light of divine consciousness that resides within all of us floods our bodies, both physical and, nonphysical resulting in greater connection, clarity, and synchronicity.

When our awareness expands in this way, our consciousness moves beyond the maya or density of the third dimension. This third dimensional experience is wrought with karma: pain, struggle, and suffering. However, at this juncture of time and space and planetary consciousness we can expand beyond this limitation and evolve from the perspective of joy and the dimension of creating life experience from effortless intention.

LETTING GO, THE EGO AND TRANSFORMATION

DNA Infinity healing is profound. It will change your life, and requires a "death" of the old. This may sound intimidating, and yet it is the quintessential portal of liberation. The ego, and the old ways of being must fall away, so the new you may be birthed. Just as the phoenix regenerates cyclically, your evolution requires a complete letting go of what no longer serves you, in every way—your health, your relationships, your career, your diet, and other habits – ALL of WHO YOU ARE!

TRAUMA BLOCKS IN THE ENERGY FIELD

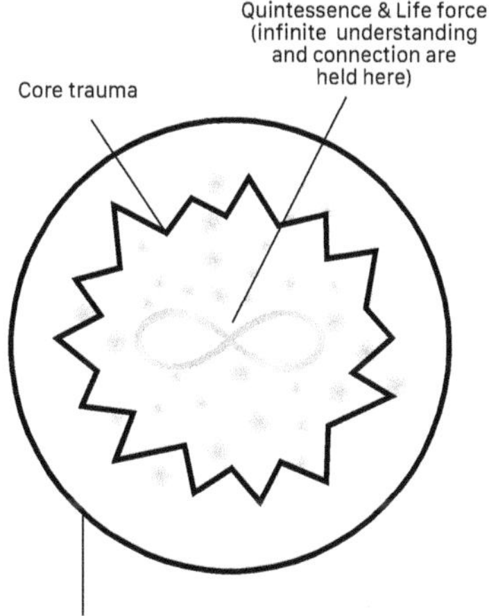

All the old thought patterns, beliefs, emotions, images, and energy will rise to the surface to be cleared. Welcome and release them as they do, be in the flow, and continue to remind your monkey mind that a higher dimension of experience is unfolding within and all around you. Use your essential oil and herbal formulas to anchor and assimilate this process. Connect into your heart, and the zero-point field at the very center and breathe in a great sense of gratitude: thank the teaching from your ancestry as the divine consciousness integrates the trauma through its own cyclical journey, illuminating greater wisdom, consciousness, and the unlocking of higher degrees of your own quintessence held ready to be set free.

TRANSFORMATION OF TRAUMA

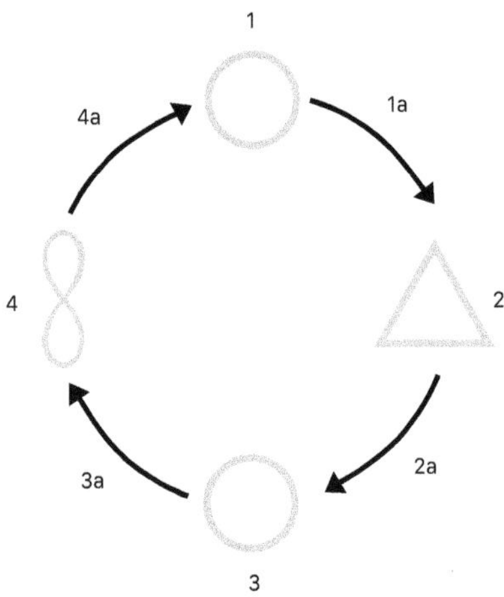

1. Trauma held in the DNA and Auric Field.
   1a. Healing - new awareness - increase in emotional intelligence.
2. Comprehension of Soul level teaching.
   2a. Assimilation of wisdom.
3. Consciousness expands.
   3a. Quintessence fills the cells and floods the system.
4. Connection deepens to infinite intelligence.
   4a. Elevation in consciousness imprints on web of life and expands planetary consciousness.

This brings us back to the microcosm of the macrocosm of the infinity symbol, whereby every degree of quantum shift we make transforms the cosmic, collective consciousness and lifts the planetary frequency, in turn per the greater design for Mother Earth. Gandhi spoke of changing ourselves to change the world. We can transform and elevate the consciousness of the planet one by one, and when we heal and shift our perspective and expectation of life and relationship, both areas change around us. This new you may seem foreign: this is OK and natural.

As this next iteration of yourself emerges, you may notice different habits, taste in clothes, food, music as your system redefines your environment both internal and external. By letting go of old patterns, we make way for the new healthier, habit patterns to form. You can liken this to the simple practice of cleaning out your closet, removing what you no longer wear, love, or desire to "fit into" again. This creates the space and vacuum from the universal perspective to new, beautiful clothes to fill it.

MEDITATION – INFINITY ACTIVATION FOR TRAUMA RELEASE

To access the meditation please go to www.zenergymedicinals.com

- ∞ Get comfortable, take a deep breath in. Inhale your cistus trauma release synergy for thirty seconds while you focus on the clarity of your intention.
- ∞ Envision a golden pyramid. The pyramid as a form of sacred geometry is a very powerful archetype that represents the universal law of manifestation, and the opportunity that we have here from a human perspective to self-actualize or achieve self-mastery. One side of the pyramid represents the child's consciousness. Another side represents the feminine and then the next the masculine. We all have these aspects within us. The male and female represent our personality aspects, our DNA, and everything genetically that comes through our lineage from our mother and our mother's mother and all the way down. And then the same for the masculine side. The child consciousness represents every unresolved experience in our early childhood, seeded with our treasure map so to speak of why our soul has come here to learn, grow, and evolve.
- ∞ In this meditation today, we invite the intention to release all energies that no longer serve us, including our old story so we can come into a new relationship ourselves from a place of empowerment, vision, and the ability to manifest our life experience from a place beyond limitation.
- ∞ Invite your intention to connect deeply into the core of the Earth, to draw upon the great abundance and protection that is held here.
- ∞ Invite the intention to open the third eye, by which you see before you the brilliance of a great being of light. Out of her left palm emanates a platinum light, which beams into your third eye. As this light is pulsating platinum rays to the third eye, she moves her hand down and beams the platinum light into your heart and high heart center.

Cleansing, clearing with an invitation for you to let go of all that no longer serves your highest truth.

∞ As this platinum light pulsates in your heart center, she moves her hand down to your belly, your sacral area, and beams the platinum light inviting you to release all judgement of self, all limitations, all the emotional burdens that you've carried through this life and many, many others.

∞ Letting go of all the places where you've felt separate from the Earth, from your body, from mother Earth, mother of all mothers. A golden light begins to pour down upon you filled with sacred symbols and geometry.

∞ On the next breath in, bring your intention back to the bright being before you that is igniting memory and healing sequences into the strands of DNA. In her other palm, now you see an emerald light, emanating, pulsating, and she holds this light in front of your heart, beaming it directly into the places of child consciousness that are still frozen.

∞ This healing is for your ancestors who carried this pain and struggle. It is for you and the courage of your soul to bring it into the light in this lifetime for transmutation. Golden light beams into every cell and molecule in your body and actualizes to a golden infinity symbol.

∞ At that concentric point, within the infinity symbol, breathe into that zero-point field of limitless potential as your DNA is repairing.

∞ We call forth for an activation, the divine seed blueprint, perfected by the Creator, the invitation of your I AM presence to guide this activation. Bringing back the soul fragments bathed in light, return to wholeness, anchoring this into the cellular consciousness now.

∞ Allow now a recalibration of your soul triad, purifying through the genetic line, mother and father bloodline. And a holding of the sacred child within and all children to come, all who have come. We offer this healing for the Earth and all kingdoms of life: plant, mineral, animal, human. All that is seen, unseen, past, present, still unfolding. Bringing this frequency of light all the way through the timelines, through all time and no time, all aspects, all dimensions, all realities.

CHAPTER 4

Opening to the Blessing Stream of Abundance

So, you might be asking yourself, "Why is there a chapter on abundance in a book regarding health and well-being?" Great question! Abundance is completely connected to your health and we are asking you to not just think of abundance as a monetary value but of all the abundance that flows through your life. Financial stress is one of the major contributors to disease and family problems. But we are wanting you to dive deeper with your thoughts around abundance. It's a dynamic part of our lives so how do we receive and allow the unlimited abundance to enter our lives and EVERY part of our DNA?

Now strap up and hold on because the abundance is going to start pouring into your life in ways you never imagined. In fact, open up the key to your unlimited imagination and dream big, baby!

Now let's talk about our friend, Jennifer.

Jennifer is a middle-aged woman who has experienced great levels of abundance in her life. Her ancestors on the father's bloodline had experienced vast levels of financial abundance, but only to ultimately lose most of it. She presented to us with the intention to exponentially increase her abundance, lifting her financial glass ceiling consistently. Although her physical health and energy levels were a concern, the sacred energy spoke primarily to past relationships with money on the father's line and deep disappointment, betrayal, sadness, and frustration on the mother's line. All healing is spiral in nature, and like an onion. As we heal one layer another comes to the surface to be cleared. Even so there are times where "quantum healing" becomes possible and multiple layers come to the surface, all connected in nature, like the lattice work of an intricate root system. Healing cannot be forced; our higher self and I AM presence guide our journey of transformation in perfect divine time.

Since this is meant to be a planet of evolution, a schoolhouse of sorts to create the conditions for our soul growth, our expansion and ultimately remembrance of our divinity, it is imperative to make the connections or points of realization within our experience to be able to assimilate the wisdom and unlock greater levels of our "quintessence", aka superhero power, sacredly held in our DNA.

When Jennifer did not achieve her monthly goal, she would experience deep disappointment, then frustration and all-out anger. The intensity of this emotion would pull her out of alignment, and she would become depressed, pick up a cold or a flu bug, and her bank balance would further dwindle. Deep within her cellular consciousness and DNA was the expectation of loss and failure at the intended financial goal based on past experiences in her bloodline, cementing belief systems and perpetuating the pattern as the vicious cycle would repeat itself. Once she was able to make the connections in her life and family patterning and hold a place of compassion for herself, we were able to clear the layers.

When we pull ourselves out of alignment, with our thoughts, emotions which are all responding to our belief system, we close off from the pathway of abundance that was on its way. Furthermore, our ability to receive deeply and consistently is directly correlated to the level of what we have cleared and what we are ready and open to allow in. Otherwise, the abundance can only come in so far and then just doesn't stick.

Jennifer was ready to let go of the old and receive a new experience of life. She was open. When we align with effortless intention, we are anointed with grace. The resistance melts away and surrender propels us forward to the next greatest iteration of self, that person we have always somewhere known we can be, that we are meant to become.

When we speak of clearing, or detox from this perspective, it is as if we are stripping away the layers of emotion, experience, wounds, and trauma that are held in the DNA. It all seeps from your bones, bone marrow, and blood to be cleared to make way for the new energetic configurations to nourish the cells and to imprint and activate throughout your system holographically. Symbolically, from the level of DNA in the cells, the entire physical body and all the layers of the energy body shift as well. Since we are in human form our physical body is our "tool" for creation, gauging our levels of vibration and consciousness through its health and vitality. We can be spiritually awake, purposeful, and physically and wholly alive, resonating at the zenith of our potential. An exception to this is when we are experiencing a physical health crisis, which is in fact the body's way of communicating truth and opportunity for healing and soul growth.

We all can live a life of magic, vision, and abundance beyond what seems possible to our mind and limited thinking. Even when we have experienced pain, struggle, negative patterns, disease, and dross, our higher nature coaxes us to find the resources to shift, heal, grow, and RISE.

When we look at the energy consciousness of abundance in our lives, we must view it from all perspectives. Abundance is more than monetary in nature, although it certainly is that too. Abundance also takes many forms: Love. Vitality. Energy. Thought. Inspiration. Clarity. Creativity. Passion. Health. Support. Nourishment.

ABUNDANCE AND OPENING TO MIRACLE CONSCIOUSNESS

Intention:
I AM OPEN to receive the grandest experience of ABUNDANCE that this multidimensional life can offer me. I call upon the highest vibration, patterned perfectly for my being. I invite and allow all streams of abundance into my sacred human heart, to its very core, to the zero-point field of limitless creation where the DIVINE resonance and sentience can create far greater than I can rationalize. I align with miracle consciousness, which is my birthright. I allow miracles to flow to and through me and I recognize myself as a DIVINE being of LIGHT.

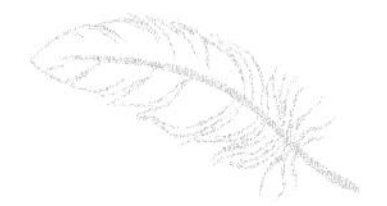

Miracles are not just for avatars. Miracle consciousness is accessible to each one of us that walks the face of this Earth. Take a moment to see how this statement resonates with you. Does it strike a chord of truth? Or does it feel like a sheer impossibility? Or even stronger – sacrilege? No need to judge your response, simply welcome it. Listen for what you believe to be true.

Remember, perception is nine-tenths of reality and the precursor to creation. Your beliefs tied to abundance and miracles are not entirely your own. Your entire lineage, your mother and father bloodlines, experiences, and beliefs are held within your DNA. This energy often holds antiquated intentions to protect its line from the pain and struggle of the past. The current juncture of time and space allows us the ability to quantum leap and shift these patterns, dissolving the limitations of the past to create our own experience of Heaven on Earth. In this moment, let's take the step forward together and invite in the potential for a life of greater abundance than you have ever dared to imagine. Breathe in the vibration of miracle consciousness allowing it to ease its way into the cells and all the particles of our being.

As you continue to explore your relationship with abundance and miracles, watch to ensure that you are open to grander possibilities and avoid words like revenue, money, top line, bottom line, profit, or phrases that limit or constrict the flow. When we expand beyond a framework of third dimensional reality, our mind does not have a framework to engage with the limitless nature of the universe. We can let go of every limiting factor in our DNA, from our experience and through our bloodlines, in every moment and every breath.

AW Close to my thirty-first birthday I was exhibiting at a body–mind-spirit show on Cape Cod, Massachusetts and happened to cross paths with a beautiful, brilliant woman and spiritual teacher. We exchanged products and services and I left our meeting with a sense of gratitude and humility. Frankly, I was overcome with her generosity … the generosity of her spirit, her gifts, her loving presence, and her light. After our meeting I had a sense that some of the pieces of my life were really beginning to fit together. The following month my first husband and I moved from South Florida to a part of Massachusetts that was very near to her home.

The apartment that my spouse and I lived in served like a womb for me and a haven for my relationship that birthed anew. We worked with a prayer grid that the spiritual teacher had given us. In about a week or so after that was complete, I telephoned her to see if she wanted to get together. I decided that since she offered spiritual readings I would very much like one for my birthday. We chose a time and then advanced the schedule based on her guidance.

As I walked up the pathway to her home that cold January day, I was struck by a sense of peace and safety I felt there. There was something just beyond my grasp: was it familiarity? Her home was like a temple, beautiful statues of gods and goddesses throughout. There was a sense of ease and sweetness between us, knowing each other's soul. She informed me they were moving the following week to California. I was shocked and a bit disappointed to hear that this new ally would be leaving. She explained that her guidance had told her that a spiritual family would be the next occupants of her home and expressed her wonder, "Is it you?"

As much as I wished that to be true, I told her my husband and I were not able to purchase a home right then, especially one that was so lofty. Renting was also out of the question as we had just signed a lease and we were paying quite a nominal fee.

There were several synchronistic events that took place while we were together that day. More than once I was struck by the most beautiful aroma of lilies when there were none in the house. Photos of spiritual teachers filled her home: Mother Meera, Sai Baba, and Amma, and I experienced a sense of comfort, of beingness and wholeness while I was there.

During her spiritual reading, she gave me homework to make a list of all the qualities in a home that I wanted, and to bring it back for a meeting the following week. Also, synchronistically, my husband and I had just created that list before we moved to Massachusetts. I left her home that day in a sense of bewilderment and in knowing that there was magic at work. I stayed in a semi dream state until our next meeting.

I returned with my homework in hand, and it became clear that we would live there. The guidance was to surrender and to trust, and the assurance was there that this was the best that could possibly happen for all involved. This woman, this new ally who was now presenting me with an opportunity to live in her home went on to tell me that she knew that very first day when I came that I would be the woman who would be the next occupant of the home. She was also guided to rent us the home at a very affordable rate, far beneath market value for the property until my economic situation changed within the next few months.

Suddenly, so suddenly, it was this blessed beautiful home that had every single element contained within it and around it that had been included on our list we created some months before … and better. It even so happened that our particular neighborhood has a "grandfather" exemption clause to run a business directly out of your home. Divine perfection.

The time that I spent preparing to move felt like packing up and jumping off the cliff into the great beyond – terrifying, exhilarating, filled with fear and uncertainty. Yet the guidance was clear and the signs plentiful. I realize that I was being drawn to the very edge of my comfort zone and pushed beyond that point. Thoughts ran through my head: "What the hell am I doing, have I lost my mind?"

At one point as these thoughts were running through me, I stopped to pump gas and looked down, and there in an ice filled puddle was a gold Israeli coin. Later, I found out that that type of coin is symbolic of significant abundance and spiritual synchronicity. It was in those moments that I tasted the sweetness of surrender and the opening of my heart to receive love, support, guidance and abundance in ways greater than I thought possible.

I was filled with the expression of gratitude and humility beyond what any words could express. Simultaneously it brought me deeper into my personal commitment, into my work of service, in love and light and divine truth. I was struck by how palpable miracles can be, how possible they can be, and how they exist beyond any sense of limitation of the third dimensional realm. How they are completely multidimensional in nature and if we open our heart to the possibility, to the potential of something far greater than we are, and simultaneously working in conjunction with us, with our own sense of divinity and our humanness amazing things happen. When we open our hearts to receive what may be considered a miracle, life can unfold beyond our wildest dreams.

This is our prayer and intention for you, a life of your wildest, most vibrant dreams. For you. Your children. Your children's children, and so on. What is possible today may simply not have been part of the grand design yesterday. Carpe diem.

DISCOVERY DIVE – GARDEN OF PLENTY AND PLANTING THE SEEDS

Set aside some time for this exercise. You may want to have some colored pencils or other artistic implements and perhaps even a larger paper than this to work with. This exercise is best done between the new and the full moon.

You may enhance this experience by inhaling the Abundance Blend formula for 30–45 seconds and making an invigorating cup of Garden Tea.

Abundance Blend

- ∞ 1 drop Carrot Seed essential oil (*Daucus carota*)
- ∞ 3 drops Wild Orange essential oil (*Citrus sinensis*)
- ∞ 1 drop Clary Sage essential oil (*Salvia sclarea*)
- ∞ 1 drop Geranium essential oil (*Pelargonium graveolens*)

Blend into 1 tablespoon carrier oil (jojoba, coconut, sweet almond, etc.). Apply sparingly to the palms of your hands, inhale and then apply to the heart center inviting in the greatest experience of abundance that this life can offer you.

Garden Tea

Ingredients:

- ∞ 20 g Green tea – *Camellia sinensis*
- ∞ 6 g Chrysanthemum – *Chrysanthemum morifolium*
- ∞ 3 g Calendula – *Calendula officinalis*
- ∞ 3 g Ginkgo – *Ginkgo biloba*
- ∞ 3 g Helichrysum – *Helichrysum italicum*
- ∞ 3 g Honeysuckle – *Lonicera periclymenum*
- ∞ 3 g Spearmint – *Mentha spicata*
- ∞ 2 g Ginger root – *Zingiber officinale*

Combine all ingredients: Infuse 1 tablespoon of tea for 4 minutes in 236 ml of water.

Add a little sweetener if you like. Sip and enjoy!

To access the meditation please go to www.zenergymedicinals.com

- ∞ As you breathe in, envision yourself as a master gardener. You have as much land as you wish to cultivate. The sun is bright, the air warm and sweet, and the sacred Earth around you is pulsating a vibrant green. The more that you gaze upon it, the more you realize this is the brightest shade of green you've ever seen; it is alive and filled with the pulse of all creation. On your next breath in, invite the intention for the soil to be perfectly tilled, cultivated, and nutrient rich for your seeds to flourish.
- ∞ You may choose to see rows, or you may envision rings of soil prepared for your seeds. Allow your vision to unfold in its own organic manner. As you gaze down now, you see a golden basket in your hands. It is filled with seeds of all shapes, sizes, and colors. Some seeds may represent changes in your physical health, your weight, fitness level, healthy digestion, healing from a specific disease process; some may represent a new love or a rekindling of a current flame, others could be a renewed sense of peace and calm, while some may be planted for a new career or revitalized passion for the one you have; yet others could be for a healing within the family, your children, a new home or travel: the opportunities are as endless as your creativity flows.
- ∞ Notice as you decide what each seed is for, if there is a voice or feeling or blockage that stops you from going further. Jot it down to fully honor your process.

Now envision yourself walking your garden in a state of open heartedness, planting your seeds gently and purposefully into your sacred soil. As you lovingly cover the seeds with soil, contemplate how you will nurture and care for them from germination to harvest and all the beauty in between. Now envision each seed as a fully actualized intention; allow yourself to experience all the emotions that would flow with each manifestation in your life. Then breathe in a sense of gratitude for the full cornucopia of bounty … Thank and bless Mother Earth for this beautiful co-creation.

- ∞ You may choose to sketch out your garden and any thoughts and feelings that arose during this process. We love to add photographs of plants into our personal journals to deepen the connection to the natural world.

DISCOVERY DIVE – FAMILY ABUNDANCE TREE

FAMILY ABUNDANCE TREE

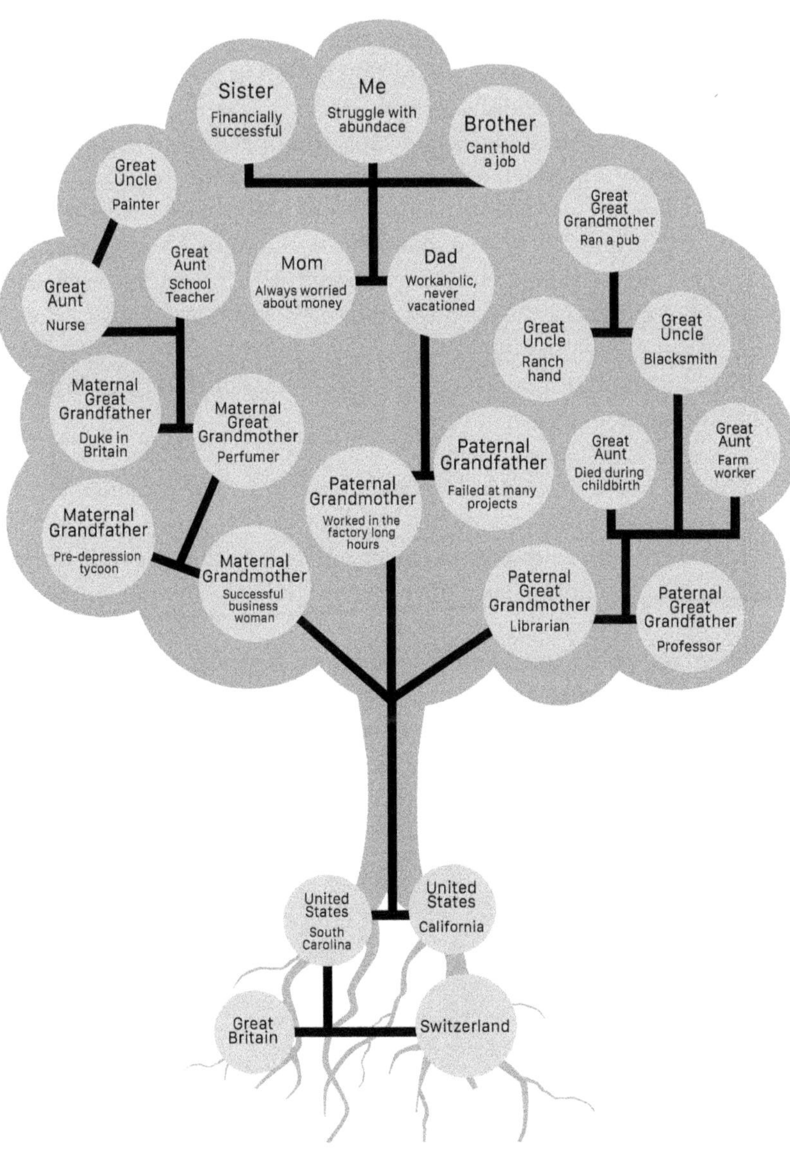

Our ancestors' experience of wealth and abundance or lack thereof is held within you holographically, from the auric field down to the level of DNA. Those patterns, belief systems, and images mold your perspective and current relationship dynamic with money are often tied into cultural collective experience. For example, the subconscious experience of the Irish potato famine runs along the DNA with those who carry that bloodline. Those of the Persian descent often experience the polar opposite, coming from a tradition rooted in great opulence.

Both the cultural consciousness and our specific genetic lineage affects our relationship, understanding, and openness to abundance.

Consider your parents' relationship to money, and specifically what they believed to be true about wealth and abundance. Did they have to work hard for it? Was it unattainable or plentiful? Was there joy or disdain about spending? Were they spendthrifts or penny-pinchers or somewhere in between? Was debt an issue?

Consider your cultural descent and what relationship it has to wealth and abundance.

How has this impacted your belief and experience of money?

Think about these questions and query your family as far back as possible to better understand the effects of the past on your life today.

Fill out the worksheet Family Abundance Tree, to see the connections and moments of realization that you have about your family genetic history of abundance. If you find areas you don't know about, it might be a good opportunity to do some family "digging."

FAMILY ABUNDANCE TREE

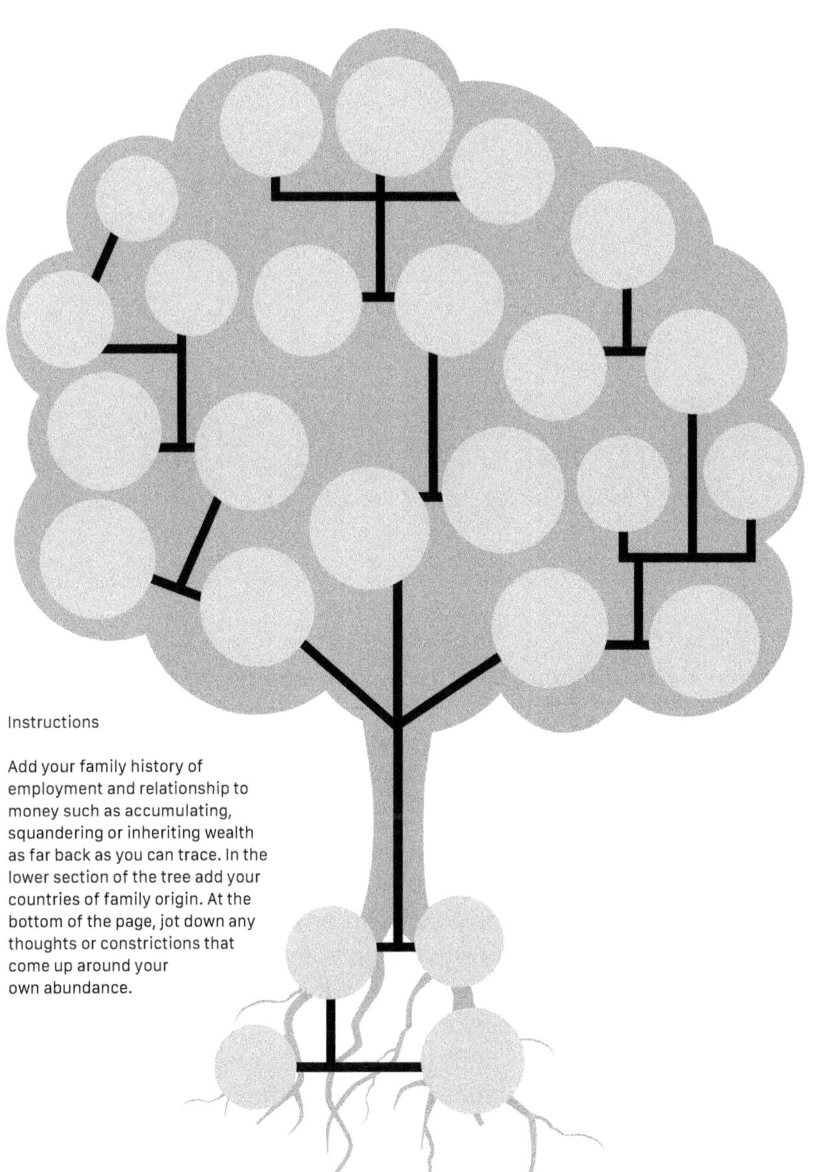

Instructions

Add your family history of employment and relationship to money such as accumulating, squandering or inheriting wealth as far back as you can trace. In the lower section of the tree add your countries of family origin. At the bottom of the page, jot down any thoughts or constrictions that come up around your own abundance.

MEDITATION – OPENING TO ABUNDANCE

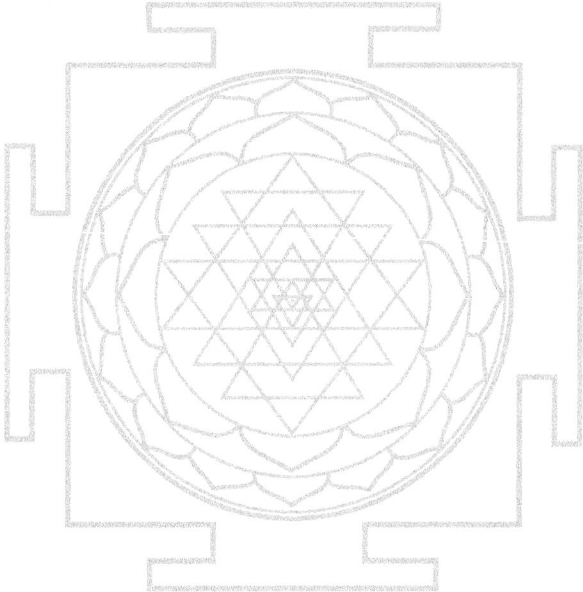

To access the meditation please go to www.zenergymedicinals.com

Breathe in your Abundance Blend and allow this intention to open to greater abundance to expand into every area of your life.

"I receive the highest potential of 'blessings' from all sources, known and unknown, seen and unseen, in form and still unfolding."

- ∞ Breathe into the center of your heart space. As you do this, invite in the presence of your spiritual guides, teachers, guardians, angels, your teams of light, your highest self, and your deva of abundance and the DNA Infinity team of light.
- ∞ Envision a pink ray of light that begins to ease its way into your heart space. This pink light is filled with coding to connect and commune with your cellular consciousness to activate the frequency of abundance, the template of miracle consciousness.
- ∞ Envision the horizontal and the vertical infinity symbol, merging at the very center of your heart into the dimension known as the zero-point field: The dimension of limitless creation. Breathing in

light into the concentric point at the center of your heart and the center of the infinity symbols, filling this point which is also a dimension at the very center of the cell. Activating additional strands of DNA in accordance with your I AM presence.

∞ Breathing in with the knowing that this light and healing is moving through your entire genetic line, the bloodline from mother, father, both pathways of creation. All the way to the origin point. Breathe in. Infinite light is filling your field as the lotus petals of the heart continue to open … love, compassion, and gratitude.

∞ Allow your cells and your energy field to reconfigure to this frequency as you invite in the biggest and brightest intention of abundance, of miracle consciousness for your life. Opening and allowing the full spectrum of abundance of light, of love, support, resources, money, health, vitality, nourishment, support, pleasure, friendship, sensuality, creativity, laughter, harmony.

∞ Take a few minutes to envision your deepest longings for this life. And when your intentions are fully clear, when you've seen, felt, imagined each one coming to fruition, allow yourself to experience the feelings, the emotions that you would with each one of your intentions fully manifest, fully actualized, fully alive … all around you. Take that feeling into each cell, each molecule, particle, subatomic structure, into the blood, in the bones. Invite that feeling into the crystalline structure of your body.

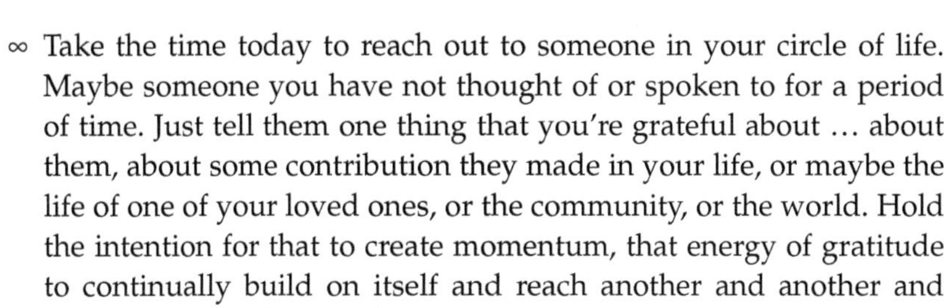

∞ Take the time today to reach out to someone in your circle of life. Maybe someone you have not thought of or spoken to for a period of time. Just tell them one thing that you're grateful about … about them, about some contribution they made in your life, or maybe the life of one of your loved ones, or the community, or the world. Hold the intention for that to create momentum, that energy of gratitude to continually build on itself and reach another and another and another. In great love, so be it.

ABUNDANCE AFFIRMATIONS

Karmic Release

- ∞ I release all past debts that are no longer honoring me.
- ∞ I release all strands of DNA in my genetic line of abundance that are entangled with loss, lack, poverty, and abuse.
- ∞ I release all vows of poverty, entitlement, and dark energy around money.

Deva of Abundance

- ∞ I call upon the deva of abundance to surround my being with the healing green and pink light of abundance.
- ∞ I am in the flow of a blessing stream of abundance.

I AM Open to Receiving Abundance

- ∞ I am open to receiving the abundance of the universe.
- ∞ I receive a consistent and abundant flow of money.

GOLDEN FEATHER GUIDANCE

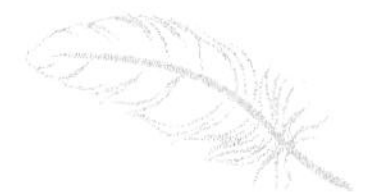

Immerse a crystal in a bowl of water during the full moon and leave out overnight to charge the stone and use it in your daily abundance meditations.

Envision a waterfall of liquid light falling upon your energy field, cleansing all the distorted beliefs and past relationships with money.

CHAPTER 5

Freedom Photon Wheel

What is it that you have come here for? To be? To create? What have you brought into this world to transform? What gifts are still waiting to be unlocked in your DNA?

The Freedom Photon Wheel is an essential adjunct to your personal process journey. It holds the keys to unlock YOUR freedom as each element activates within you the ability to open a doorway to accelerate the unlimited healing. These elements are to be used together as they create a quantum and magical level of healing at the deep core of your cellular DNA. This chapter explains each element in detail: what it is, why you are using it to unlock the DNA, and how it will elevate

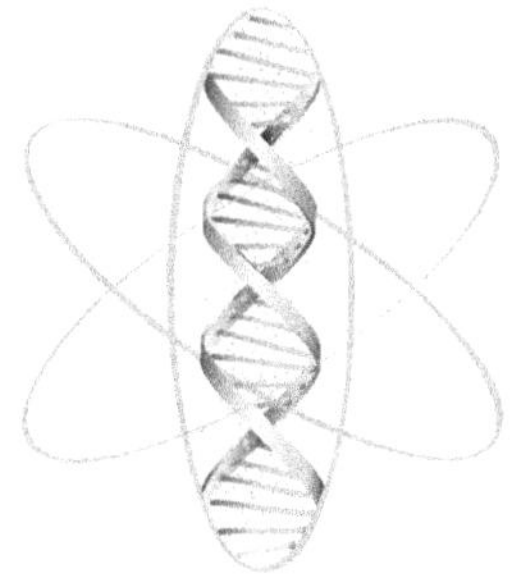

and expand your healing. You might not be familiar with some of these elements, this is totally OK. Get to know them and think of them as your new friends on this magical journey of healing.

So why did we choose the photon as the medium for transmission? The photon is an electromagnetic form of light passing through the frequency of the elements and into you. This allows the light frequency to anchor into the cellular genetic consciousness at a quantum rate that is now possible. It creates a magnetic path of transmission so you can experience the light ray of photonics and birthing of the ancient wisdom within. Ah ha, we just activated this within you. Boom! That's how easy it is. This is also where the holographic healing activates and is ignited within all your layers, physical and nonphysical.

The Freedom Photon Wheel, FPW, is designed to bring in all the archetypes into one dimension or intention to stimulate the innate healing power within. The wheel is divided into eleven categories each opening or creating a doorway into the DNA of the cells in the body, mind, and spirit.

When using the photon wheel for cellular healing, there are several ways to use and pick the archetypes. One, you can use the FPW that has been designated with the major element in each category to amplify the healing. Two, as you become more familiar with the archetypes, you can use your intuition or a pendulum to pick different elements to create your own Freedom Photon Wheel.

As you move along your own healing spiral, that which evolves over a lifetime, you require the support of elements along the way to assist you in the clearing, balancing, and assimilation process. The journey of awakening and accelerating your consciousness allows you to move through *Survive to Thrive Triad* and to ultimately bring healing to your own individual trinity: that of your masculine, feminine, and child personality aspects. Once you achieve a certain degree of understanding and self-transformation, you can actualize your life purpose. We are each destined with a unique gift that resonates and vibrates at a certain level of individual frequency. The elements on the wheel will activate your own essence and attune you to *Detox, Nourish, Activate* each organ system.

We know you have chosen this book because you are ready for transformation and change: maybe your old mantra was, "I can't do this anymore." These elements will help you shift not only your physical and emotional bodies but also your belief systems. We know this transformational journey might seem exciting and even scary, but we have been in your shoes and know that you can do this. "We believe in you," you truly have everything you could ever need within you. It's important as you use the *Freedom Photon Elements* that you are gentle and loving with yourself. Please see the *Golden Feather Guidance* tips throughout the book to support, nurture, and to embrace your self-care.

TRANSFORMATION AND SUSTAINABLE HEALING

Have you worked with several healing modalities and gained short bursts of relief only to find yourself seemingly back to square one? Well, you are not alone. Let's take a closer look at what happens when we ignite the flame of healing but don't follow through.

First, we want you to be certain, every moment in your life has led you perfectly here and now. Know that and trust this certainty just like you will take your next breath.

Take a moment to view the feather and infinity images. The golden feather is your key to transformation through self-care. As you nurture your inner being through the Freedom Photon Wheel you are connecting to an infinite and expansive quantum field of healing.

GOLDEN FEATHER GUIDANCE

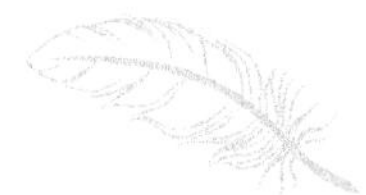

Love and nurture your inner self with a gift. A treat you have been longing for that truly makes your heart sing with joy. Something that you have never done before, maybe even been a little scared to do, that will help you jump on the wheel of release so you can fly with your wings spread and embrace your superhero within. Let your spirit fly!

For sustainable healing at the DNA level, we must approach our alchemical elements from both pathways, internal and external, physical and nonphysical. Take the infinity symbol, representing two ellipses or pathways that converge in the middle and access the zero-point field. The zero-point field is an unlimited space of limitless potential that moves in all directions around you yet brings you back to a place of centeredness or grounding, bringing the heart and mind together where you experience a deep feeling of oneness and connection. This place of safety and love assists in releasing core wounding of separation from source or how you refer to your higher power. Have you ever experienced a sense of deep longing? As if your heart just aches with each breath but you are not sure why? This is the soul's longing we are inviting you to connect into at this moment. Take a deep breath in and know that you are deeply loved.

It is with specific intent that we offer eleven variations of alchemical elements, the Freedom Photon Wheel, for your healing and metamorphosis. Each one of you carries a unique light and a set of messages, preserved perfectly in your DNA, and you each have a specific *Freedom Formula* if you will for optimum health – and it will change and evolve with time as you do. When you move beyond the third dimensional matrix of density to a five-dimensional vision and beyond, with a collective of powerful interventions, you can source what synergies will be effective and will perpetuate a quantum leap of sustainable health.

You will experience a greater sense of self awareness and elevation of your consciousness along the pyramid of self-realization and the actualization of your higher purpose. Each of the eleven elements, in our Freedom Photon Wheel, will focus on a different level of consciousness. Remember, a synergy will always be more effective than the singular: in this case working with more than one of the elements will accelerate your healing process.

Remember to listen to your body, to the rate and rhythm of energy and physical responses to determine if you should hasten or quicken your Freedom Formula. Your specific Freedom Formula is your magical mix of diamond force where YOU are listening and intuitively selecting the elements for your system shift (the organ system). The number of elements is up to you. Remove and release all constriction and let the force flow freely in your choices.

Throughout the book the golden feather tips help you nourish yourself with deep self-care.

THE FREEDOM PHOTON WHEEL INTENTION AND RITUAL

In the three body system chapters of this book, the interventions have been divided into major and minor archetypes. The major archetype is the plant or element that has the highest connection to healing the specific system, Detox, Nourish, Activate. For the major archetypes, you will see many different medicinal actions for several systems and the minor archetypes will only have medicinal actions pertaining to that system.

Once you have picked the archetypes and are ready to begin the healing process, we suggest you designate an area for your FPW. If you don't have the actual element, don't worry, the element will still be charged with your intention. You can also place pictures, candles, flowers, or anything else you feel called by to connect your sacred space. Once you have created the cherished space, read and listen to the meditations for further integration. How long should you use the same intention or FPW? We recommend changing the wheel's archetypes and intention at least once per week as the cells of your body are forever changing and healing.

You can add to the FPW wheel any other items that are supportive to your process. At the end of each chapter, you will be guided with a ritual for integration. Break out those pens, markers, glue sticks, stickers, or whatever kindles your inner artist. Here are some suggestions of other items you might want to use but remember there is NO LIMIT to what you can use. For example, a trip to the beach might spark you to bring back shells, sea water, and sand to add to your wheel as you are invoking a feeling of freedom and connecting into your adrenal glands. So, get creative and have fun with your healing. It is after all your pathway to freedom and the fullest expression and experience of life ready to be created!

Here are a few ideas to add to your sacred space and Freedom Photon Wheel: feathers, oracle cards, poetry, journal entries, artwork, images of spiritual teachers, guides, nature, and family members – both those ancestral allies and those here on the physical plane, talismans or amulets, pranayama, music, mantras and affirmations, candles, chocolate, sage, incense and resins, flowers, and other sacred items you love and bring your joy.

Freedom Photon Wheel Ritual

The Freedom Photon Wheel Ritual allows you to assimilate and integrate the sacred medicine of each system holographically throughout your physical and nonphysical bodies down to the DNA level for sustainable shifts of healing and consciousness. The ritual itself offers a ceremonial aspect to our healing to symbolize points of shift and honor our journey of transformation. This process is not about erasing our history. We change our history through the process of understanding how the past affects our present now and future. The light of understanding combined with letting go and intentions for something greater pave the path for our new story to unfold.

Print your blank FPW to prepare for your ritual. We recommend finding a place of solitude in your home that can consistently be used as your sacred space for meditation and ritual. This will continue to strengthen your positive intention and force field for self-mastery and create more significant momentum in your healing journey.

As you prepare for your ritual choose your core grouping of archetypes: aromatherapy, botanical, crystal, and sacred geometry, then place them on your FPW. We recommend choosing the preceding four interventions to get started, but you can add more as you wish. Feel free to revert to this chapter as you prepare for your first ritual.

FREEDOM PHOTON WHEEL™

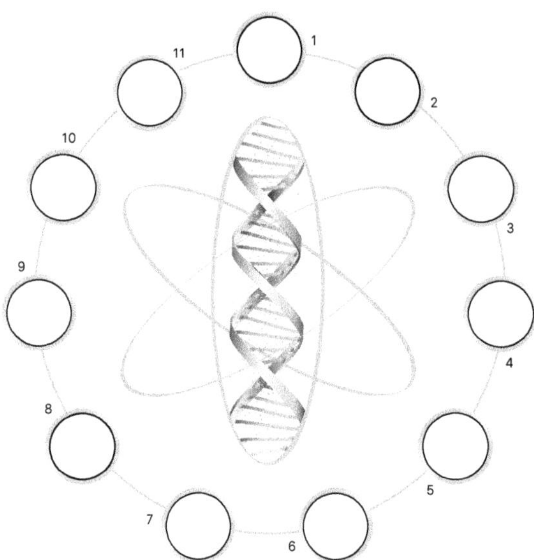

1 Alchemy Animal
2 Aromatherapy
3 Botanical
4 Light Wheel
5 Crystal
6 Photon Vibration
7 Flower or Gem Essence
8 Intention
9 Meditation Mudra
10 Sacred Geometry
11 Nutrition

ALCHEMY ANIMALS

Each animal has its own unique wisdom and knowledge to help you on your path to freedom. Take time to tune in to the animals that call out to you, knowing and trusting that this animal is here to support you and hold in your journey. You will find that different animals will be called to you at different times as you revisit this aspect of healing again and again. The creature connections, in each section, are affirmations to call forth the innate power within each animal to support you on your path to freedom. The animal kingdom is extremely potent and dynamic for cellular healing due to animals' innate connection to the human DNA. Did you know that you share DNA with all the creatures on this beautiful planet? For example, we share 44 percent of the same DNA as a bumble bee, amazing huh! So, what does this mean exactly when it comes to healing the DNA and using the alchemy animals? Well, when we share the DNA of so many elements on the planet, it's easy to connect in with their energy and ask them for assistance in a more profound healing. Sometimes as humans, we just need to let go of our enormous ego and experience something different for a change to get us out of our rut or pattern of dysfunction.

BOTANICAL MEDICINE AND CELLULAR IMPACT

INVITATION TO THE PLANT KINGDOM

We are taught to learn. To read books (even this one), memorize data, believe the experts (ourselves included), pay heed to every do and don't in the realm of safety data (we are not at all refuting safety), YET we are often not educated on the importance of and the how-to of listening to the plant, the bearer of wisdom, medicine, and healing. We have culturally and geographically not often had the chance to pick up the plant in our hands, showing our gratitude for the enormous amount of effort that went into each seed's germination, nurturing, harvest, and subsequent processing. Moving into this energy, or frequency of gratitude, openness, and humility, teaches us that the plant has volumes to speak. Its heritage, its wisdom, its magic and power are a service to all of humanity. After all, what could be more potent than messages that come directly from the heart of nature? We encourage you to begin to explore the beauty and wisdom of building intimate relationships with the plants, to hear their medicine and messages for your specific healing and evolution. Cultivating your clear connection to your inner "wise one" voice is the most valuable of practices. That voice, direct from our higher self, or divine self, speaks only truth, holds the answers to every question we may ask, even if we aren't yet ready to hear the response.

PLANT KINGDOM INVOCATION

I open to the wisdom of the plants, I intend for their full spectrum of medicine to be activated, for the original intent from the SOURCE to be actualized, and for humanity to receive deep healing and restoration of the perfected blueprint for us all.

We call upon the deep lost wisdom of the ancient plants of this planet and of the other worlds to bring in their wisdom and knowledge: Frankincense, White Angelica, Juniper, Bristlecone Pine, Fungi, Mosses, Seaweeds and Ferns. We call forth the plant spirits of all the flowers, spices, roots, seeds, woods, fruits, resins, herbs; come sing, shine, and illuminate us to the greatness of healing potencies you offer, remind us of our divinity and light and innate ability to heal and come together in great love as ONE.

How do plants have a cellular impact? Did you know that the cellular makeup of a plant cell and an animal cell is very similar? They have the same organelles, such as a nucleus, mitochondria, rough endoplasmic reticulum, and Golgi apparatus. Plants are also like humans in needing water, sunlight, and a form of energy (food) for survival. These similarities grant the ability for acquiescence between the two organisms. For example, several studies have been done involving turmeric, and it has been shown that the influence of the constituent polyphenol found in turmeric is profound at apoptosis or cell death. This archetype is used in the brain and nervous system photon wheel to clear unwanted cellular debris and DNA from the system.

AROMATHERAPY

Why do we look to aromatics as such a pivotal and primary alchemical element in the Freedom Photon Wheel? From a vibrational perspective, they hold a full spectrum of vibration and sacred geometry. When this energy is invited into the body, the cells, and the auric field, it brings a pattern of recognition to the human system. This ignites the spark of divine consciousness and actuates restoration within the system on every level: physical, mental, emotional. As the "quintessence of the plant" essential oils are a most potent form of alchemy, encoded with ancient earthly and cosmic frequencies to clear, awaken, align, and activate our innate healing spirit throughout the DNA. Furthermore, passing through the blood and brain barriers, essential oils have certain effects on all systems of the body including both the primitive and more recently developed aspects of our brain. The limbic connection is powerful, as is the synergy of working holographically with the nervous system to clear trauma. We will explore more on this in the brain chapter, yet for the here and now let's explore some key information for your foundational understanding and ability to formulate your own alchemy at home!

Aromatics have been prized for centuries for their therapeutic, spiritual, and esthetic benefits. The ancient Egyptians used aromatic herbs and infused oils such as myrrh and cinnamon for mummification, specifically for their antibacterial, antiviral, and antiseptic properties. One blend called Kyphi was formulated with more than fifteen different aromatics including frankincense, juniper, and cardamom. This blend was used medicinally, ceremonially, and as perfume. The Greek philosopher Plutarch had this to say about Kyphi: "It's aromatic substances lull to sleep, allay anxieties, and brighten dreams. It is made of things that delight most in the night."

The term "aromatherapy" itself was not coined until 1937 by the French chemist and perfumer René Maurice Gattefossé. Yet it was not until the 1950s that aromatherapy took another shift in its meaning when the French biochemist Marguerite Maury began to study and apply the use of essential oils and cosmetology. Maury also advocated for a holistic approach to well-being, postulating that, "for each individual there is an individual remedy." Aromatherapy, in its truest form, is the practice of blending on an individual specific basis, facilitating the body to activate its own innate healing ability.

WHAT ARE ESSENTIAL OILS?

Essential oils are products of plant metabolism. Composed of chemical constituents, essential oils mediate between the plant and its environment, attracting, repelling, and communicating to achieve homeostasis. Each essential oil may have well over 100 constituents yet is only one of several that impart odor and taste. True rose oil comprises over 250 chemical constituents, yet only 2 percent create the aroma, making it one of the most difficult oils to replicate synthetically. Essential oils are stored in various parts of the plant, for example, flowers (rose), roots (vetiver), fruit (orange), and heartwood (sandalwood). Essential oils are extracted solely via distillation (steam/water), citrus oils via expression, and absolutes via enfleurage and solvent extraction. Many factors contribute to the quality of the essential oil produced including cultivation, environment, type of herbage used (fresh, dried, organic), harvesting methods, as well as type and length of distillation.

HOW DO THEY WORK?

The most effective method is inhalation. When inhaling an essential oil, the molecules travel through the olfactory system to the brain, specifically the limbic system, which regulates much of our physiology and specifically mood, memory, and emotion. Just as a familiar melody can evoke a particular event or period in our life, scent may be perceived as the key that unlocks our past.

Essential oils are also absorbed into the skin, traversing the bloodstream to various organs and it is certain that the absorption time differs with each essential oil as well as other determinants. Aromatic massage is an effective method when working through the skin and because it increases circulation, essential oils are absorbed more readily into the skin. Aromatic massage offers more than a general sense of well-being by toning, detoxifying, and balancing much of the body (i.e., lymphatic, circulatory systems, muscles, organs).

Essential oils also work in a powerful yet subtle way when used with the auric field surrounding the physical body as well as the chakra system, or light wheels. The psycho-spiritual use of essential oils often perpetuates an immediate response. This form of subtle aromatherapy seems to clear, activate, and foster a pathway of release. As we begin to work in the realm of the intangible, the journey of our soul illuminates with clarity and purpose. We strive ahead with renewed vitality and dedication and ultimately the remembrance of our own true divinity.

See Appendix A: Aromatherapy Safety and Formulations for information on how to make your own aromatherapy healing remedies.

Due to the increasing methodology available for adulteration, it is imperative to purchase from trustworthy and knowledgeable sources, creating a demand for efficacious and superior quality essential oils. Otherwise, we must accept both the uncertainty of results produced using, and the responsibility of fueling the demand for, inferior quality essential oils.

Over 90 percent of the essential oils produced are supplied to the fragrance and flavor industry and because of this many are standardized to improve the scent quality of the oil. In view of the holistic paradigm, we see that for an essential oil to be pure and natural, it needs to be whole. Even minute compounds alter not only the chemical makeup of the essential oil but the application and effects as well. One can support holistic aromatherapy by purchasing non-standardized essential oils. Insisting on organic, biodynamic, and sustainable wild crafted sources honors the trinity of the plants, the Earth, and the resultant medicine for the healing of humanity. Some of the essential oils included here are endangered and should be used reverently and sparingly as their medicine is still potent alchemy for healing at the cellular, DNA, and soul level. You will see an asterisk to designate these plants both in the aromatherapy and botanical medicine interventions in the book.

BOTANICAL MEDICINE

THE HISTORY OF HERBAL MEDICINE

Botanical medicine has been used for healing purposes long before recorded history. Ancient writings of the Chinese and Egyptian cultures describe medicinal plants used in their daily life and rituals. The indigenous cultures used herbs in their healing ceremonies, while other cultures developed advanced plants systems we use today (e.g., Ayurveda, Western Herbalism, and Traditional Chinese Medicine). Many different cultures still around have a long-lost history of using herbal medicine and the same plants for similar purposes. So why has this precious part of our healing been lost and even buried. As humans living in the twenty-first century, we want everything to be a quick fix and an immediate answer. Plant medicine is a more powerful method of healing but developing a relationship with the plant is a different and more profound experience. Our hope through this book is that you will personally begin to develop a greater connection to the plant kingdom, igniting the long-lost wisdom of healing within yourself and your community. It takes a change in your community to make a lasting change on the planet.

HERBAL MEDICINE TODAY

Recent information from the World Health Organization estimates 80 percent of people on this beautiful planet are using some aspect of herbal medicine for their health care. As more of our society becomes dissatisfied with the side effects, cost, and efficacy of prescription medications they are turning to herbal medicine for solutions. One of the aspects that have hindered the use of herbal medicine is the lack of evidence-based testing. But if we look back at the history of herbal medicine and its many, many uses, isn't that enough? Archaeologists can trace back the use of herbal medicine to 60,000 years ago! Wow, plants have such a deep, ingrained healing intelligence within, now we just need to tap into it.

HOW DOES BOTANICAL MEDICINE WORK?

Botanicals contain many ingredients and constituents that they work synergistically to produce therapeutic effects. Many factors can affect how effective the constituents of a medicinal plant will be. For example, the type of environment in which a plant is grown can be beneficial or toxic. FYI, some toxic environments can make a plant stronger but we don't recommend using these plants because they can also have some toxins in their DNA and environment. In addition, how and when it was harvested and processed will also influence the quality of the resulting herbal extract.

See Appendix B: Botanical Formulations for information on how to make your own botanical healing remedies.

LIGHT WHEELS

Born of the ancient Indian culture and sacred language of Sanskrit, the chakra system, that you will see listed as light wheels herein, provides a powerful intervention for personal growth and empowerment.

Through becoming acquainted with this system, we can begin to understand our own innate areas of power as well as those areas to develop and strengthen within our own lives.

There are seven major chakra centers (see diagram) or light wheels that are held within the auric or energy field. This energy field comprises seven major levels. It is a hologram for our experiences, past, present, and many still unfolding. The most known are the emotional body, the astral body, the mental body, and the spiritual body. This auric field holds all of our life's experiences. The chakras are the main centers of energy, or prana, and information transmitters and receivers if you will, that correlate to specific physical, psychological, and spiritual health and well-being. They can indicate whether a person is prone to digestive disturbances, a lack of confidence, or a fear of speaking up and out.

DNA LIGHT WHEELS

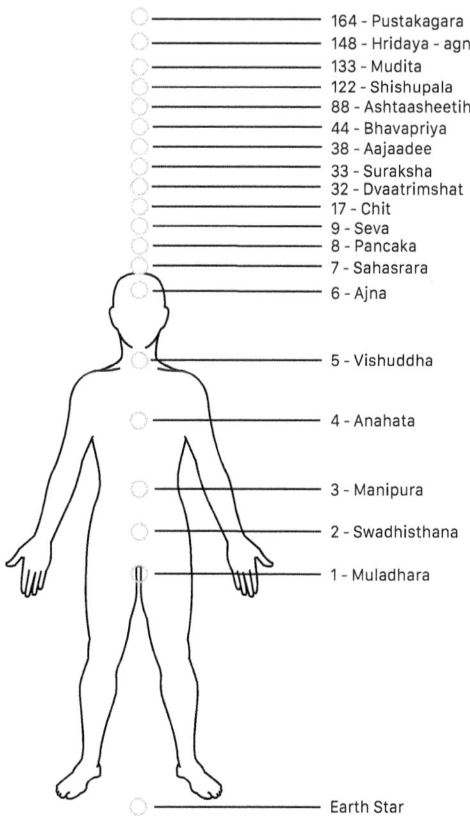

There are also five other chakra centers which connect beyond the primary seven chakras located in the physical body, bridging to the Earth and, the gateway chakras to our soul or inner being. We have also included higher number chakras for higher realm integration. Honestly folks, some of these haven't been widely discussed but we have added them in the book to align specific chakra centers within you, the planet, and the universe.

The hara point, or dantian, which resides below the navel (not to be confused with the sacral chakra) is the power point that integrates the lower three chakras and facilitates our connection into the Earth. Along this hara point lies the sushumna or hara line. This is the central current from the heavens or cosmic consciousness that runs down through the "chakra tube" grounding into the center of the Earth. The Hara line also known as the line of intention stands as our connection to our life's purpose, a specific blueprint that each soul is born with to accomplish throughout their life here on Earth.

There are two additional energy lines that start at the root chakra, the Ida (yin or feminine in nature) and the Pingala (yang or masculine in nature). As these energies intertwine, their intersections create vortexes at nerve ganglia (accumulations of nerve fibers) along the spine. These vortexes are known as chakras, or light wheels.

Although there are primarily seven light wheel centers, there are thousands of other sub vortexes throughout the body. The palms of the hands and the soles of the feet serve as some of the most significant sub centers. When these centers are open fully, we have greater capacity to let the life-force energy or prana flow through us and outward to all that we contact, such as our families, colleagues, strangers, pets, plants, and of course the Earth in general. These vortexes serve as "two-way tunnels" allowing energy to flow through each of the subtle bodies that make up the auric field, that is, physical too emotional to mental to spiritual. When there are blockages within these chakras, physical, emotional, and spiritual disease can begin to manifest indicating that there is work to do to bring the whole self back into a state of harmony.

Essentially, the intention is to first become aware that these centers exist and are a direct mapping system to our physical, psychological, and spiritual health and well-being. Then we can begin to personally identify and address our own areas for development and take the practical steps that lead to personal growth and empowerment.

Remember that color is a powerful vibrational healing tool. By wearing the color of the chakra, or eating food that is that color, we bring that resonance or specific vibrational support into our auric field for balance and healing. Essential oils, herbs, crystals, sacred geometry, and sound are also wonderful interventions to Detox, Nourish, Activate the chakras.

HOW CAN CHANGING THE VIBRATION HEAL THE DNA?

Our DNA is not only physical in nature, but it also has a holographic, energetic form. Our energetic DNA runs through the entire chakra system and all levels of the auric field and is influenced by our emotions and vibration. This might be easier to understand if you think about your aura. The aura is an energetic image, ever changing, a reflection of the chakras and their color and the energy that surrounds all living things. This reflection has a DNA imprint that connects the aura to the physical being and amplifies the message of the DNA and RNA. These cellular strands of DNA connect forming a shimmering, sparkly field of light. By activating or turning on the chakras, the DNA can be easily repaired and shifted. This is the essence of holographic healing.

CRYSTALS AND STONES

INVOCATION TO AWAKEN THE CRYSTAL ELEMENTALS

Guardians of the Earth we call upon you to bring forth the knowledge and healing wisdom of the crystal elementals. May we hear your guidance, feel your protection, and heed your assistance in the reprogramming and restructuring of our DNA. We ask for the ancient crystals from this world and other worlds beyond to be activated and be with us now: moldavite, diamond, emerald, obsidian, pearl, amber, chalcopyrite, ruby, tektite, peridot, and the meteoroid. Awaken within us the remembrance of our own crystalline consciousness and potential. May we remember how to work in tandem, receiving your healing potencies, your healing vibration to activate the full DNA sequence within our human form. May the full vibration of your light and healing perfected from the mind of the Creator be activated and united upon this great planet.

Crystals and stones are the flowers or keys of the Earth's crust and crystalline grid which are on the planet to assist us in many ways of cellular healing. This *Webster's Dictionary* definition of crystals is key to how we use the crystals to activate our DNA and cells: "A body that is formed by the solidification of a chemical element, a compound, or a mixture and has a regularly repeating internal arrangement of its atoms and often external plane faces." Since a crystal has an electrical arrangement of atoms, our body both physically and energetically can recognize and assimilate the crystalline information. Crystals also have piezoelectricity where they communicate via electricity or light. As humans we are made up of 99 percent atoms which gives us easy access to the energetic message communication from the crystalline world and the ability to use this energetic form to alter our DNA. By working with and wearing crystals, we can activate our original blueprint for crystalline structure in our cellular and energy bodies.

SO HOW DO WE USE CRYSTALS TO HEAL TRAUMA AND THE DNA?

The electric charge of the crystals has a similar composition to the electrons and water in our body. Since water is a conductor, our body is a receptor for the vibration and sound waves of the crystals. This vibration, or sound wave, penetrates the phospholipid bilayer of the cell membrane and emits an electric charge to the nucleus and the mitochondria of the cell.

Masura Emoto (2005) discovered that human consciousness influenced water and stated, "Water records information, and while circulating throughout the earth distributes information. This water sent from the universe is full of the information of life …" The crystals of the Earth function much in the same way: they can keep the energetic records of time and space in their crystalline form.

When using the Freedom Photon Wheel, it is important to initiate this archetype to activate the inherent message and cellular imprint of the crystal with your intention. Some of the crystals suggested in the book are rare so you can print out a photograph or set the intention to connect with the cosmic consciousness and vital life force of the crystal in your Freedom Photon Wheel. Each system offers a crystal grid attunement to Detox, Nourish and Activate healing.

PHOTON VIBRATION

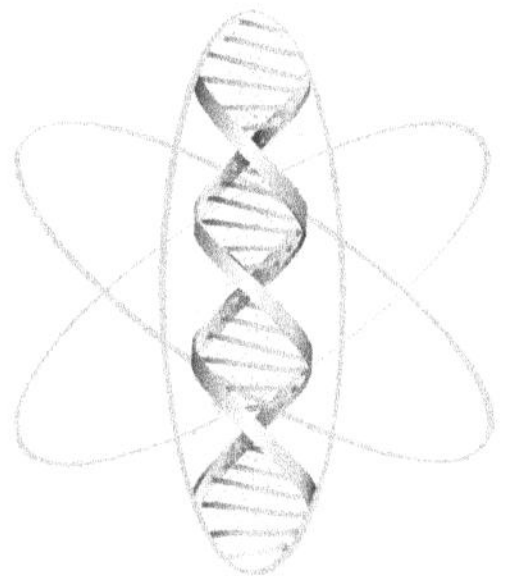

As we discussed earlier, the photon is a particle of light, carrying magnetic force and energy that allows greater transmission of vibrational and holographic healing. The more light your cells can absorb and carry directly affects your vibration and ability to create the life of vibrancy you were meant to live. Each of the chapters in the book divided into Detox, Nourish, Activate has a photon symbol with a dot designated for each system. This dot represents the moment in time and space where you have focused intention and empowered it with your elected alchemical element.

We choose these dots and locations specifically to awaken and vibrationally charge your DNA as you work through each system in the book. To enhance the energetic attunement of each location you can place a crystal, we recommend a clear quartz crystal, on the photon vibration circle as well as one on the specified dot. The quartz crystal will help magnify and amplify your thoughts and align them with the true intention of your soul or soul purpose. The quartz is recognized as a conduit stone and will enable you to receive information more clearly during your healing sessions and while reading this book.

VIBRATIONAL HEALING METHODS

Known by a myriad of names, vibrational healing encompasses a vast number of variations and techniques. These different terms share an expanse of common ground. All require the specific intention of the healer to invoke or channel the universal life force, known as "chi" in China, "prana" in India, and "reiki" in Japan. These modalities seek to energize and balance in a holistic manner, addressing physical, emotional, and spiritual queries. Just as a mother instinctively places her hands on her child after a fall, these types of healing provide the comfort of caring touch as well as healing energy.

Oftentimes the question arises, "But how does it really work?" To answer this, we first turn to science. As we began to move away from the principles of Newtonian physics, such as separation and finite law, the early nineteenth century found new concepts upon which to explain the human dynamic, such as field theory and the theory of relativity. These groundbreaking discoveries introduced us to the idea that matter and energy are interchangeable. All matter is energy and therefore this energy is all around and within us. Scientific research has been conducted around the globe in support and further expansion of these ideas. This measurable energy that surrounds and interpenetrates the human body is often called the aura or the human energy field. This field carries the beliefs, thoughts, emotions, and experiences of each individual; when healing energy is applied to this human energy field physiological changes occur.

Historical reference and modern-day implications, including case studies can be found in Barbara Brennan's international bestseller, *Hands of Light, A Guide to Healing Through the Human Energy Field*. Brennan, a thought leader and pioneer in the realm of energy medicine is the founder of the Barbara Brennan Healing School, a four-year, accredited educational facility that leads the professional development of healers worldwide and is unparalleled in its professional, grounded approach to vibrational medicine to transform physical and emotional health termed Brennan Healing Science™.

Vibrational medicine speeds up holographic healing by addressing our whole health. Whether initially concerned with a physiological, emotional, or spiritual imbalance, vibrational healing can shift the energy of our trinity and clear, balance, and restore on all levels down to the cellular consciousness and DNA to heal at quantum levels.

We have developed a technique called *Essential Oil Based Tapping* that combines tapping specific meridian points with a system specific essential oil. EOBT assists us in healing at the cellular level by synergistically combining specific essential oils, meridian or other energetic points with the intention for vibrational shifts in the energy and emotional field.

This is but a few core vibrational healing modalities of which there are a myriad of offshoots. We will offer you both practical and innovative techniques in the coming chapters to introduce you to or deepen your experience of vibrational healing. Explore and vet what resonates for you wherever you are on the transformative healing journey.

FLOWER AND GEM ESSENCES

Flower and gem essences are vibrational remedies made from either the gem or flower. Essences can be made through intentional practices of anchoring the cosmic consciousness and vital life force of the gem or flower into water or a carrier oil. The benefit of working with the intentional infusion is that they can be shifted to different potencies, depending on the level of the miasm the individual is working to bring healing or increased light and life force to. The higher the homeopathic potency, the more self-adjusting the essence is.

Flower essences can also be made from the physical representation of the plant or mineral, like in the case of Bach Flower Remedies. Flower and gem essences work in the realm of the subtle bodies and levels of consciousness, which lends their benefit to core level healing and balancing and clearing the emotional bodies.

Everything is crystalline in nature whether it's manifest or not. When using the flower and gem essences, it's helpful to use them for twelve months to cleanse and balance the emotional and etheric bodies and with that holographically impact healing at the cellular and DNA level.

THE POWER OF INTENTION, GUIDING AFFIRMATIONS, AND MANTRAS

Intention is perhaps the most potent intangible element that we can work with along the Freedom Photon Wheel. Where our intention and therefore attention go, our energy flows. This is where it becomes imperative to be clear on our intention: positive, negative, and effortless. Increasing your awareness to the places where your negative intention lurks in the shadow is critical to shifting your power from a place of negative, lower self-creation.

You are a powerful creator, and energy does not distinguish between negative and positive creations. Self-responsibility fuels your ability to witness and evaluate how and where positive and negative intention creates experience in your life. What is effortless intention? As we release our subconscious "blockages" of trauma, we move to a clarity of intentional creation, allowing effortless intention to flow as the main source of creating life experience. Interested? You will experience more and more of this synchronistically as you move through the pages ahead.

Affirmations

- ∞ I have everything I need within me to heal on the deepest levels. I AM THAT I AM.

- ∞ I unlock the DNA in my timeline and free my truest potential.
- ∞ MY DNA IS FULLY ACTIVE AND FUNCTIONAL.

Mantras

Mantras invoke the names of the Divine. When working with mantras or chanting the divine names, it allows for a higher realization of ourselves to permeate our being. It's through this process that we can anchor the energies of our highest self, create safety and protection around our energy field, and liken our vibration with our true god self or true divine nature. It allows us to move through the lower or more negative vibrations, helping us to reduce depression, anger, and negative emotions.

Mantras allow us to focus on the divine versus our lower selves or ego. They enhance the power of our concentration and pull our higher selves to merge with our personality aspects. An example mantra is Aum, a sacred sound that originated at the beginning of time and can be used to connect to the seventh or crown chakra and our inner being or higher self.

Mantras can be spoken out loud, whispered, or said silently in the mind within the inner plane. Mantras are a sacred practice. They are devotional. Another mantra is Elohim, which means literally all that God is. So, when you are using the mantra, you're attracting that energy, that vibration, and that consciousness to yourself into your intentions. If you have mantras that you leave on while you are sleeping that's beneficial in programming your subconscious. Mantras build spiritual forces. They purify, cleanse, and heal the energy bodies.

When you are chanting the mantra or name of the divine, you're programming the blueprint of perfection from the mind of God into your system, into your cells, into your energy bodies. It helps to elevate your consciousness to align with your true god self. When you have a practice of working with mantras as you go throughout your day, every single person you encounter benefits from the energy of the mantra and the sacred vibrations of benevolence that surround it.

MEDITATIONS AND MUDRAS

The alchemy of meditation is multidimensional and serves as a practical reminder that we can tap into divine consciousness at any and every moment we choose. From a spiritual perspective, meditation allows our energy fields to easily align and ground with the Earth to find stillness through the chaos of the world around us. From a more esoteric perspective it assists us in assimilating the higher vibrational frequencies available to us through this evolutionary process.

There are numerous physical and emotional benefits from cultivating a consistent meditation practice. It calms the mind and offers greater mental clarity. From a perspective of healing, it allows an intimate connection to form with our inner authentic self. Harnessing the monkey mind accesses the inner voice of knowing and wisdom. We can explore our emotional trigger points and responses, and review and untangle our thought patterns.

Our thoughts and in particular our emotions create a chain reaction from the brain and nervous system to molecular and neurochemical processes. By bringing mindful awareness to our emotional natures, we can better steer and navigate the trajectory of our responses and consciously command our creative and healing processes, leaving behind the victim persona and any patterns that no longer serve us.

Meditation also allows the opportunity to feel our physical discomfort and pain that often goes unnoticed for far too long. We can investigate the dark crevices of our shadow to find the area of fear, anxiety, and the propaganda of our lower selves. There is a profound comfort and presence that can be found in stillness. Consistent daily practice – we recommend at least fifteen minutes per day – gently encourages heightened emotional resilience. It also allows us to feel connected easily and harmoniously with others, a paramount planetary teaching during this time of evolution.

Mudras are movements and formations of the hand that synergistically connect the physical body with the spiritual body. They allow the doorway to open for communication of our soul and the spiritual world to engage our brain, nervous system, and cellular consciousness. Our fingers and hands have motor and sensory nerve endings, and the mudras create a channel for the brain to transmit healing to the body.

In each meditation DNA section, there is a mudra on the Freedom Photon Wheel. Rooted in ancient Indian tradition, mudras are hand gestures that direct specific vibrational frequency to the physical and nonphysical body. Mudras stimulate certain aspects of the brain and physiology for energy flow and empower our physical, mental, emotional, and spiritual healing. Combined with the meditations and other alchemical interventions in the Freedom Photon Wheel, the mudras will create greater synergy and momentum for your holistic healing.

There are two ways you can use the mudras for your FPW. First, add the mudra to your daily meditation practice – you don't need to hold it the whole time, this might be too taxing on your energetic system, but instead you can work up to holding the mudra for longer periods of time. Second, when you are activating your FPW and setting system healing intention, you may use the mudra for your activation ceremony.

SACRED GEOMETRY

Historical thought, attributed to Plato, speaks to the creation of the universe by a divine geometric plan. Nature exemplifies this concept in numerous ways, such as from the nautilus shell, which naturally forms in a logarithmic spiral. Honey bees form hexagonal shells to store their honey. The Platonic solids, the five core building blocks of matter, hold a perfect symmetry and are the third dimensional representation of the ethereal in physical form: tetrahedron, octahedron, cube, icosahedron, and dodecahedron.

Sacred geometry intertwines art and science, the esoteric to physics; it lights up and lines up both hemispheres of the brain as well as the connection and pathways between Heaven and Earth and in infinite elegance articulates the pulse of all life throughout creation.

Sacred geometry allows you to bring information and intelligence from the cosmic perspective down to the individual self. Through increasing our awareness of the life pulse of expansion, contraction, and stasis, you can tune in and enhance your multidimensional nature's ability to receive new information, energy, and experience through a broader perspective. You can then funnel the new frequencies down through all your energy bodies to your cellular consciousness and DNA. It is only through the stillness of stasis that integration can be fully anchored, and it is here that we are invited into the "rapture" of unity consciousness to expand a greater understanding of our humanity in the context of the cosmos.

Infinity Symbol

This form of sacred geometry is a potent actuator of shift. It invites multiple paradigms of intelligence and opportunity from all time continuums into the present moment. From one angle, we see the microcosm and the macrocosm; for sustainable healing, we must activate both pathways from the external using vibrational healing elements like aromatherapy, sacred geometry, and crystals to internal pathways, like botanical medicine and whole foods; then both circuits meet in the middle, intermingling and creating a synergistic harmonic to change. All pathways of the infinity symbol come back to the center: the zero-point field of limitless creation.

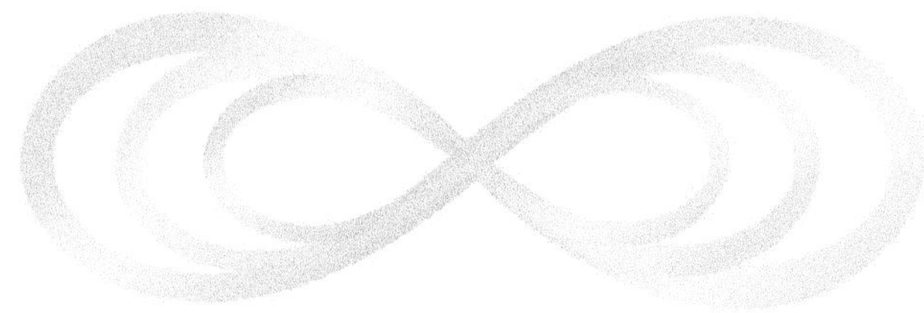

Vesica Pisces

The Vesica Pisces holds the frequency of creation, and the merging of the first two cells at procreation. It also represents the origin point for the flower of life. This variation also depicts the configuration of the trinity, or triad as mentioned previously, an intrinsic aspect of creation in this reality.

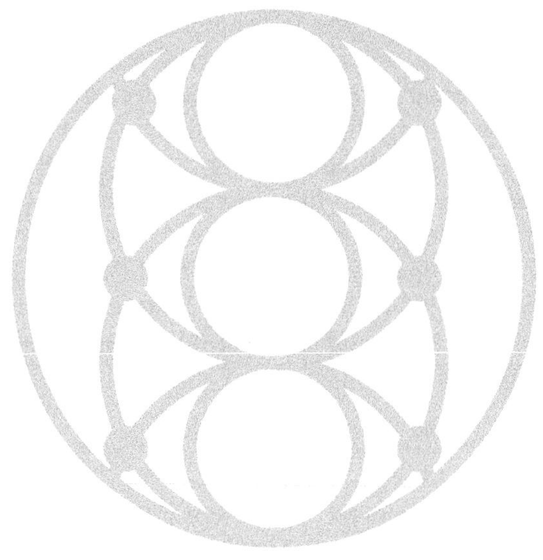

Flower of Life

The Flower of Life activates the cellular memory of harmony and unity. It can be meditated upon to bring healing to core relationships and to restore the original blueprint for humanity through the DNA and mother and father bloodlines.

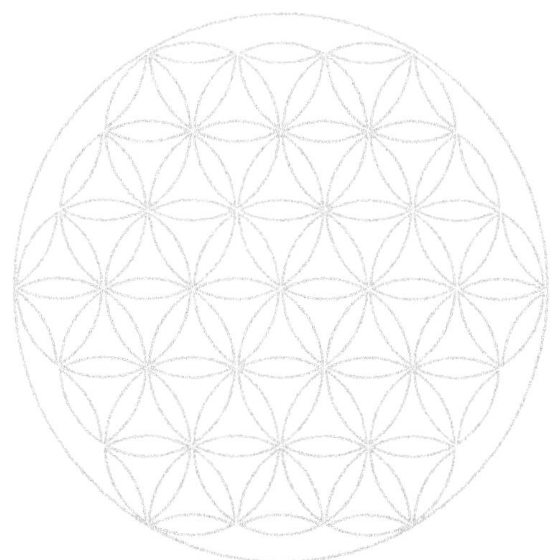

In each system section of the book, you will discover the major archetype sacred geometry symbol on the Freedom Photon Wheel diagram. This main archetype has been chosen to align or tune your vibration to the organ (heart, adrenals, and brain) and then to specifically Detox, Nourish, Activate. We invite you to search or source through your own hand and heart more sacred geometry symbols as you begin your own self-discoveries of healing, to use on your blank Freedom Photon Wheel.

Ways to incorporate sacred geometry into your daily life and rituals.

- ∞ Infuse your water with sacred geometry by adding a sticker, drawing, or picture to the outside of a bottle or glass. If you have a metal sacred geometry symbol you may place this inside the water but make sure the metal won't' degrade and put toxins into the water. When you drink the infused water, the water will be able to penetrate or be absorbed more easily into the cell membrane and other structures of the cell.
- ∞ Wearing sacred geometry, as jewelry, brings your electrical charge or field into a closer vibratory alignment with the symbol and helps achieve energetic shifts at a much faster pace. Remember, as with all vibrational healing, drink extra water to facilitate assimilation and clearing of the physical and psycho-spiritual bodies.
- ∞ Hang artwork featuring sacred geometry designs in your meditation space or around your altar to increase your healing intention.
- ∞ Tape or post a picture of the archetype on your mirror in the bathroom or bedroom. This will activate your aura with the symbol each time you look in the mirror and help clear imbalances in the chakra system.
- ∞ Meditate on the symbol by holding the archetype in your hand and visualizing the image at the top of the head and below the feet to create a clear channel of energy through your chakra system and physical body.
- ∞ Change the wallpaper on your phone or desktop to sacred geometry. Not only is this powerful for frequent energetic awareness but will also help to block electric and magnetic fields (EMFs) from your field.
- ∞ Grids: As discussed in earlier in Chapter Five, creating a crystalline grid can raise the frequency and power of your intention. For the sacred geometry, place a picture, drawing, or actual metal symbol

in the grid for amplification. For example, if you were doing a heart DNA centering grid, you could pick one of the sacred geometry archetypes from the section along with emeralds, malachite, and atlantisite, and to fully charge and engage the healing power of the grid place the symbol under the stones. This is a very powerful healing and not to be taken lightly so we recommend keeping some notes in your journal during this transformative healing phase.

NUTRITION

Nutrition and whole foods are among the easiest access points to shifting the DNA, very similar to aromatherapy and botanical medicine. Whole foods are easily digested, absorbed, and assimilated since we have been ingesting them as a species for thousands of years. Our bodies recognize the genetic pattern of coding that has been imprinted onto the cell either from first ingestion or from a long forgotten genetic memory. Therefore, when you eat a food you may not have ever eaten, it tastes so good and yummy. Has that ever happened to you?

In the organ system chapters of the book, you will find a major archetype food on the Freedom Photon Wheel, or FPW as well as other suggestions for each system. The nutritive foods might seem familiar or maybe obscure. We suggest adding the foods into your nutritional plan while you are working with a specific FPW. If you have a sensitivity, place the food or picture of the food on the FPW. You will still reap all the benefits of the cellular calibration.

What if your system is not absorbing nutrients from food? Will you still have benefits for the DNA? Yes, you will still absorb the nutrients but not at the same nutrient dense level. If you think you are having a cellular imbalance from a digestive imbalance or toxic overload this might be a good opportunity to dig deeper into the root cause of the disturbance. Your body will still absorb nutrients to continually shift the DNA but at a much slower or diffused rate. Also, please listen again to the DNA meditation in Chapter Two to assist in cellular and DNA balancing.

WATER

Water is also an important component of the food and nutrition photon wheel. Water has so many benefits to the physical body: it detoxifies, hydrates the skin, lubricates the joints, helps efficient digestion and assimilation, enables nutrients to move in and out of the cell membrane, and improves cellular function for genetic replication. We recommend you drink at least half a pint of water per day to assist in bodily function, and when you are working with the FPW drink extra water and electrolytes or add a dash of salt to assist in cellular function. Also place a small glass of water on the FPW to energize with the vibration of your intention and then make sure to drink the water afterwards to Detox, Nourish, Activate all the cells.

WHOLE FOODS

As we move forward into the realm of genetically modified foods, our planet and your body will be making shifts to align with these new foods. Our recommendation is to consume the highest quality, organic, non-GMO foods – but we know this might not always be possible, especially in this time and planetary shift.

There are a few easy ways to prepare for and cope with these upcoming changes. One, grow your own food and medicine. There are SO many benefits to having your own garden – delicious food, nutrient dense, lower carbon footprint, support for the bees, butterflies, and birds, self-care (nurturing YOU), and more. Two, wash your vegetables and fruits you buy at the store in a cool bath of lemon water to clean and remove toxins. Three, create a crystal grid in the fridge and on the counter to nullify genetic alterations. Four, choose an intention to begin each meal: "This food nourishes each cell of my being," and "My body loves this food," "This food activates my DNA and energizes my body," or "My body digests, assimilates, and absorbs all the essential nutrients from this meal."

How does food shift our relationship to trauma? Many of us use food as a comfort when dealing with past or current trauma. Addictions and disorders are very common in food relationships. The deeper question here is what was the trauma that stemmed this initial relationship and how can this relationship change? In Chapter Three, we discussed trauma and the many ties it has to our physical and psycho-spiritual bodies. When it comes to food, the trauma trigger needs to be eliminated from the nutritional plan for at least ninety days to enable your hormonal system to recalibrate.

CHAPTER 6

Loving Yourself Inside and Out – The Heart

The heart is the seat of self-love and the point of connectivity for relationships and generating joy. Through this chapter, you will discover how healing this system releases deep rooted trauma and frees the spirit. On a physical level, the heart is the root of circulation and when this system is blocked or stagnant it causes physical disease throughout the body limiting the movement and functioning of other organs. On an emotional level, all healing begins with the heart.

The heart is physically centered in the middle of your body as a gateway between the two aspects of yourself. The lower aspect of the body controls the digestive organs and communicates with the brain via the channel of the heart. You might have heard of the brain/gut connection—this is what we are referring to here. Your body relays pertinent information to the digestive organs as well as the corresponding nerves along the spine via a communication pathway or nervous system pathway. Trauma plays a specific role in the change of this communication pathway.

Let's use the telephone game as a great example of how this works. Your brain functions like an operator or hub of information going in and out. The messages then are traveling through the magnificent pathway of the heart either out to the body or back up to the brain.

As this pathway becomes toxic with trauma and disease, or burdened from overwork, the messages become garbled and unclear for the entire system. The Freedom Photon Wheels, to Detox, Nourish, Activate the heart, will empower you with the knowledge and understanding to open the heart up fully and to re-establish connections in your body.

Self love is a portal for great transformation. It is a bridge for your highest, wisest, and most vibrant self to evolve across. It is a crucial component to creating and nurturing the healthy, joyous relationships you desire. Our relationship with ourselves and our history defines the relationships we have with all those we encounter through projection and transference. Our inner landscape is filled with peaks and valleys of past experiences which continue to project reality and experience in our current day to day life. The valleys of unresolved emotion and trauma held in the subconscious filter our perception of reality and our ability to relate to ourselves and others in emotionally healthy ways.

Inner reflection: Take some time out to reflect on your core relationships. Consider how kind, gentle, and loving you are with yourself. What about your patterns of self-care and self-talk? This speaks volumes on how you model your expectations and judgements of those around you. Next, take an honest assessment of your primary dynamics in relationship with your significant other, children, parents, siblings, and colleagues. We can begin to see our own patterns popping up for better or worse among these bonds, all present in our lives for a reason, to teach and transform our inner landscape.

Personal Insights with Adora

My journey is chock full of lessons around self-love and countless opportunities for both self-forgiveness and profound gratitude. My tendency to overwork, overdo, overcompensate, over-caretake, over-give, and full on overexert would often bring me to states of resentment, sadness, and exhaustion where I would find myself desiring to escape from a deep ocean of depression and isolation. In turn, my expectation of others was off the charts unrealistic, and I would find myself perpetually disappointed to the point where I would stop expecting anything and begin the cycle again. Even now, I must continually train myself to leave the chatter of the drill sergeant by the wayside, and to be gentler and more loving, allowing for downtime and fun as part of my own intentional practice.

Many years ago, I heard the story of Dr. Hew Len and Ho'oponopono. It is potent alchemy.

In a nutshell, Dr. Len is a Hawaiian psychologist who views well-being from the perspective that we are 100 percent personally responsible for our life experiences and their resultant outcomes, from our personal health to that of our relationship to others, finances, career and self-expression.

He worked as a therapist in a Hawaiian state hospital, specifically with the criminally insane, yet he never saw a patient in person. He would sit with their files and photos with the express intention of cleaning the energy with self-healing and a powerful practice of self-love.

With the perspective that we are responsible for everything we witness and experience in life—he would reflect inward, bringing healing to the point within himself that created that person or circumstance and silently repeating, "I'm sorry. I love you. Please forgive me. Thank you." As he cleaned this energy within himself, his patients healed.

As we heal the places of pain and disease within ourselves, those around us heal. It is a universal principle and a facet of alchemy. It allows the concept of "right relationship" to flow and breathe life into our hearts and those that surround us. The one thing we want more than anything, whether we are aware of it, want to contemplate or even admit it, is to love. To love ourselves, even when we cause our own pain and suffering, to learn how to love others in healthy ways, based on who they are as individuals vs. who we want them to be, and as important, to learn how to allow ourselves to receive love! This practice allows us to bring that love and compassion deeper into ourselves and then to merge it with the divined force of creation, producing a potent synergy for healing at the core DNA level.

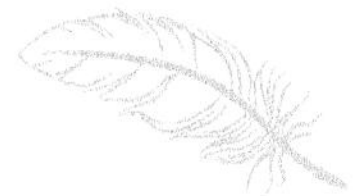

When am I using my superpower to the best of my ability?
When you LOVE yourself, no matter what!

HEALING THE TRAUMA OF THE HEART

The heart holds deeply rooted seeds of trauma and to move forward on your path to freedom the journey needs to begin with a deep look inside. Take a moment to close your eyes and take a deep breath in. How does that breath feel in your chest? Is there tightness? Is there constriction? Do you feel freedom of movement here? Do you feel joy? Love? Expansion? When was the last time you felt truly loved? Do you love yourself? What does love mean to you? These are deep and emotionally provoking questions you might want to explore more in your journal or on one of the Discovery Dives you will find in this chapter.

As you move through each section of this chapter, please take your time and practice the golden feather guidance suggestions to further your expansion of the heart. Be gentle with yourself and explore with a sense of love and trust as you go deeper into healing. Remember, YOU chose this book because YOU are ready for the healing to begin.

GRATITUDE

Gratitude as a practice is powerful. Gratitude with the precursor of forgiveness is exponentially powerful. To be clear, the focus here is on self-forgiveness. The practice of forgiving others has more complexity. It cannot be conjured through conscious, mental work and is multifaceted. Start with freeing yourself first. Allowing your release from the prisons created through shame, guilt, self judgement, self-betrayal – all those moments where you have fallen. You are perfectly imperfect and always can up the level of your game of personal growth. Compassion fills the stream of consciousness that is forgiveness and is a critical life lesson to be assimilated in the hero's and heroine's journey. It allows your heart to remain open and expand.

FORGIVENESS

You are the blooming rose of summer, the seed planted deep within your heart. The intentional practices of forgiveness and gratitude allow the bloom and fragrance of your heart to fully unfold. When you leave out these two fundamental components, it is like having an unattended garden cluttered with weeds and the bountiful fruits, still on the vine, ravaged by pests.

Om Mani Padme Hum: "Pay homage to the compassionate one, yourself."

THE INNER WORKINGS OF THE HEART

∞ To access the physical heart healing meditation please go to www.zenergymedicinals.com

In your self discovery of healing, it is key to learn about the physical nature of each organ. You might be asking why this aspect is so important. To really dive deep into the body on a cellular level and heal the DNA, you need to have a basic understanding of where the organ is located and its function. Imagine if you got in the driver's seat of a car and you were asked to drive but had no knowledge of a car?

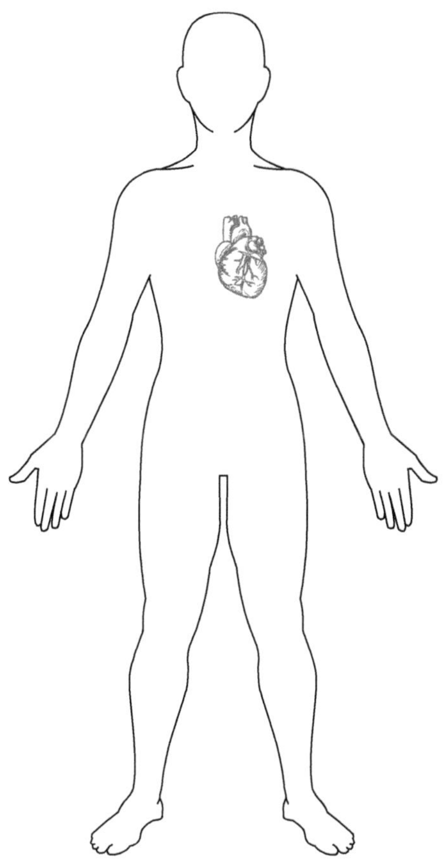

You probably wouldn't go very far or fast but with a quick overview you could be zooming down the road to fun and freedom. We will also be referring to specific anatomical locations in this chapter and we want YOU to be EMPOWERED!

ANATOMICAL LOCATION

The heart is a large pumping organ located along the body's midline in the thoracic region or center of the chest. Physically the heart is located more on the left side of the body than the right and the ribs provide a physical protection or barrier to the outside world. The top of the heart, known as the heart's base, connects to the great blood vessels of the body: the aorta, vena cava, pulmonary trunk, and pulmonary veins.

CIRCULATORY LOOPS

There are two primary circulatory loops in the human body: the pulmonary loop and the systemic loop. The pulmonary loop transports deoxygenated blood from the right side of the heart to the lungs and the blood picks up oxygen and then returns to the left side of the heart. The systemic loop carries highly oxygenated blood from the left side of the heart to all the tissues throughout the body. The systemic circulation then removes wastes from body tissues and returns deoxygenated blood to the right side of the heart.

BLOOD VESSELS

The blood vessels are the body's pathways allowing blood to flow accurately from the heart to every region of the body and back again. There are many sizes of blood vessels which allow the blood to flow, ranging from very thin capillaries to thick arteries.

CORONARY CIRCULATION

The heart has its own set of blood vessels that provide the myocardium, muscular tissues of the heart, with nutrients and oxygen necessary to pump blood throughout the body.

FUNCTION OF THE HEART

The cardiovascular system has three major functions: regulation of homeostasis, protection, and transportation.

Detox: The heart maintains homeostasis of several internal conditions. The blood vessels assist the body in regulating body temperature by controlling the blood flow to the skin, to balance pH, and the albumin in the blood plasma helps support an isotonic environment.

Nourish: The cardiovascular system protects the body via the white blood cells. White blood cells fight pathogens and clean up cellular debris that has invaded the body. Red blood cells and platelets prevent microorganisms from entering the body and liquids from leaking out.

Activate: The blood distributes nutrients and oxygen and clears away any waste and carbon dioxide to be processed or removed from the body.

REGULATION OF BLOOD PRESSURE

Many functions of the cardiovascular system control blood pressure. Nerve signals and hormones from the brain affect the rate and strength of heart contractions. The contractions and rate of the heartbeat also lead to an increase in blood pressure. The amount of blood in the body also affects blood pressure. The body will raise blood pressure when there is a higher volume of blood in the body which in turn increases heart rate.

CARDIOVASCULAR DISEASE AND DYSFUNCTION

Why is cardiovascular disease so prevalent in current global health? On the physical level, it's easy to see that lack of nutrition and exercise are contributors, but there are exceedingly more reasons as we will examine with a different perspective lens. Have you heard the expression "wear your heart on your chest [or sleeve]"? During the Middle Ages, the knights would wear a token of affection on their sleeve or chest as a symbol of their love. This was a time when, as a society, we were much more open about our emotions and able to display our deepest feelings on the outside for all to see. As time has evolved, we have become more closed, more private, and more protective of our feelings not only for others but for ourselves. We are now moving into a time of elevated awareness of our feelings and expression, and this book is going to activate forgotten memories in your DNA of love and self-love as well as those of the planet to instill heart healing.

Our hearts are deeply affected by physical trauma, and emotional trauma can also cause physical ailments. For example, a person experiencing high levels of daily stress and anxiety can experience physical symptoms such as palpitations and rapid heart rate. These and other physical cardiac symptoms can also occur intermittently from a previous traumatic event which you might remember or not have any recollection of. As you are working through the Discovery Dives in the book, pay close attention to emotions manifesting as physical conditions. These are areas requiring considerable healing and exploration.

The DNA of the heart is a complex yet simple concept. This system supplies and supports the entire body and unless problematic, is mostly silent. Your past genetic history has brought you into this moment and now we would like you to shift your focus to your genetic future. First, we want you to breathe in this concept. YOUR DNA IS ABLE TO CHANGE AND SHIFT.

Currently most of the scientific thought is that our DNA changes and even more commonly it's called a mutation. Now shift that old thought paradigm with this affirmation.

"The DNA of my heart easily heals, transforms, and adapts to my ever-evolving being."

As you begin to observe the changes in your heart through the Detox, Nourish, Activate practices, some things might be so subtle at first you might not recognize them. We want to emphasize the importance of keeping a journal as you work through the book. This will allow you the ability to reflect on who you were when you started this book. Trust us, you will not be the same person at the end!

Golden Feather Tip

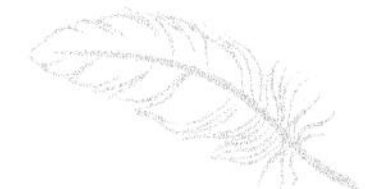

Your greatest superpower is loving yourself unconditionally.

PSYCHO-SPIRITUAL ASPECTS OF THE HEART

HEART SYSTEM PSYCHO-SPIRITUAL PATHWAY

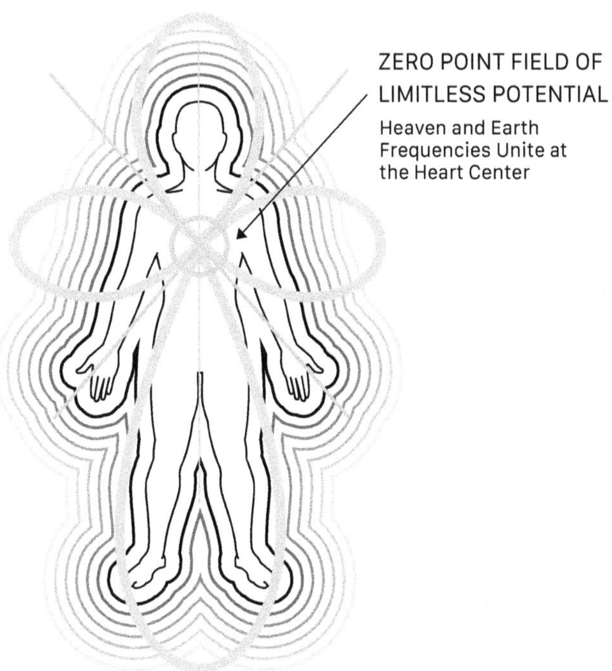

The vertical and horizontal Infinity sacred geometric formations converge in the center of the heartspace accessing the zero point field of limitless creative potential. This sacred dimension holds all infinite possibilities. The co-creative ability to actualize intention from the perspective of wholeness and unity, beyond conflict (personal and otherwise) is directly correlated to the degree of healing at the subconscious and DNA level of the individual.

What is it about the heart and love that engages us at every level? Self. Other. Tribe. Planet. Cosmos.

Our hearts unite Heaven and Earth, they bridge our higher aspects of being to our deeply rooted earthbound selves. They can sing the sweetest songs of love, joy, and the promise of worlds of fulfillment. They can also ache and break for love or love lost to a profound abyss of pain and grief that at points in our lives seems inconsolable. And then there are places in the middle where we feel numb, closed off, disconnected, and alone as if we were floating on an iceberg of isolation, frozen in a state of turmoil.

Energetically, our hearts represent our gateway to the astral body, the shamanic realm. Past life memories including energy blocks in many forms are held on the astral level. Emotionally we hold tremendous energy here that relates to our ability to give and receive love and the holding of loss, betrayal, anger, resentment, and disappointment for those relational experiences that have gone awry. Our emotions are indicators as to how we feel about specific experiences and represent the opportunity to heal and assimilate the lessons of life. In a positive light, the heart is our portal to experience the immense joy that is possible. The emotions are beacons of light that when open emanate the most beautiful of frequencies, that of love and compassion.

As we move into the experiential portion of the heart, ask yourself how much joy you allow yourself to feel daily? Is it hampered by the pains of the past, or the stress and overwhelm of mundane life?

Our hearts are portals of connectivity, uniting us with all of humanity and every other kingdom of life. When we reach a certain point of spiritual awakening, our hearts can vibrate unconditional love for ourselves and for others.

Ultimately, there are the moments of nirvana that are elusive yet attainable, where through the opening of the many-petaled lotus of the heart, we can experience the greatest sense of connection, understanding, and bliss that is possible in human form. Imagine a moment where everything you have ever questioned, misunderstood, or felt hurt or betrayed by within yourself, your family, the world, and even the universe, danced in complete meaning, comprehension, and unity.

Moments like this are possible and are fruits of the journey of healing, awakening, and the desire for evolution along your personal path. Meditation and the other interventions in these pages, along with your deepest soul longings and intentions can illuminate quantum shifts in your consciousness and hearts that will imprint and shift your life in ways that your mind may not be able to comprehend in this moment.

When we look at the energetic physiology of the heart, we can begin to witness the complexity of human nature. From the relational perspective, every dynamic and expression of love that we experienced and witnessed is held here. Relational cords to our mother and father and every person we are in relation with or have ever had a relationship with are also present here. The health of those cords, or connections, is in direct correlation to the harmony of our relationships.

Exploring our genetic and personal past and recurring patterns allows us to make the energetic, mental, and emotional connections that drive our present. It is only then we can shift that energy through transforming our old story into a newly engaged and empowered life story. These stories are the signatures of our cell's DNA, and it is only we that determine what story we want to tell, feel, and ultimately live, now and in the future.

DETOX THE HEART

Welcome to detoxing the heart! You made it! We know you are excited for this journey through the layers of the heart to unfold. Get ready to let go!

DETOXING THE HEART – THE PHYSICAL PERSPECTIVE

Physically there are many signs for the communication signals your body gives you that it needs a cardiovascular detox. The question is, are you listening? The body has a specific way it communicates and sends signals and after a certain time, if you are not listening, it switches gears for another message – hopefully one you will listen to this time. It's usually at this stage that you have begun to experience more signs or clues of dysfunction. Let's look at some examples of signs your body might be sending you – pay attention to me!

You might be experiencing:

- ∞ cold hands and feet
- ∞ swelling in the extremities
- ∞ thick blood or excess clotting
- ∞ abnormal urinary pH
- ∞ clogged arteries
- ∞ sluggish blood flow
- ∞ decreased oxygenation
- ∞ shortness of breath
- ∞ high or low blood pressure
- ∞ genetic dysfunction

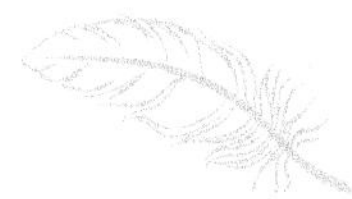

We suggest you get out your journal and start making a list of messages your body is sending you in relation to detoxing the heart.

DETOXING THE HEART — THE PSYCHO-SPIRITUAL PERSPECTIVE

When we contemplate detox from the psycho-spiritual aspects of the heart, the big key is letting go. Our thought forms, feelings, and beliefs mold our external reality and until we can move through and clear many layers of distortion, we continue to perpetuate the same patterns—in relationship, career, health, finances, and so on. In this chapter, you are invited to come into some of the deepest places in your heart and surrender. We all have been hurt, betrayed, lost ourselves and loved ones through various means. We have all experienced some level of abuse, rage, desperation, and fear. You are not alone and yet your experiences are unique and have different meanings based on your own soul's journey.

Letting go of the pains of the past allows the heart to open. We do not live fully without our hearts being open. As if deeply loving and connecting with another is not enough, our hearts are also portals of creation.

AW

At forty-five, I found love. The type of true love I had always dreamt about. And for years and decades written about him in multiple journals, intentions about his character, passions, intellect, his ability to love and understand me with all my imperfections.

It was not all rainbows and butterflies. There was a period where it literally felt like a crowbar was forcibly ripping my heart open. It was physically painful. Deeply. I would sob uncontrollably, for what seemed no reason. My heart was opening. I could feel in ways that I had never experienced before. In one aspect, I was shocked. I had thought my heart had been opened for years, that I was completely emotionally available, and that deep intimacy was easy for me.

I had spent a good chunk of my time and energy blaming the past men I had been romantically intertwined with. The truth is, they were reflections of parts of me that were screaming out for healing. They were places of grief, disappointment, and terror. I could not connect with another person in the way I longed to until my own healing journey deepened. The depth of relationship I have now is one of the greatest blessings of my life. In the beginning it often felt like a roller-coaster ride. I recall a time at a Six Flags theme park, with a great fear of heights, I sat alone in the front of the coaster, which at that time was one of the largest in the US. I remember feeling exhilaration as the coaster slowly made its climb to a high peak. Just about the time it neared the top, I had a panic attack. I was certain I was going to die and attempted to leave the safety harness so I could make my escape.

This is how I felt off and on for a long time. It was a dance of push and pull. Every time this popped up was another opportunity to let go.

Letting go of all the times I had been hurt, felt abandoned, been abused both physically and emotionally and psychically. I had to let go of the places where the voices from those in my past that said I wasn't good enough, smart enough, strong enough, worth enough became the voice inside of my head. Our internal voices create molecules in our bodies. These can be molecules of health or lack thereof, but they are indeed molecules of emotion. When we let go of the old ways, we have the space for something entirely new and delightful to fill it.

HEART DETOX FREEDOM PHOTON WHEEL

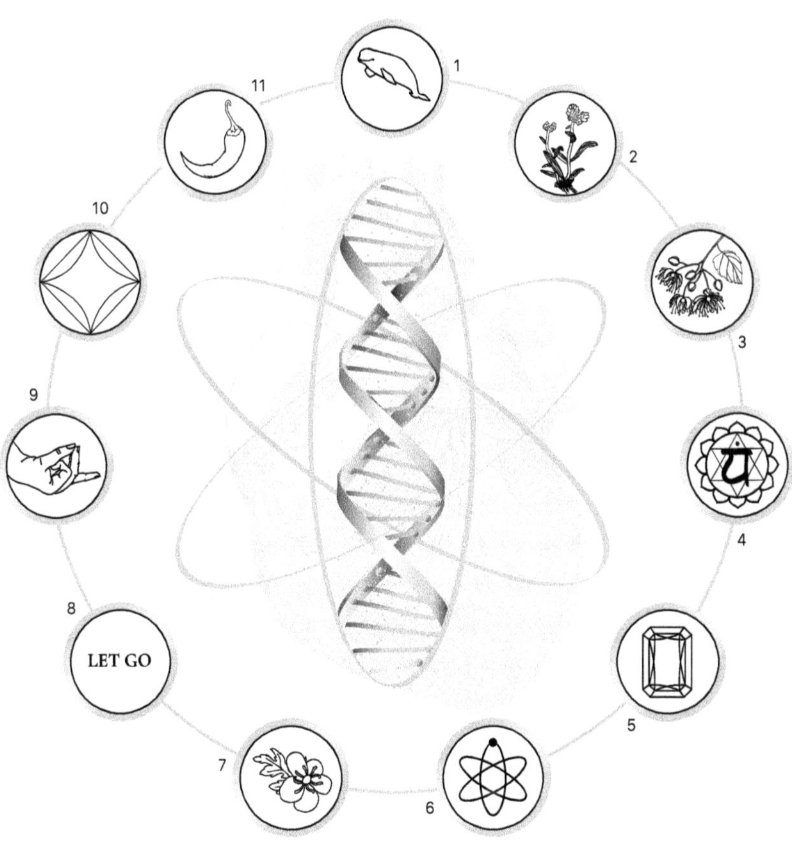

1 Alchemy Animal: Beluga Whale
2 Aromatherapy: Spikenard
3 Botanical: Linden
4 Light Wheel: Anahata
5 Crystal: Emerald
6 Photon Vibration
7 Flower or Gem Essence: Hawthorn
8 Intention: Let Go
9 Meditation Mudra: Hridaya
10 Sacred Geometry
11 Nutrition: Cayenne Pepper

HEART DETOX
INFINITY INFLUENCERS

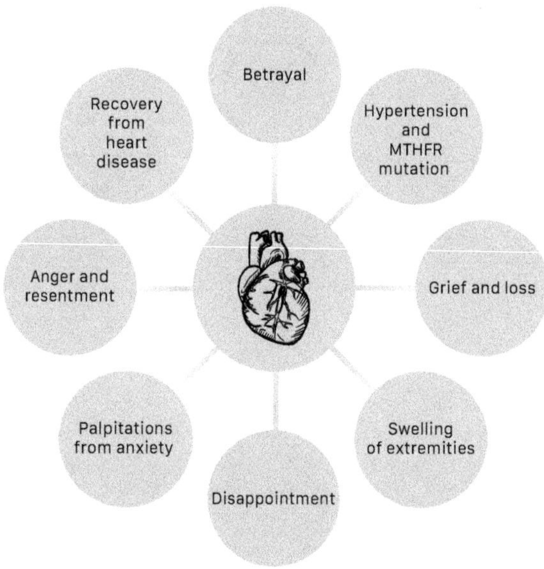

DETOX THE HEART – ALCHEMY ANIMALS

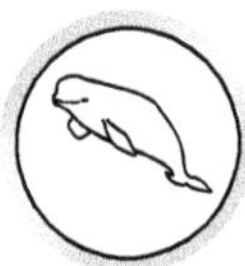

The detox alchemy animals of the heart help to support you in the process of letting go. Let's be real – letting go can bring up old patterns to deal with and we are not saying that letting go is always the easy road – but IT CAN BE! These animals, as you will see, are strong and powerful.

MAJOR ARCHETYPE

BELUGA WHALE

The beluga whale is an animal of ancient wisdom, freedom, creation, and song. If you are resonating with this beautiful whale it is time to open, let go, and sing a song of joy. This glorious creature travels the planet singing a sound of love to awaken the healing within. As your body is detoxing the beluga whale connects to your cellular wisdom and helps you conserve energy, as letting go can be a depleting process. The sweet chatter of the beluga whale can also help you release ruminating thoughts and clear the mind to create a deeper connection to the heart.

Creature Connection: "I embrace love deeply within my heart with the vibration of music and song."

MINOR ARCHETYPES

Coral Snake

The coral snake is a reptile of tremendous healing, wisdom, and transformation. The snake comes forward as an alchemy animal to help us shed elements that are no longer serving us both physically and emotionally. You can picture the snake as it sheds its skin as a time of rebirth and transition. The snake helps us to transform poisons or toxins from the body which can lead to striking healings and rebirths by increasing blood circulation.

Energetically the snake has long been associated with kundalini energy and a rising of energy from the root chakra and the Earth up through the spine and activating all the chakras. This kundalini energy can help open, and release buried emotions and move them up and out of the body. If you are working on releasing repressed anger the coral snake helps to connect for self-compassion but to having a deep compassion and forgiveness for others.

Creature Connection: "I embrace the transitional power of the coral snake, let go of my defenses, embrace new opportunities, and call upon my inner wisdom for a great healing to begin now."

Harpy Eagle

The harpy eagle is the biggest and most dynamic of all the species of eagles possessing a great power of enlightening the spirit and creating new dreams. The Native Americans have long used the sacred feathers of the eagle in ceremonies to connect with the great father sky and cleanse the energetic field or aura. When the harpy eagle is an alchemy animal in your life, it is a great time to receive a message from your inner self or spirit, so open your heart and connect inward. The eagle also can soar high above, connecting to the energy of the sun giving a greater sense of perspective and purification of situations or illnesses that we have lost sight of.

When you are called to the energy of the harpy eagle, it is a time to reflect on times that you may have caused hurt to yourself or others and to call upon this magnificent bird to help you speak truth. It is also a time to conserve your energy for there is coming a time when you will need to draw deeply on this reserve. Draw upon the deep sense of knowing that you have a greater purpose and responsibility to yourself and the planet – breathe!

Creature Connection: "I call upon the tremendous strength, power, and sight of the harpy eagle to allow me to see all situations with a new perspective and light so that I can fly easily into the next chapter of my life."

ANIMAL ADDITIONS

- ∞ Dove
- ∞ Horse
- ∞ Polar bear

DETOX THE HEART – AROMATHERAPY

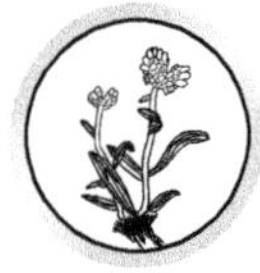

MAJOR ARCHETYPE

SPIKENARD – *Nardostachys jatamansi*

Part Extracted: The rhizome and roots

Core Properties: Anti-inflammatory, antispasmodic, calmative, cardiotonic, carminative, digestive stimulant, neurotonic, phlebotonic
Safety: nontoxic, non-irritant

Spikenard carries a beautiful resonance with the heart. Its ancient aroma of moist earth and decaying wood carries the frequency to ease into the depth of our trauma in a rich embrace. Also known as nard, this sacred oil is revered in the biblical story of the high initiate Mary Magdalene anointing Jesus prior to the Last Supper. Spikenard can access our own "Holy of Holies," our innermost sanctuary where the Light of the Divine is constant within us and to carry its profound aromatic molecules and healing energy into the cellular consciousness.

This oil has a unique ability to ease us into a space of letting go by strengthening the connection to our soul and higher self. It is also a potent oil for bringing light and healing to the relational cords of our ancestry through the DNA. Spikenard is vibrationally encoded to support DNA level clearing of the dogmatic attachment to the religious philosophies perpetuating fear, patriarchal hierarchy, and avarice, to allow the true essence of the spiritual teachings to be communicated. Specifically, spikenard can bring to light areas of wisdom that have been passed down through your mother and father bloodlines.

From an emotional perspective, spikenard has an anchoring ability to stabilize erratic emotional peaks and valleys.

AW At different points of my life, when I have felt myself slipping back into an old pattern of closing my heart and isolating myself to avoid the grief and disappointment I "just knew" was right around the corner, spikenard became a great ally. Those patterns ran deep through my DNA, specifically on my father's bloodline. The women on this side of the family suffered financially and emotionally, often raising children alone in economic hardship. This clearing and healing has been an enormous part of my own healing journey to allow myself to give and receive love and to deeply trust another.

For those who tend to irrational thought processes, nard has a balancing and centering effect on the mental body and is particularly beneficial to those who tend to hyperactive and anxious thinking as well as those with a tendency to spend an excess of time and energy in their mind, disconnecting from the heart center and physical body. As an excellent anti-inflammatory and antispasmodic, spikenard calms uncertain and frenetic energy in all levels of the auric field. This is one of the most potent and versatile essential oils to have on your team.

Detox the Heart – Spikenard Medicine to Connect with Ancestry Wisdom

Apply 1–2 drops of essential oil to your left palm, raise your hand to the heavens and invite the light and grace of your ancestors to encircle you with their loving energy. Breathe in the aromatic molecules of spikenard deeply into your heart space as you connect in with each heart of the beings around you. On your next breath intake, state your intention to receive a message from them regarding one or more of the gifts passed down through your lineage. This may come through a message conveyed to you collectively or by them individually. Be open and allow what comes through. Close with a blessing of gratitude and any other message from your heart to theirs.

Eucalyptus – *Eucalyptus radiata*

Part Extracted: Leaf

Core Properties: antibacterial, anti-catarrhal, antifungal, anti-infectious, antirheumatic, antiviral, decongestant, expectorant, febrifuge, immune tonic, insect repellent, rubefacient
Safety: nontoxic, non-irritant

Eucalyptus is a powerhouse of a remedy. Although the globulous species is the most known, we adore the radiata species as it has a gentler nature, which makes it more tolerable for younger ages. This also allows for greater ease and efficacy in working with the psycho-spiritual aspects of healing to access trauma at the cellular level and through the calcified energy or "blocks" of trauma in the auric field. This species is also known for its antiviral potency.

Eucalyptus is a fast-growing tree, and this is a parallel of its level to quickly shift energy in the spiritual, mental, and emotional bodies. Inhalation of eucalyptus immediately opens and expands the chest, clearing the pathway for release and increasing awareness to the greater possibilities of life. This oil carries the vibration of expansion and freedom and is particularly helpful for breaking up old patterns of energy that have been entrenched and difficult to let go of. This is one of the best oils to clear stagnant energy and emotions. In addition to clearing and opening the heart, eucalyptus is supportive in freeing the spirit from places of constriction and confinement so that it can reconnect with the soul and heart space. This oil is also known for its respiratory and immune support, as well as its powerful antibacterial properties.

Detox the Heart – Cleansing the Pathways
Eucalyptus Heart Spray

- ∞ 22 drops Eucalyptus essential oil (*Eucalyptus radiata*)
- ∞ 9 drops Geranium essential oil (*Pelargonium graveolens*)
- ∞ 3 drops Lemon Verbena essential oil (*Aloysia citrodora*)

Blend into a 60 ml spray bottle of distilled water and shake well before use.
Mist energy field, inhaling deeply. You can also mist home, office, and car.

Clary Sage – *Salvia sclarea*

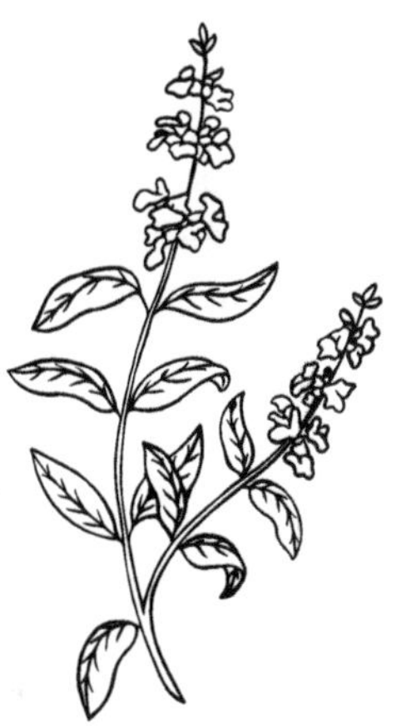

Part Extracted: Flowering tops and leaves

Core Properties: antibacterial, antidepressive, antifungal, anti-infectious, antispasmodic, astringent, carminative, neurotonic, phlebotonic, stomachic, uterine tonic
Safety: nontoxic, nonirritant, avoid during pregnancy

Known for its curative properties, clary sage brings a sense of softness to the heart and other bodily systems.

AW I first came to know clary sage in my early twenties while navigating the very painful disease process of endometriosis. The path of healing and ultimately learning from it was a profound aspect of my personal journey. Clary sage was a critical ally along the way. There were many moments when the pain was excruciating and the voices it carried within it of "being too emotional" or that it was "all in my head", as if being too female contributed to the pain, were so loud it was difficult to breathe.

With the wisdom of a sage, this oil engages those places of imbalance within us with its hypnotic aromatic melody to elicit quiet and stillness. Clary sage allows our cellular consciousness to relax and rest, two necessary components in letting go. If you have witnessed this plant growing in nature, you will be struck by how gentle it appears.

Its softness, layered with the resource strength of a bottomless well, allows the vibration and aromatic molecules to encircle the sharp edges of emotions, specifically grief, rage, disappointment, and fear and dissolve them. It is important to note that there are times when the emotions we feel do not belong to us. They are energies that we have absorbed, consciously or not, from other people, places, and things. This can be confusing, particularly for those who are empathic by nature. Creating healthy boundaries is a practice and skill that takes time to cultivate and comprehend. You will find more practices throughout this book to enhance this teaching.

Clary sage is particularly beneficial for those that tend to use judgement of others to avoid the deep pain and separation they feel within themselves. Somewhere within us, we all have the pain of not being loved in the way we wanted or needed, juxtaposed with the search for finding perfect love. Judgement is a way we avoid feeling that pain. Clary sage can allow us to embrace our judgements of self and others to come into a softer place within our hearts, where we can connect with our own sweet innocence once again.

Detox the Heart – Clary Sage Bath to Soften Emotional Edges

The bath as a refuge offers us great restorative properties. The element of water by its very nature is cleansing and healing to all levels of our auric field. It is crucial for our hydration and health at the cellular level. It deeply nourishes and soothes our emotional nature. The bath is sacrosanct, our own healing spa that we can immerse ourselves in daily for healing and rejuvenation.

Add 7–10 drops of clary sage essential oil to your bath with one cup of Epsom salts and enjoy.

Essential Oil Additions

∞ Rosewood – *Aniba rosaeodora*

HEART DETOX AROMATHERAPY
DNA BLUEPRINT BENEFITS

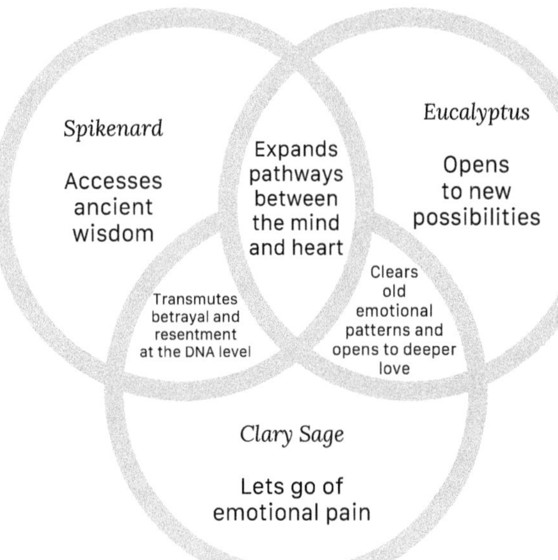

DETOX THE HEART – BOTANICAL MEDICINE

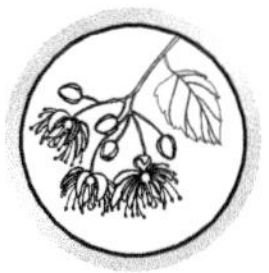

MAJOR ARCHETYPE

LINDEN – *Tilia cordata*

Parts Used: Flower and leaf

This beautiful tree has a leaf shaped like a heart, symbolic of its healing cardiovascular properties. Linden wraps you in a warm blanket of love allowing you to slowly let go not only of cellular toxicity but also emotional grief and loss. It is a relaxing herb indicated when you are feeling so wound up emotionally you are in a state of hysteria. It's especially indicated for conditions of the heart when anxiety and stress are the underlying cause. When the heart is aggravated with palpitations and hypertension, linden's soothing quality allows the physical heart to slow down and emotionally to de-stress.

Linden's ancient plant medicine is a tree of protection, lovers, and friendship. It opens the doorway to the fairy realm connecting to the sweetness and playfulness of the fairies and your inner child. In sacred ceremonies and your FPW, this is the herb to turn to for inviting in love and romance.

Detox the Heart – Linden Physical Uses

Detox: Oxygenates the blood and opens the doorways for cellular detoxification
Cardiovascular: Hypertension, arteriosclerosis, and palpitations; diaphoretic and diuretic
Nervous System: Tension, stress, hysteria, and insomnia
Adrenals: Anxiety and restlessness
Musculoskeletal System: Antispasmodic – migraines and nervous headache
Immune System: Antiviral – influenza, infections, colds, flu and fever
Integumentary System: Itchiness and fungal rashes

Detox the Heart – Linden Emotional Uses

Calms an anxious heart
Opens emotional blocks – enables surrendering to love
Soften and soothes a broken heart

Detox the Heart – Linden Energetic Uses

Protects when you feel challenged to express your truth
Neutralizes negative thought patterns
Aids in communication with the fairy realm and the trees

Detox the Heart – Linden Dosage

Infusion: Steep 1 tablespoon of Linden in 236 ml of hot water for 10 minutes – drink one cup 3x/day
Tincture: 30 drops 2–3x/day

Detox the Heart – Linden Cautions and Contraindications

None

Detox the Heart Linden Tea
Freedom to Rest

Ingredients:
16 g Linden – *Tilia cordata*
8 g Chamomile – *Matricaria recutita*
8 g Meadowsweet – *Filipendula ulmaria*
4 g Lavender – *Lavandula angustifolia*

Directions:
Combine all ingredients in a small bowl.
Infuse 1 tablespoon in 236 ml hot water for 10 minutes.
Drink 1 cup before bed for serenity and sweet dreams.

MINOR ARCHETYPES

Motherwort – *Leonurus cardiaca*

Part Used: Aerial parts

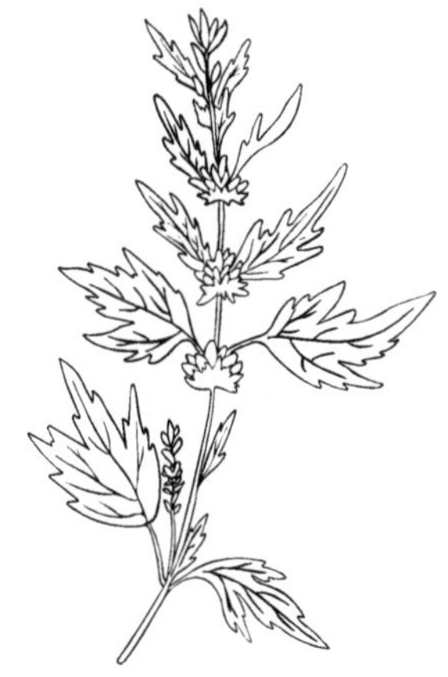

The botanical name, *Leonurus cardiaca* comes from the Greek *Leon* = lion, *ouros* = tail, and *cardiaca* refers to the heart. We often think of this plant for women who are frustrated with their life, angry, and see no way out of their current circumstance. Motherwort fights your battles for you. She is the fierce yet gentle warrior within who you have been longing to fight your battles.

Physically motherwort calms an anxious heart, mind, and spirit. It's helpful for any health conditions resulting from a nervous or anxious state of mind. It strengthens the heart in weakened health conditions without putting too much strain on an already weakened state of vitality. It also has a great affinity for the reproductive organs, aligning them with the circulatory system to filter stagnant blood flow.

Detox the Heart – Motherwort Physical Uses

Detox: Protects the cellular membrane from toxicity and pathogens disrupting the harmony
Cardiovascular: Hypertension due to stress, inhibits myocardial cell firing, increases coronary perfusion, tachycardia, and palpitations
Nervous System: Anxiety, nervousness, restlessness, calming irritability, delirium, and unrest
Adrenals: Supports recovery from adrenal burnout
Women's Health: Emmenagogue, amenorrhea, improves mesenteric circulation of the uterus, menstrual cramp, and unrest due to menopause
Thyroid: Hyperthyroidism
Antiaging: Longevity and immortality

Detox the Heart – Motherwort Emotional Uses

Used for melancholy and restlessness from emotional and physical ailments of the heart
Strengthens the heart emotionally

Detox the Heart – Motherwort Energetic Uses

Promotes inner trust and confidence for the future
Protective herb, especially in ceremonies
Designed to protect pregnant women and their unborn children
Place around the home or above doorways to keep away unwanted energy or unwelcome guests

Detox the Heart – Motherwort Dosage

Liquid Extract: 20–40 drops 1–4 x/day
Infusion: 1 tablespoon per cup of water
Topical: use over the uterus for suppressed and painful menstruation

Detox the Heart – Motherwort Cautions and Contraindications

May cause stomach upset in larger doses
Pregnancy

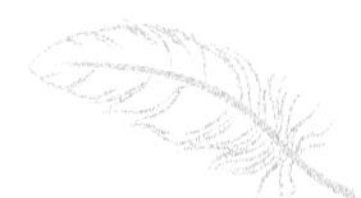

Detox the Heart – Motherwort Freedom to Love Cordial

Ingredients:
57 g Motherwort – *Leonurus cardiaca*
28 g Damiana – *Turnera diffusa*
½ cup Blueberries
1 tablespoon Lavender – *Lavandula angustifolia*
½ teaspoon Cinnamon – *Cinnamomum burmanni*
Vodka, brandy, or pure grain alcohol
Sweetener: honey, maple syrup, or glycerite
Note: use fresh or dried herb dependent on availability
Directions: See Appendix B
Serving Suggestions: Mix with iced tea or carbonated water or use as a dessert topping. To drink as is, serve cordial in a small glass – or in your belly button for some romantic fun or party tricks.

Astragalus – *Astragalus membranaceus*

Part Used: Root

Astragalus has been used since ancient times in traditional Chinese medicine as a warming tonic. It works like an antioxidant protecting the heart from free radical damage and it also increases red blood cell production helping with recovery of cardiovascular diseases. It also protects the heart from free radical DNA damage. Astragalus promotes discharge of fluids promoting urination, reducing swelling and eliminating toxins. When combined with other cardiovascular herbs, it is a wonderful cardiovascular tonic increasing stamina, endurance and warms the blood.

Detox the Heart – Astragalus Physical Uses

Detox: Preserves integrity of the cellular membrane
Cardiovascular: Cardioprotective, strengthens capillaries, improves anemia, vasodilator, hypertension, and antioxidant
Nervous System: Stress and increases stamina
Adrenal System: Fatigue especially form immune dysfunction
Immune System: Antibacterial and antiviral, autoimmune disease, cancer prevention, anti-tumor, post-surgery or major trauma
Musculoskeletal: Anti-inflammatory
Urinary: Diuretic
Reproductive: Hormone balancing, increases sperm motility
Vitality: night sweets, antiaging and cell regeneration

Detox the Heart – Astragalus Emotional Uses

Release painful memories of trauma
Lightens a heavy heart
Uplifting, balancing, and protective

Detox the Heart – Astragalus Energetic Uses

Time travel to different dimension
Keep the dried root in a sachet on your sacred altar to promote physical health and peace
Plant on your property or around for family protection

Detox the Heart – Astragalus Dosage

Tincture: 2–5 ml 3x/day
Decoction: 1 tablespoon dried herb in 8 oz of water 3x/day

Detox the Heart – Astragalus Cautions and Contraindications

None

Detox the Heart – Astragalus Freedom to Surrender

Make a decoction of 14 g Astragalus root to 236 ml of water. Steep for 10 minutes.
Drink prior to the sacred ceremony to release painful memories.

BOTANICAL ADDITIONS

∞ Cardamom – *Elettaria cardamomum*
∞ California Poppy – *Eschscholzia californica*

HEART DETOX BOTANICAL MEDICINE
DNA BLUEPRINT BENEFITS

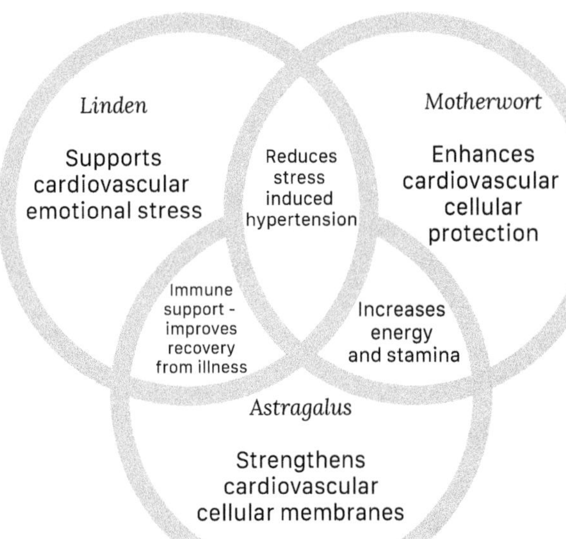

DETOX THE HEART – LIGHT WHEELS

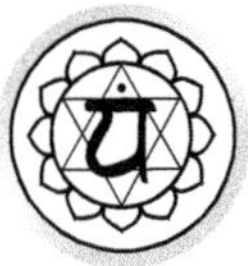

Some of the light wheels or chakras may seem new to you. The power of your intention is one of the most potent alchemical interventions you have at your disposal. You can simply invite in this light wheel to connect, open, expand, and balance for your highest good.

MAJOR ARCHETYPE

THE 4th LIGHT WHEEL, Anahata

The fourth light wheel is the seat of the celestial soul and the gateway to communication with your inner being. It is connected to the heart and the creation of dreams. You know the feeling when you are watching the sunrise on the horizon or you see a rainbow in the distance. This is the love of your heart.

This light wheel opens you to the sweetness and tenderness of your inner child. It is through reuniting the passions and dreams of when you were a child to the visions of today that this light wheel is enlightened. Anahata is also about complete and unconditional love of yourself. Having compassion for your self growth – which is not always the easiest journey. This light wheel also represents all relational cords and holds the emotional dynamics and patterns from our core relationships.

Anahata is connected physically to the heart and the thymus gland, the gland of immune defense. When this light wheel is fully functional the circulatory and lymphatic systems will drain excess toxins and cellular debris clogging clear circulation.

MINOR ARCHETYPES

∞ The 2nd light wheel, Svadhisthana

Svadhisthana is the sacral light wheel and connects the seat of sexuality with the heart. This light wheel aligns with the water element creating a flow of sexual energy up from the base to the heart. Svadhisthana releases walls of pain or hurt you may have put up around you as a defense mechanism from sexual trauma or violence. When this light wheel is activated you will feel the power of true self-expression and intimacy. This light wheel also supports us to release emotions that have been denied and depressed deep within the auric field and the physical body.

COLORS

MAJOR ARCHETYPE

PINK

Rose pink is the color of the heart detox system and physically releases dysfunction of the cardiovascular system that might further manifest as serious disease. It is the color of cardiac prevention. Emotionally and spiritually pink helps us release old relationships deeply seated in the heart. Pink reminds us that love can be soft, gentle, and without conditions.

COLOR ADDITIONS

∞ Chartreuse green
∞ Salmon
∞ Emerald green

SOUND

∞ Yam

Yam is the note of F sounding like "yarm." Use this sound frequency and vibration by either playing a recording or by saying it aloud in repetition for 5–10 minutes. You can also use it in conjunction with detox the heart mudra for extra attunement. Yam helps quiet the heart and mind allowing you to open to the immense vastness and stillness within.

DETOX THE HEART – CRYSTALS AND STONES

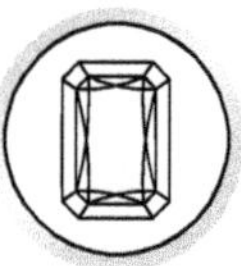

MAJOR ARCHETYPE

EMERALD

The emerald engages the human heart with the resonance of unity and connection, vibrates with the heart of humanity, and allows for greater ease with the Earth connection, letting go of the anger and frustration towards your human brothers and sisters. Emerald's alchemy heals deep trauma and clears the personal and planetary injustices against each other from war, racism, and tribal power struggles.

The emerald, with its crystalline green, is the stone of greatest energetic connection to the fourth chakra of pure love, joy, and compassion. This crystal opens the doorway of our heart enabling pure, honest communication with our true self and others. Emerald also assists in clearing the astral body of thought forms and past life energetic structures. It also allows us to connect to the greater love of the universe and our higher selves, while simultaneously enhancing and expanding our connection to the Earth.

When worn or placed on the heart center, the body is infused with a brilliant green ray of light clearing out stagnant relationships, sexual trauma, and past life rejections, and encircles the energetic body or aura with a light of abundant love. Infused with the energy consciousness of grace, emerald also works intensely with the emotional body processing abandonment, scarcity around love and money, and surmounting feelings of unworthiness. It clears the energy of resistance connected to self-love and the ability to give and receive it too.

The strength of emerald physically helps to recover and rebalance cardiovascular disease and illnesses promoting vitality. It will bring the physical body into a state of hemostasis where all the cardiomyocytes are working in harmony. Wearing the stone close to your heart can also help with acute cardiac arrhythmia, palpitations, and high blood pressure.

MINOR ARCHETYPES

∞ Unakite Jasper

Unakite is a powerful stone eliminating toxins in the heart and releasing damaged cellular buildup from cardiovascular disease. When releasing old trauma, it works subtly on the emotional body in small waves to help prevent the shock of releasing repressed emotions too quickly. You may notice as you are healing and detoxing the heart many feelings of anger will surface to be released. This is normal but can be challenging. Unakite will help soften this release as if you were lying on a soft cloud gently sailing through the blue sky. Jasper also invigorates vital life force, assisting the meridians and nadis to open to receive more light. The auric field balances and we can reconnect with a sense of trust in opening the heart with this stone.

∞ Lapis Lazuli

Lapis lazuli is an ancient stone connected back to the time of the great pharaohs of Egypt and often placed in the tombs of royalty. This ancient energy still carries through the DNA and energetic vibration of this crystal, reviving the long-lost knowledge of power and healing within you.

It draws a connection between the heart center and the eighth chakra, the electromagnetic field, surrounding your being and creating an aperture into the soul and enhancing spiritual insight. Lapis activates the wisdom of sacred mysticism and esoteric memories of the healing arts and high sensory perception, reawakening the third eye.

Lapis recharges the cellular and emotional system and nourishes the sixth level of the auric field, the celestial body with the remembrance of spiritual love from all transcendent light beings.

DETOX THE HEART CRYSTAL GRID

Place a bright green cloth, cotton or silk is best, on the floor. Lie down on your back on top of the cloth, with your head facing north. Additionally you may choose to add the soap stone, pistachio opal and or opalight - see the image for placement. Relax for 15-30 minutes. Note - By lying in the full sun for this healing session you will receive the most benefits. Drink a glass of water with added spirulina or chlorophyll after the treatment to realign cellular communication and accelerate detoxification. Immediately after the treatment cleanse the crystals and stones. (See Appendix A)

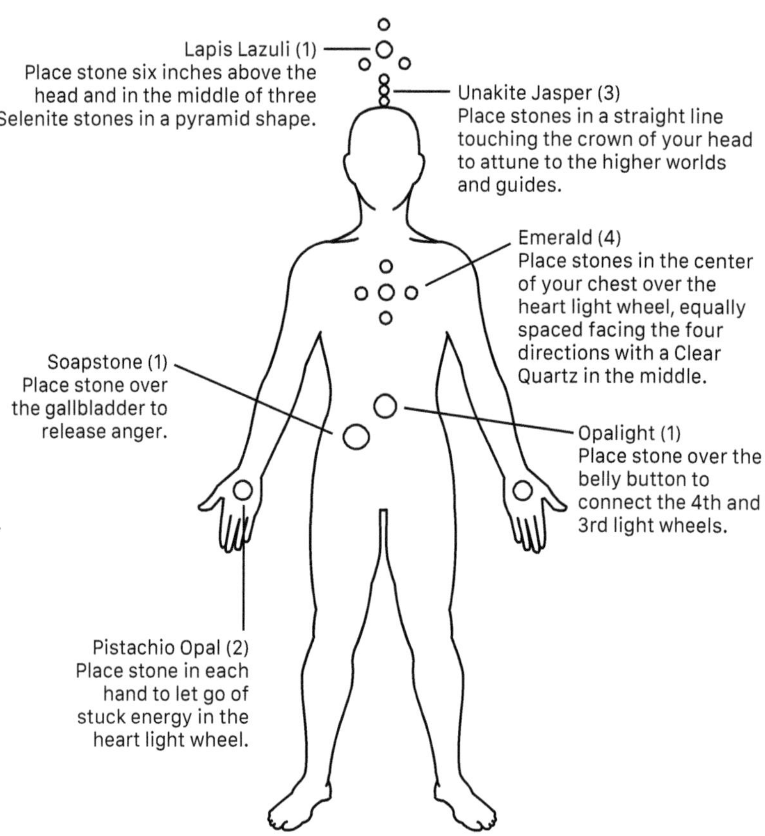

DETOX THE HEART – ENERGETIC AND VIBRATIONAL TECHNIQUES

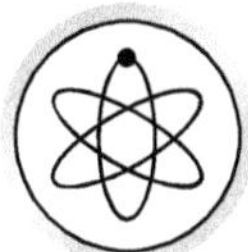

MAJOR ARCHETYPE

DETOX THE HEART HYDROTHERAPY

Ingredients:

- ∞ 170 g Pink Himalayan Sea Salt
- ∞ 340 g Epsom Salt
- ∞ 3 drops Spikenard essential oil (*Nardostachys jatamansi*)
- ∞ 1 drop Eucalyptus essential oil (*Eucalyptus radiata*)
- ∞ 1 drops Immortelle essential oil (*Helichrysum italicum*)
- ∞ 4 drops Clary Sage essential oil (*Salvia sclarea*)
- ∞ 7 drops of Hawthorn flower essence

Directions:
Add salts and essential oils to warm water. Choose a crystal from the detox heart section and add to bath. Best to be done at night before bed.

MINOR ARCHETYPE

Detox the Heart Water Ceremony

This form of vibrational alchemy imprints the vibration, life force, and specific healing energy of the crystal into one of the most nourishing and restorative elements, water. Taken on an empty stomach in the morning allows for a rapid cellular response and often a tangible feeling of shift of emotional energy and awareness.

Take your cleansed and programmed crystal and add it to a glass or pitcher of fresh clean water. Wrap your hand around the vessel and align your intention to infuse water molecules with the consciousness of love, gratitude, and the desire to release anything that limits your experience of love and joy. To enhance the alchemy of the intervention, infuse with a pink colored light. After 20 minutes, remove the crystal, thank it for sharing its vibration and drink the water as desired. NOTE: Remember to strain crystal prior to drinking and enjoy with the intention of allowing the spectrum of vibration to permeate and heal at the cellular level.

Needed:

- ∞ 1 piece of Unakite jasper
- ∞ 1 vessel of water

Infuse as instructed above and drink throughout the day. Refrigerate unused portions for later use.

Detox the Heart EOBT

Place one drop of spikenard essential oils between the first two fingertips of the right hand, inhale deeply, and tap the Heart-6, Yin Cleft, Xi Cleft point of the heart meridian for 30 seconds with the intention of letting your heart release all that no longer serves you.

Location: On the palmar side of the wrist. Run your finger from the pinky side of the wrist over the tendon (flexor carpi ulnaris tendon) and fall into the valley 1/2 inch below (proximal to) the flexure of the wrist.

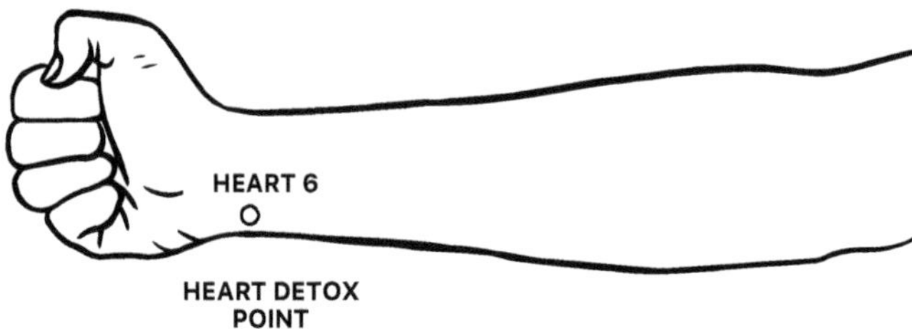

DETOX THE HEART – FLOWER AND GEM ESSENCES

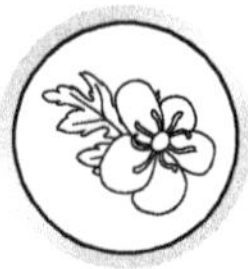

FLOWER ESSENCES

MAJOR ARCHETYPE

HAWTHORN

Hawthorn calls you to own your emotional strength to create. It invites you to shape-shift your creative process with clear, intense conviction by raising your frequency to transform anger and frustration into compassionate creative action. Hawthorn reminds you that each experience is a growth opportunity, a way to hone your spirit and your wisdom. Whether you are working on an art, business, or garden project, or want to recreate your life, hawthorn will be your ally.

MINOR ARCHETYPE

MOTHERWORT

Motherwort flower essence works through the front of the heart chakra to help you feel/sense that your heart is connected to the matrix of ALL, the spiritual life force of the universe. It invites you to experience the expanded nature of your heart that is grounded in the present moment. This engenders deep peace and quiet. Motherwort essence promotes the heart chakra to spin with an open and stable flow and clears the area where the heart chakra moves through your personal physical, emotional, and mental energy fields. It encourages love and compassion for yourself and soothes the sense of emotional boundary violation by another person.

FLOWER ESSENCE ADDITIONS

∞ Linden
∞ Raspberry
∞ Strawberry

GEM ESSENCES

MAJOR ARCHETYPE

DIAMOND

As a master healer, diamond essence contains the vibrational structure of utmost clarity. It clears core imbalance at the cellular and DNA level, as well as every level of the auric field. Supportive to releasing negative patterns and memories, diamond connects us to higher dimensional frequencies to facilitate awakening to our divine nature. It assists in opening the heart to transmit love and higher vibrations. Diamond essence is excellent for lending vibrancy to the skin as well as optimizing cilia function. Its potent transmutational nature assists us in clearing energetic constructs of limitation to connect with the infinite limitless potential of the zero-point field. This is a prime essence to increase abundance. Diamond is also good for clearing the spinal fluid, the cerebrospinal fluid and clearing the lymph system. Diamond is also great for opening the crown, opening to higher dimensions, connecting with the great central sun.

DETOX THE HEART – INTENTIONS

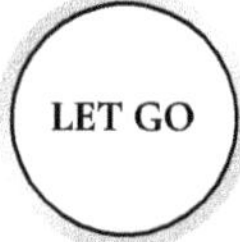

MAJOR ARCHETYPE

LET GO

MINOR ARCHETYPES

∞ I let go and trust that there is a greater force at work in my life.
∞ My heart and being are fully free to give and receive love.
∞ I release the old pattern and programming that I am unlovable.

ADDITIONAL INTENTIONS

- ∞ I release and let go the cells of my heart and blood that are no longer serving me, and I allow in fully functioning and healthy red blood cells.
- ∞ I honor healthy boundaries in my relationships.
- ∞ I open myself to a new, happier, and healthier experience and expressions of love with myself and others.

DETOX THE HEART – MEDITATION MUDRA

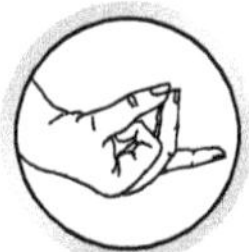

Hridaya Mudra

I open and surrender to a life filled with love and joy.
I let go of my past and embrace the true lightness within.

Hridaya mudra opens the doorway to your heart and allows the release of pain and suffering and invites in a feeling of freedom. It will envelop and wrap you in a sense of safety and trust because it is through this connection the true essence of healing begins. This mudra encourages the lungs, chest, and heart to open fully and release toxic trauma holding you back from your full healing potential. As your heart opens further, your racing mind and ego will reset and release physical tension and emotional pain. This mudra also activates the fourth chakra, Anahata, the center of unequivocal self-love. As you work with this mudra, notice the feeling of lightness as if a great weight has been lifted off your chest.

Hridaya Mudra Alignment

1. Place your hands in front of your heart center and face the palms together with the fingertips pointing upward.

2. Interweave your fingertips together and with the index finger closest to your heart center.
3. Touch your thumbs at the tips forming the shape of a heart.
4. Take a deep breath, let your body relax.
5. You may now either do the meditation below or 10 minutes of *Heart Breathing* (see Detox the Heart Energetic and Vibrational techniques).
6. You may also use this mudra at any time you are feeling tension in your chest or emotionally pent up to release and let go.

Detox the Heart Meditation Mudra

∞ To access the meditation please go to www.zenergymedicinals.com

∞ Take a deep breath in, inhaling one of the Heart Detox suggested oils or a synergy you have created for 30–45 seconds.

∞ Hold the Hridaya mudra and take several breaths to align and attune to your inner heart. With each breath, feel the expansion of your heart, chest, and lungs allowing your blood to fully circulate and cleanse your body and mind.

∞ Feel the vital healing energy coursing through your body and heart as waves of pink light, embracing a sense of peace and openness. Repeat the intention three times either silently or aloud: "I open and surrender to all feelings of love and joy. I let go of my pain and embrace the true lightness within."

∞ This meditation is for letting go. Letting go of the past and all that no longer serves the truth of who you are. Invite a pulsating pink light into the very center of your heart.

∞ Connect with the core Earth crystal receiving the amber life force to nourish your cellular matrices, particle, wave particle, all the atomic structures within the physiology, the bone, the blood.

∞ Envision a three-part flame of pink, amber, and gold in the center of your heart. Allow this flame of light to fully ignite and expand within your heart space.

∞ Release all energies and attachments to all people, places, and things, all karmic attachments, all lower vibrations that pull on your heart strings. Now invite in a cleansing and clearing of your relational cords. The first from adulthood, where you sit in this moment of time and space, and we're going to invite this cleansing and clearing to move back along your timeline, backward in time, letting go of the pain of all relationships where you didn't feel seen or heard for who you truly are, where you weren't witnessed in beauty and respect and honor. Letting go of past betrayals, disappointment, sorrow, and grief. Allowing the emotions of rage, anger, fear to dissolve. Of all the times you felt you weren't enough, letting go. Surrendering the heaviness you felt in your heart in this life and continuing to move all the way back through all the levels of your adulthood, young adulthood. Inviting the precious energy of your inner child's consciousness to come into your heart space. Breathe in until you can envision yourself at a particular age or time and invite your child self to be held within the arms of your adult self. Fill that younger version with the presence of unconditional love, safety, and support.

∞ Invite the vibration of unconditional love to come in through the cellular portal into the DNA in mother and father bloodlines. Clearing these frequencies through your genetic heritage. We invite this clearing through all time and no time, through all aspects, all dimensions, all realities … back to the origin point of this soul. Breathe in and allow the recalibration to take place on all levels.

DETOX THE HEART – SACRED GEOMETRY

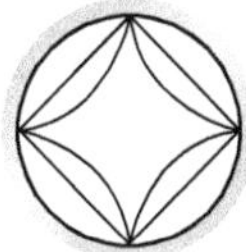

MAJOR ARCHETYPE

DETOX THE HEART SACRED GEOMETRY

Our intentional and original depiction of the Detox the Heart sacred geometry invites you to reconnect with the center of your heart space, to align with the zero-point field, the dimension of limitless creation. The diamond shape frequency supports the letting go of all the old patterns, emotions, and ways of being throughout your whole being, represented by the circle and through the cellular levels of DNA in the family bloodlines.

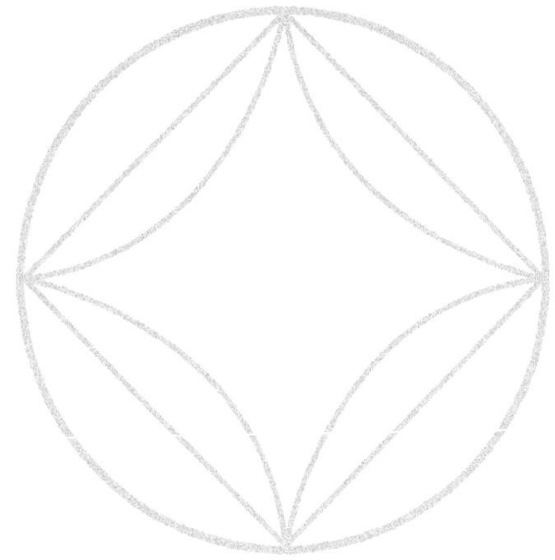

DETOX THE HEART – NUTRITION

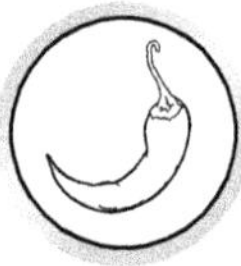

MAJOR ARCHETYPE

CAYENNE PEPPER

The cayenne pepper or chili is a powerful cardiovascular stimulant. It has the key constituent, capsaicin, which activates circulation and digestion. It encourages the removal of toxic wastes and debris from the cells and emunctories by its invigorating heat. It can be added to culinary dishes to help with headaches, arthritis, neuralgia, and cardiac disorders with cold extremities and poor blood flow. It also helps stimulate digestive enzymes and hydrochloric acid reducing gas, bloating, and can help with some cases of diarrhea.

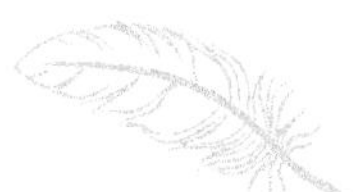

For poor circulation, add a pinch of cayenne powder or chili sauce to each meal. If you don't like spicy foods, dilute the cayenne pepper in a glass of water and honey to kill the heat.

MINOR ARCHETYPES

Cranberry

Cranberry is a little fruit with a power pack chock full of antioxidants fighting off free radicals causing damage to the DNA and cell membrane, especially the cardiomyocytes. Cranberries contain polyphenols which studies have shown prevent cardiovascular disease from developing by reducing systolic blood pressure and improving levels of HDL cholesterol (Battaglia, 1995).

Garlic

Garlic is a pungent superfood. It lowers blood pressure, reduces cholesterol, and decreases blood sugar. Its amazing microbial constituent, allicin, is a natural antibiotic and an excellent food for bronchial conditions. It's a nutrient dense food rich in vitamins C and B, manganese, phosphorus, and calcium. Note of caution: it is a natural blood thinner so use with care when taking blood thinning medications or other nutraceuticals (Gerber, 2000).

NUTRITIONAL ADDITIONS

- Fig
- Red peppercorns
- Tomatoes
- Kidney bean
- Artichokes

DETOX THE HEART – DISCOVERY DIVE – FORGIVENESS AND LETTING GO

Forgiveness is a process with its own timing. It cannot be rushed, forced, or coerced into action.

When it is authentic, it is one of the most potent and rapid transformational interventions. Forgiveness allows you to set yourself free and those you hold captive to your pains of the past.

True forgiveness offers the ability to garner new levels of awareness and understanding of the soul's path and how history repeats itself until fully encompassed and embraced with the full spectrum of love available to you in moments of transcendence.

Letting go of what holds you back and binds you to the past will set you free. Some aspects are held in the conscious mind and some in the subconscious. Be gentle with yourself. Everything comes to the light in its own perfect timing. The "letting go" opens the pathway for new beginnings to unfold and for the grace of divine flow to enter and engage with our highest selves.

Your openness, honesty, and freedom to explore and allow this discovery process to unfold springboards your evolution with ease and greater velocity. This Discovery Dives can illuminate core themes and patterns that you have come to heal. Embrace the answers from a place of compassion as they bring insight and consciousness to your journey.

Remembering to invoke your highest self, I AM presence, and support teams of light with this and any Discovery Dive to create a supportive container for your personal explorations.

Where and how have I felt betrayed in my past?

Are there patterns of abuse in my past? Physical. Emotional. Sexual? When and by whom? Was there abuse in your family of origin?

How did my parents express their love? To me and my siblings? To each other? Was the love I received consistent? What were the conditions? How was I bad? Not good enough? How did I shine in their eyes?

Have you experienced infidelity? You or your partner?

What similarities exist between your past partners and your parent of the same sex? The parent of the opposite sex?

What am I "white knuckling" or over controlling in my life? Where did this pattern stem from in my past?

Is it easier for me to give or receive love? Do I over give? Do I take more than I give?

How do I experience shame and guilt in my life? Sex? Food? Addiction? Religion? Where is it stored in my body?

FREEDOM PHOTON WHEEL™

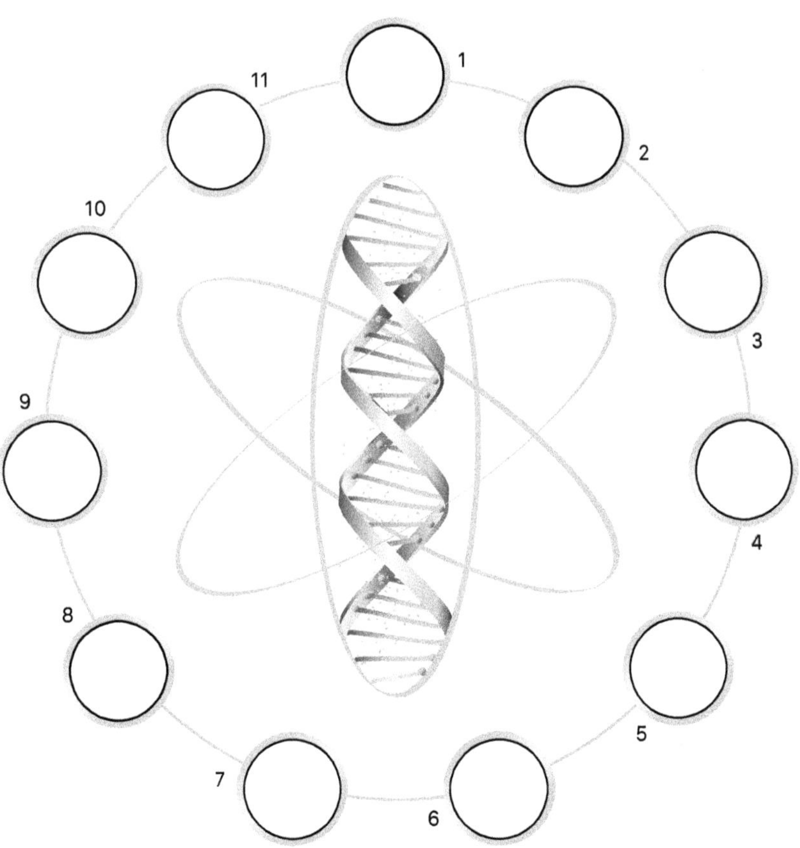

DETOX THE HEART
YOUR PERSONAL FREEDOM PHOTON RITUAL

Moon Phase

It is best to perform your ritual when the moon is waning from the full moon to the new moon, to align with the phase. However, the power of your intention and momentum is key so if you are inspired at another time, go for it.

Intention

"I let go all energy, emotions, patterns, and beliefs that no longer serve me with ease, grace, and faith down to the level of DNA and my genetic lineage."

Select, Align, and Activate

Select your interventions according to the instructions in Chapter Five. Inhale and apply your chosen essential oil for 30–45 seconds. Use your botanical tincture or tea as directed. You may also listen to the meditation and use the mudra from this chapter while attuning your FPW.

Affirmation

"Divine consciousness assists me in dissolving and letting go (see below) of all that I have carried through my lineage, my mother and father bloodlines so that I allow the fullest experience of giving and receiving love.

Letting Go

Struggle. Scarcity. Limitation. Slavery. Abuse (of self and others). Tyranny. Betrayal. Loss. Blocks to giving and receiving love. Isolation. Suffering. Memories of pain.

NOURISH THE HEART

Nourishment is a critical component to our existence. Food and water can provide sustenance, yet to fully thrive we require nourishment in many forms: emotional connection and support, the exercise of our mental faculties, and spiritual communion to inspire our innate curiosity and longing to understand our incorporeal nature.

Nourishing the heart allows all the places of grief, trauma, betrayal, and disappointment to be filled with love. We wrote earlier about the deep desire within the child consciousness for perfect love: those same aspects within us are always searching for the love we did not receive or that we feel we did not receive when we were young. Remember, perception is nine tenths of reality. Until we understand fully that we need to fill ourselves with that love we see and experience life with blinders on.

Part of the challenge here is that this is not just a cognitive knowledge, it must be a visceral understanding for sustainable healing and empowerment. AND when we are triggered in emotional reaction, which is inevitable, we forget. Within this challenge lies the exciting opportunity to shift. That is the beauty of evolution, having the compassionate realization of just how much you have transformed your life through your physical, emotional, and spiritual health and well-being.

Sustainable healing, the kind that leads to quantum leaps along your sacred spiral of transformation, aka superhero journey, hungers for love. As we clear out the old patterns, pains, and places of suffering, the newly opened places crave to be filled. If we miss this all-important process of nourishment, it is easy for the previous habitual ways to return. Our love is the MOST potent alchemical intervention at the ready in each moment. Our deliberate intention of allowing the floodgates of our love and then divine love to fill every cell, every molecule, and every particle within us to then create the life of our dreams.

HEART NOURISH FREEDOM PHOTON WHEEL

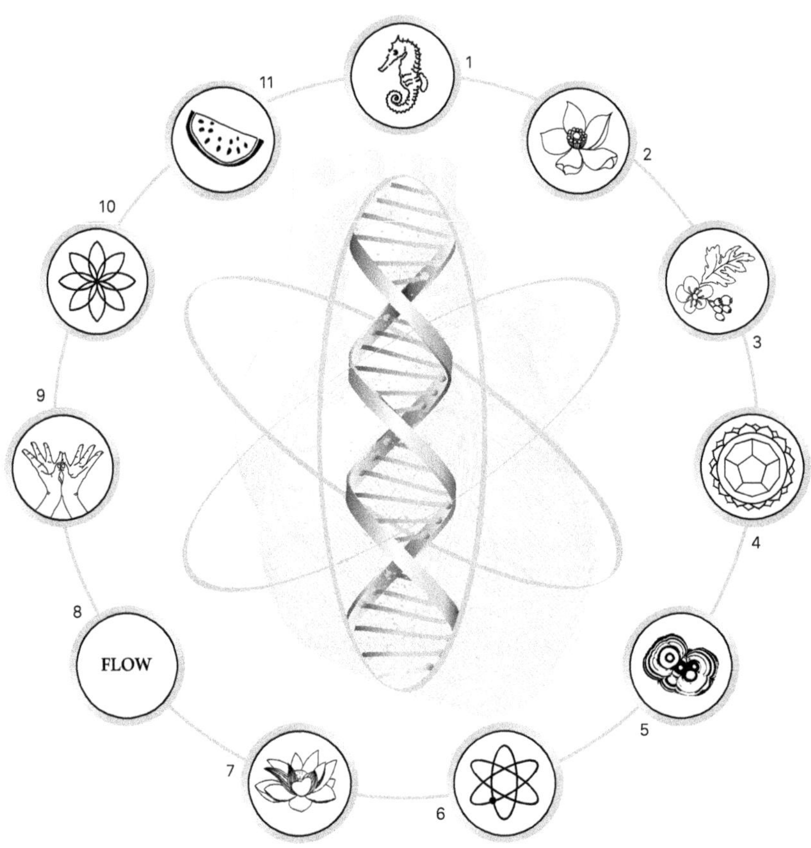

1 Alchemy Animal: Seahorse
2 Aromatherapy: Neroli
3 Botanical: Hawthorn
4 Light Wheel: Bhavapriya
5 Crystal: Malachite
6 Photon Vibration
7 Flower or Gem Essence: Pink Lotus
8 Intention: Flow
9 Meditation Mudra: Padma
10 Sacred Geometry
11 Nutrition: Watermelon

HEART NOURISH
INFINITY INFLUENCERS

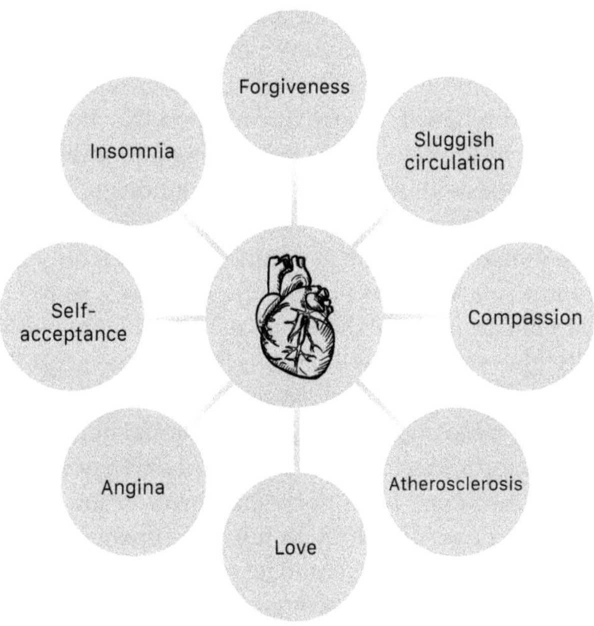

NOURISH THE HEART – ALCHEMY ANIMALS

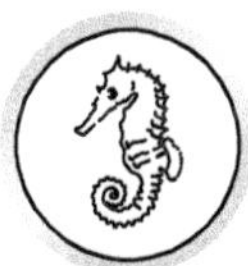

The alchemy animals to nourish the heart are your connection to the element of water. They help you to embrace and infuse the healing qualities of water: flexibility, hydration, renewal, flow, purification, and protection.

MAJOR ARCHETYPE

SEAHORSE

The seahorse is a playful and loving animal helping us to remember the joyful side of love and the free movement through the waters of love. The seahorse is connected to the ocean and invokes the power of the waves, birth, and renewal. Invoke or call upon this alchemy animal to bring you stability through the rocky waters of a tumultuous relationship as the seahorse will help with patience, kindness, and observation from a new perspective to see all sides of a situation that might seem stuck. The seahorse also is here to remind us that the only way to truly help others in a relationship is to nurture ourselves, so dive deep into the ocean of self-care and feel the waves of nourishment wash over you.

Physically the seahorse will help nourish the heart by balancing the fluids or blood pumping in and out of the heart. The boney infrastructure of the seahorse protects the internal body, especially the myocardiocytes, providing the muscle of the heart a new resiliency.

Creature Connection: "I call upon the power of the seahorse. I feel the flow of the sea coursing through my body opening my heart to all relationships. I dance with the seahorse on the waves of the ocean and light of the moon calling forth my inner child to laugh and play with the mermaids. My blood is strong and nourishes each system of my body, waking each cell with a new sense of resilience and comfort."

MINOR ARCHETYPES

Dolphin

The dolphin is such a magnificent alchemy animal of exuberance and effervescence. The dolphin has a deep connection to the sea but because of the spouting breath of the dolphin there is a cycle of life, rebirth, and creation that is the underlying current of this alchemy animal. The dolphin promotes greater oxygenation through the cardiovascular and respiratory systems and tones the cadence of the heart. The dolphins have a deep connection to the primal life force within and can help us travel back through many lifetimes and timelines back to our true and deepest selves. Note: See the breathing and sound meditation later in this chapter to connect with the deeper alchemy of the dolphin.

Creature Connection: "I breathe in the air of life. I float and play in the soul of the sea. I listen to the sound of my heart calling out my name. May I unite with my heart's truest, sacred purpose."

Parrot

The parrot is a bird of magic used in healing rituals and ceremonies. The healing colors of the rainbow connect to the nourishing rays of the sun and open the doorway to the soul. As you probably know, the parrot is quite the talker, and this archetype can shift a locked or blocked heart into one of receiving and communicating. The parrot also helps us remember the value of silence and a quiet mind. When you resonate to parrot alchemy, we suggest taking a day of silence and going inward to reflect on your relationship with yourself and others.

Creature Connection: "I call upon the majestic and glorious wings of the parrot to surround my heart with the power of the rainbow sun. I open my heart to receive all messages from my inner being and child within."

ANIMAL ADDITIONS

- ∞ Rabbit
- ∞ Koala

NOURISH THE HEART – AROMATHERAPY

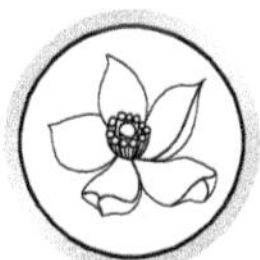

MAJOR ARCHETYPE

NEROLI – *Citrus aurantium var. amara*

Part Extracted: Flower

Core Properties: antibacterial, antidepressive, anti-infectious, antiparasitic, astringent (mild), calmative, digestive stimulant
Safety: nontoxic, nonirritant

True neroli or orange blossom oil is precious, rare, and highly expensive. This often-adulterated oil in its full and completely natural state is in one word, exquisite.

AW Although I had encountered this expression of the orange tree early in my studies of aromatherapy, it wasn't until a journey to Egypt that I fell in love.

In early 2000, my trip to Egypt was entrenched in mysticism. As it was my second journey, I was more accustomed to the culture and the ways of the people and felt much safer. The unique opportunity was to travel to so many sacred sites prior to general opening for ceremony, meditation, and toning. One of my favorites was the temple at Dendera, which is the temple dedicated to Goddess Hathor. While we were there, I had images of the temple in the earlier days, restored to its perfection, its beauty, and elaborate center for healing. Many of the rooms had healing tables that were created of stone and cutouts in the ceiling to allow for certain configurations of stars and healing energy that they would bring to the individual on the table.

I stayed at the Mena house at the foot of the Great Pyramid at Giza. The view from my balcony at nightfall was enchanting in the rarest of ways, looking out at one of the most puzzling wonders of the world, fully illuminated with the desert as a backdrop and the sweet aroma of orange blossoms filling the night air. The property had numerous orange trees and it just so happened they were in full bloom. I sat during the hot days as the petals fell and made a carpet to luxuriate on beneath me.

This utterly clear memory demonstrates the power of the olfactory-limbic connection. The essential oil becomes the anchor, or rather the key to access the memory, forever etched and accessible in your consciousness, and with it the emotional connections and experience that live and breathe there. When I inhale neroli, I envision the sweetest melody intertwining with the aromatic molecules. It is this nourishing sweetness, like honey, that gently drips its vibration into the heart and all the cellular structures of the body.

Its bright aroma lifts the spirit and speaks to the remembrance of joy and light heartedness. Neroli is highly beneficial for those who tend to be harsh and critical of themselves and can assist in shifting this energy to that of self-love and compassion. This oil assists in dissolving extreme emotions like jealousy, anger, and self-hatred. It aids in settling shock and counterbalancing PTSD.

One day of this trip, on the spring equinox and full moon, we were offered passage to the Great Pyramid. The government had closed it to all other tourists that day, and we were graced with the experience of meditation in the Queen's Chamber by candlelight. A group then encircled the great sarcophagus and the King's Chamber for a ceremony indoctrinating the ancient ways of the rites of the Rose Cross.

Old memories were activated deep within me and my heart opened as did my spiritual centers or light wheels. A place deep within my soul had been activated, or rather reconnected, if you will. I felt as though my entire auric field had opened and was breathing and connecting with the world, seen and unseen. This innate potential exists within you, too.

In a new way, tears of expansion flowed as I walked out of the pyramid. I paused after exiting the narrow corridor and began a conversation with a tour guide. As she looked intently into my eyes, she said, ah, so that is where I know you from, long ago here in Egypt, when we used the pyramid as a rite of initiation and specific alchemy. We knew each other. She went on to tell me that she felt guided to give me a message: go into the dark void and trust. You didn't do that fully last time. And you regretted it. There was a resonance of truth in her communication and our connection. And I sat with the idea of what that meant for me in my current life.

After returning home, I spent a great deal of time in nature, walking in the woods, meditating and praying. And a few months later, I felt ready to leave my corporate job and pursue a full-time healing practice and aromatherapy product business. This place of surrender and trust would not have been possible without that time of expansion in Egypt. When the heart opens, and ways of expansion for a spiritual opening as well, an alignment can occur, offering the deep mystical wisdom to bring us to the pinnacle of transformation. It is like coming to the edge of a cliff. In that moment, our free will decides whether we make that leap into the unknown. The choice is always ours.

Awakening the Mystical Heart Meditation Oil

- ∞ 3 drops Neroli essential oil (*Citrus aurantium var. amara*)
- ∞ 1 drop Sandalwood essential oil (*Santalum austrocaledonicum*)
- ∞ 1 drop Rose otto essential oil (*Rosa damascena*)
- ∞ 2 drops Patchouli essential oil (*Pogostemon cablin*)
- ∞ 2 drops Cistus essential oil (*Cistus ladaniferus*)

Blend into 1 tablespoon coconut oil and apply sparingly to palms of hands, breathing deeply for forty-five seconds and then apply to the heart and the third eye to open and expand to the mystical nature of the universe and your own inner universe of possibility and wonder.

MINOR ARCHETYPES

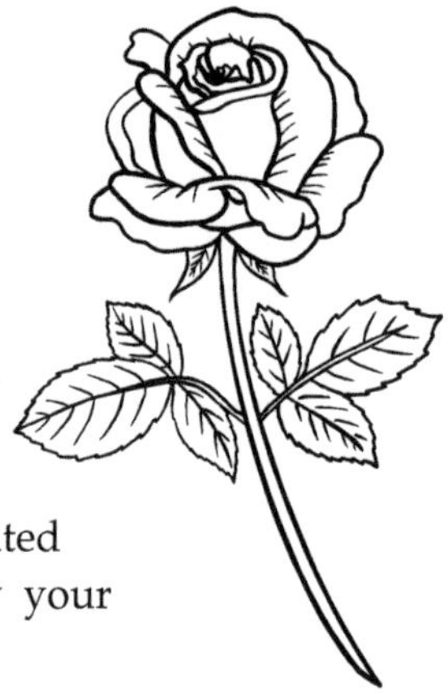

Rose – *Rosa damascena*

Part Extracted: Flower

Core Properties: Antidepressive, mildly analgesic, antiseptic, aphrodisiac, bactericidal, hemostatic, hepatic, neurotic, sedative, tonic
Safety: nontoxic, nonirritant
Special Notation: This is one of the most adulterated oils on the market. It is imperative to know your source.

The alchemy of true rose essential oil is glorious. Via inhalation, it has the instantaneous effect of heart opening when the individual holds this intention. The synergistic effect of positive intention and the rose can move mountains of stagnant emotion from the heart space. The vibration of letting go is carried within its energy signature. The cosmic blueprint for this plant is designed to move the collective consciousness of humanity forward by healing and uniting the personal heart with that of the planetary heart and that of the cosmos. This renders rose's ability to permeate the deepest places of disconnection and pain within the soul, the spirit, the heart, and down into the molecular and cellular composition of the body igniting the memory and presence of love.

The aromatic composition is created from well over 300 chemical constituents making this oil impossible to recreate synthetically. This is one of the reasons there is much black-market control of the resultant essential oil production. As we grow closer to communities based on self-reliance and sustainability, this would be a top recommended plant for home or community based growing and distillation. Rose essential oil, due to its nature as a cell regenerator, lends its ability to regenerate the spirit and to open to love again even after loss and betrayal. Its gentle strength brings hope of the future and of the resilience of the sacred human heart.

Rose offers a potent and versatile regenerative quality. It reinvigorates the spirit with the remembrance of beauty, joy, and the juicy delight of surrendering to another. Rose supports liver cell regeneration as well as that of the skin cells. It has affinity for all skin types and is one of the most profound oils for beauty, with its aromatic molecules opening our hearts to authentic beauty, emanating from the inside out, inviting us to shine that light fully regardless of the slanted expectations of the outer world.

Rose alchemy encourages self-compassion, self-love, and self-acceptance which organically ignites our inner radiance. Rose can support our natural flow of good feeling, alleviate anxiety, and lift our spirits. It is an important oil for balancing the hormones and is indicated for PMS, menopause, and disconnection for our sensual and sexual nature. Vibrationally coded within its aromatic molecules is the reminder of divine love, and the potential of opening the depth of one's being to another in the most holy of ways. The rose, particularly with its formation of petals, reminds us that the true journey is one inward and that the true quest is the reclamation of the divine light within us.

Heart Nourish – Temple of the Beloved Rose Anointing Oil

Here, we refer to the Temple of the Beloved as the portal to the Sacred Human Heart, to imbue your heart with a deep sense of divine love and wholeness.

∞ 3 drops Rose Otto essential oil (*Rosa damascena*)
∞ 1 teaspoon organic coconut oil or jojoba oil

Blend into a small bottle of your choosing.

As you hold this bottle in your hands, offer this prayer.

"I acknowledge myself as a divine being of light. I freely give and receive my love." As you invite in a greater opening of your heart, envision it being filled with pink light and add any other intentions you may have. Now apply your oil sparingly to the palms of your hands and breathe in deeply as you envision your intentions fully alive. Rub your oil on your heart and wrists and savor its rich and beautiful aroma.

Jasmine – *Jasminum grandiflorum*

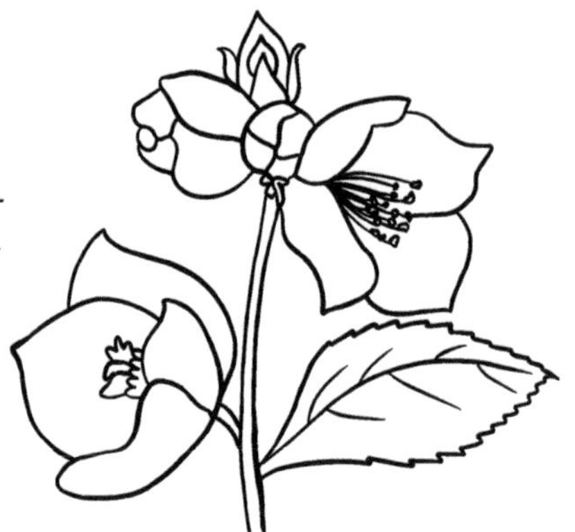

Part Extracted: Flower

Core Properties: Aphrodisiac, analgesic, anti-inflammatory, antibacterial, antiseptic, antispasmodic, anti depressive, relaxing, and stimulating
Safety: nontoxic and nonirritating, not to be used in pregnancy until delivery preparation.
Special Notation: Often adulterated

Adora's Personal Journey

Jasmine awakened my heart in India. From the flower markets to the fields to hair garlands that grace the already graceful women on the land, this aromatic had me at hello. It was in southern India that I truly began to understand and appreciate the magnificently arduous process of seed to "drop."

Like it was yesterday, I recall arriving in the fields in Mysore, joining the women to pick the flowers just as they were opening and place them in baskets, mesmerized by the heady aroma. Every flower must be picked at a particular time to encapsulate the apex of its quintessence and chemical constituents; in this case jasmine sambac only blooms from seven p.m. to two a.m. and must be picked between four and five in the morning.

It is important to note that the plant matter must be distilled within a short period of time, again to ensure the peak quality of the resultant oil. Nearly all jasmine oil on the market is considered an absolute, and is produced via solvent extraction, whereby trace amounts of solvent can be found in the absolute. Jasmine can also be produced via enfleurage where layers are placed surrounding the flower petals until their sweet aroma is infused into the fats, usually a one-to-three-day process.

Jasmine reminds us of the sweetness of life. It has the rare ability to open and align both the heart and the sexual centers, which is crucial for the fullness of sacred relationships to unfold and the true nature of tantra to reveal itself. Jasmine is indicated when there is a sexual disconnection resulting from a fear of intimacy from previous trauma, physical, emotional, or sexual. It engages a renewal in self-trust of opening one's heart, body, and soul to another.

Jasmine invites us to let go of self judgement of body image and deepen our ability to love ourselves no matter what. It helps us to release the grief when a relationship ends and encourages us to find completion and resolution for the growth and integration at the soul level.

Nourish the Heart – Sensual Jasmine Perfume Oil

∞ 1 drop of Jasmine absolute (*Jasminum sambac*)
∞ 1 drop of Jasmine absolute (*Jasminum grandiflorum*)
∞ 1 drop Amber attar (*Pinus succinifera*)
∞ 2 drops of Geranium essential oil (*Pelargonium graveolens*)
∞ 2 drops of Patchouli essential oil (*Pogostemon cablin*)

Blend into 5ml of organic jojoba and infuse with the intention to safely honor and open to your sensual beauty. Apply sparingly to wrists and lower belly and inhale the sweet perfection of this plant spirit medicine.

Essential oil Addition

∞ Gardenia monoi *Gardenia taitensis* (coconut and tiare flower)

HEART NOURISH AROMATHERAPY
DNA BLUEPRINT BENEFITS

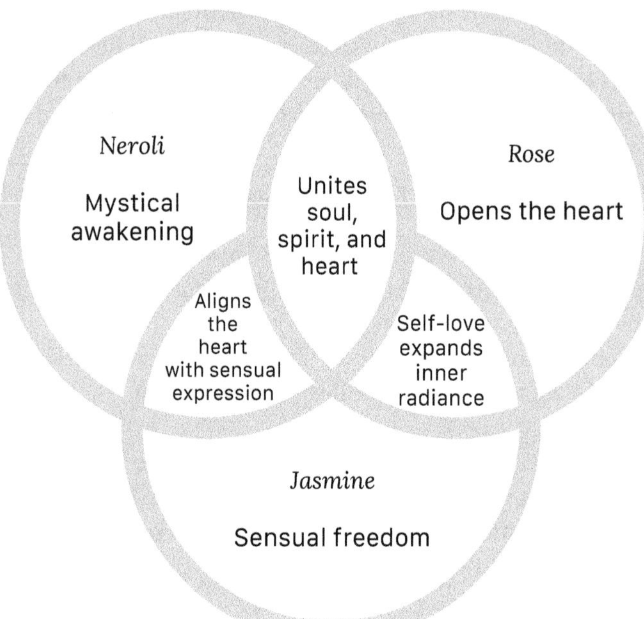

NOURISH THE HEART – BOTANICAL MEDICINE

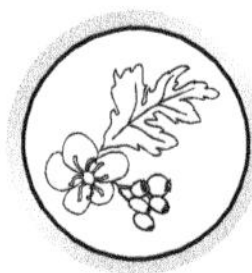

MAJOR ARCHETYPE

HAWTHORN BERRY – *Crataegus monogyna*

Part Used: Flower, leaves and fruit

One of the champion tonic remedies for the whole heart and circulatory system both physically and emotionally. It's used for many cardiac conditions including palpitations, arrhythmia, vascular insufficiency, and varicose veins. Hawthorn strengthens the cardiac muscle after overexertion from an acute or chronic condition aiding the body in recovery. Hawthorn is also an impressive fertility herb and can be used for enhancing conception and aids mothers who have had difficulties in full term pregnancies.

The red berry is high in antioxidants supplying the heart with vitamins A, C, and E, selenium, and zinc, strengthening the cardiac muscle. Hawthorn berries also preserve and nurture glutathione levels in the blood providing stability for the cellular membrane. This supreme antioxidant environment also supports precise DNA replication instead of mutation.

Hawthorn is a great mystical tree written about in books and poems for its healing magic and enchantment.

It has long been revered as an herb for the fourth chakra and emotional heart. It nourishes a grieving heart suffering from heartache and loss nurturing the soul with its sweet berry embrace. It allows you to be open and vulnerable even when it might hurt the most.

Hawthorn also has a great affinity and partnership with other heart system plants so experiment with different herbs in the heart section for your own self-discovery.

Nourish the Heart – Hawthorn Physical Uses

Nourish: Rejuvenates the cardiovascular system and mitochondria
Cardiovascular: Antioxidant, cardiac tonic, hypertension, protects against myocardial damage, peripheral vasodilator, anti-arrhythmic and diuretic
Nervous System: Sedative, stress, nervousness, and anxiety
Musculoskeletal: Collagen stabilization

Nourish the Heart – Hawthorn Emotional Uses

Emotional heartache – opens to forgiveness and trust
Healing of a constricted and wounded heart
Gives you more space to hold your emotions

Nourish the Heart – Hawthorn Energetic Uses

Spiritual heartache or a disconnection from spirit
Opens the heart to forgiveness and healing
Protection: Place above doorways to nurture broken relationships

Nourish the Heart – Hawthorn Dosage

Tincture: 4–6 ml 3x/day
Infusion: 3 teaspoons per 236 ml of water. Drink 1 cup 3x/day

Nourish the Heart – Hawthorn Cautions and Contraindications

None

Nourish the Heart – Hawthorn Freedom to Love Oxymiel

Ingredients:
32 g dried Hawthorn berries – *Crataegus monogyna*
½ scraped vanilla bean
266 ml honey
236 ml vinegar

Directions: See Appendix B on how to make an oxymiel

Dosage: 2 teaspoons per day

MINOR ARCHETYPES

Yarrow – *Achillea millefolium*

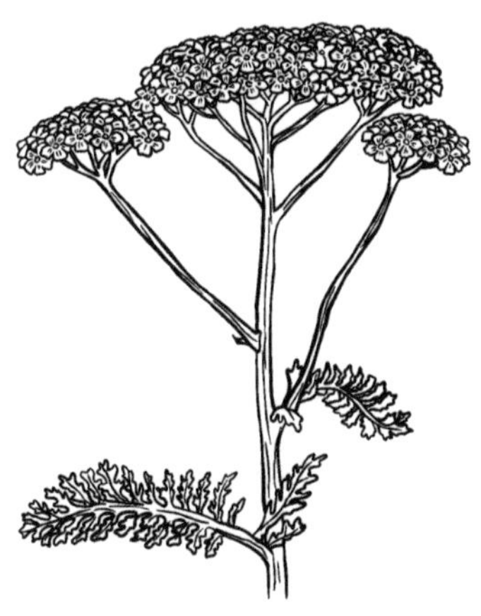

Part Used: Flower

Yarrow is a tiny yet powerful flower bringing life back into the bodily tissues due to the loss of tone or overuse. It nourishes an overworked heart and aids in recovery from acute and chronic cardiac and immune conditions especially those associated with a fever. Yarrow is an impressive antispasmodic and is used for atherosclerosis, chest pain, digestive disorders and premenstrual conditions. It also works as an astringent and hemostatic in a variety of bleeding conditions including wounds, ulcers and postpartum hemorrhage.

Emotionally yarrow is the protector of the psychic realm. It's used for recovery from traumatic and abusive relationships when a cord cutting ceremony is necessary and will assist you in regaining your power. In the similar way that yarrow works physically to stop bleeding, it works emotionally to protect and guard your precious energy and emotions from "energy vampires" sucking your vital life force. It nourishes your personal space and boundary with a white light of protection.

Nourish the Heart – Yarrow Physical Uses

Nourish: Increases speed of recovery from illness and assimilation of nutrients
Cardiovascular: Circulatory stimulant, hypertension, tones the blood vessels and thrombotic conditions
Immune System: Diaphoretic
Digestive: Bitter, stimulates digestion, liver stagnation, hemorrhoid relief
Respiratory System: Upper respiratory Infections
Urinary System: Urinary antiseptic, cystitis
Reproductive System: Relaxes and tonifies the uterus, heavy menstruation, and PMS pain
Integumentary: Wound healer – astringent and hemostatic

Nourish the Heart – Yarrow Emotional Uses

Recovery from emotional abuse
Nourish your personal space and boundaries
Nurtures a long-lasting love – find your soulmate

Nourish the Heart – Yarrow Energetic Uses

Psychic protection – stops energetic leakage
Magic of Intention – manifesting desires

Nourish the Heart – Yarrow Dosage

Infusion: Infuse 1 teaspoon with a cup of water for 10 minutes. Drink 1 cup 3x/day
Tincture: 30 drops 3x/day

Nourish the Heart – Yarrow Cautions

Pregnancy

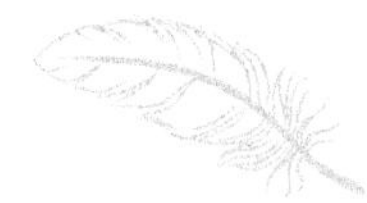

Nourish the Heart – Yarrow Freedom to Flow Compress

Compress for arterial congestion and varicose veins.
Make a concentrated infusion of 32 g of dried yarrow flowers and leaf with 236 ml of hot water.
Let cool and apply to the area of congestion 2–3x/day.

Valerian – *Valeriana officinalis*

Parts Used: Root

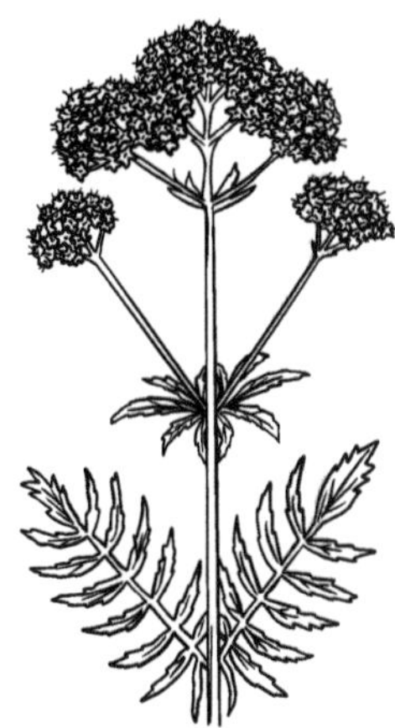

One of the most relaxing nervines available to herbal medicine since the times of the Middle Ages. It can be used safely to reduce tension, anxiety, and overexcitable states. It is an effective aid in insomnia, producing a natural healing sleep. As an antispasmodic it has a muscle relaxing effect on smooth and skeletal muscles, and will aid in the relief of cramping, neuralgias, and intestinal colic. As a pain reliever it is most indicated where that pain is associated with tension, such as in migraines. It carries no risk of dependency and does not affect mental concentration.

Valerian is most helpful for heart conditions caused by stress and anxiety. It reduces the excited state of the sympathetic nervous system and allows the parasympathetic nervous system to take control. It is most helpful for the person who is in the mode of "go, go, go" and never turns off. Can't sleep, can't focus, can't relax - the whole body is tensed and revved up.

Nourish the Heart – Valerian Physical Uses

Nourish: Clears stagnant energy from the cellular matrix
Cardiovascular System: Hypertension, tremors, palpitations, angina, and vascular insufficiency and edema
Nervous System: Anxiety, stress, depression, and insomnia
Adrenal System: Nourishes exhaustion with restful sleep
Musculoskeletal System: Muscle spasms, pain, and headache
Digestive: Abdominal spasms and colic
Reproductive: Menstrual cramps

Nourish the Heart – Valerian Emotional Uses

Grief and loss of a loved one
Irritability– anger over the loss of love
Hysteria of lost love and in argumentative states

Nourish the Heart – Valerian Energetic Uses

Connecting to the dream world and spirit guides
Aphrodisiac opening the fourth and second light wheels
Opens the fourth and sixth light wheels connecting heart to source

Nourish the Heart – Valerian Dosage

Infusion: 1–2 teaspoons per 236 ml of water. Drink 1 cup 3x/day
Tincture: 3–5 ml 2–4x/day

Nourish the Heart – Valerian Cautions and Contraindications

Caution when using with other sedatives

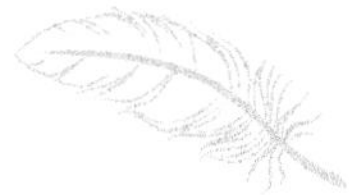

Nourish the Heart – Valerian Freedom to Unwind Tonic

For chronic anxiety and heart palpitations.
Take 5 drops of valerian and 5 drops of hawthorn tincture in water every hour until symptoms resolve.
If symptoms last for more than 2 weeks consult with your physician.

BOTANICAL ADDITIONS

- ∞ Vaccinium – *Vaccinium myrtillus*
- ∞ Milky Oats – *Avena sativa*
- ∞ Coriander – *Coriandrum sativum*
- ∞ Damiana – *Turnera diffusa*

HEART NOURISH BOTANICAL MEDICINE DNA BLUEPRINT BENEFITS

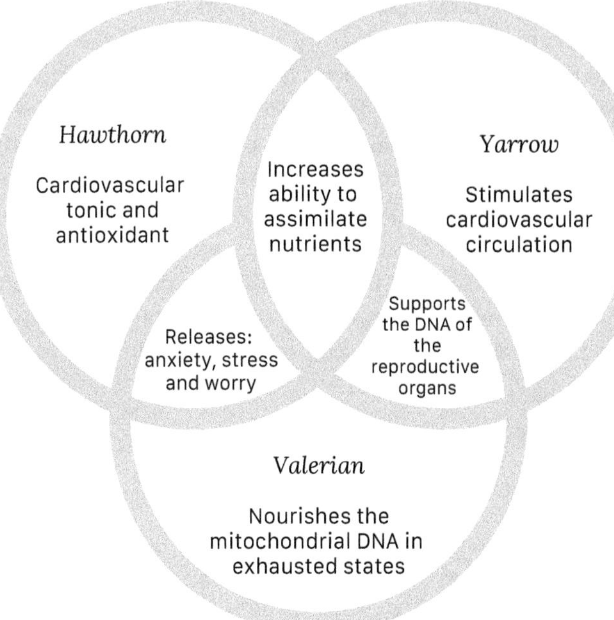

NOURISH THE HEART – LIGHT WHEELS

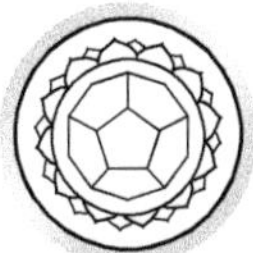

As previously mentioned, some of the light wheels or chakras may seem new to you. The power of your intention is one of the most potent alchemical interventions you have at your disposal. You can simply invite in this light wheel to connect, open, expand, and balance for your highest good. Along with this invitation, breathing in the color associated with it amplifies the alchemy.

MAJOR ARCHETYPE

THE 44th LIGHT WHEEL, BHAVAPRIYA

Bhavapriya is the opening to the fifth dimension and activates the psychic abilities and psychic language of the heart. This light wheel connects to the greater heart of humanity and helps heal the planet.

This light wheel clears this present lifetime of sexual trauma and nurtures a broken heart. It opens the heart to increased happiness and a positive outlook on life. You might think of this light wheel as the "high vibe or feel good" chakra.

Physically, Bhavapriya nourishes the cardiomyocytes with a magnificent level of vibration. Each cell radiates with the energy of the solar system and the stars, clearing the cells from any negative energy or toxicity and allowing complete absorption of nutrients and positive energy into the nucleus and DNA of the cell.

MINOR ARCHETYPES

∞ The 122nd light wheel, Shishupala

Shishupala opens your psychic powers and abilities to channel, clairvoyance, etc. It is also associated with time and astral travel allowing you to travel between realms.

COLORS

MAJOR ARCHETYPE

SALMON

Salmon is the color of nature and embodies a deeper connection to nature. This color signifies a time to nurture your relationships with family members and loved ones clearing any unresolved hurt or grief. It's easy to bury feelings of hurt when it comes to family but now is not the time to play nice: stir up the drama. Embrace the drama llama. Salmon will help you to be more approachable allowing those around you to communicate their truest needs.

How many Buddhist monks does it take to change a light bulb? Just one. But it is a long process where the monk keeps telling the bulb that change must first come from within, until the bulb attains enlightenment!

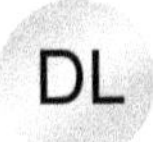

Yes, I do have a corny sense of humor, but we knew you probably needed a good laugh about now.

SOUND

Ehm

Ehm is the note of G sounding like "harm" in the back of the throat. Use this sound frequency and vibratory bija, or jewel, to invoke the fifth light wheel and create a blanket of peace around your body. After practicing this for five or ten minutes your nervous system will be settled and aligned.

NOURISH THE HEART – CRYSTALS AND STONES

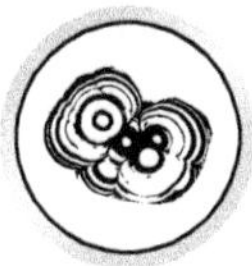

MAJOR ARCHETYPE

MALACHITE

Malachite creates alignment with every cell, wave-like motions of healing gently help to release blockages in the physical and emotional body. Malachite is a crystal of protection and envelops the heart in a shield of salmon colored light as the heart is breaking through any limitations of carrying out your deepest dreams and desires. Malachite overcomes the victimization philosophy that ties us down from moving forward in life and expanding the heart. It's so easy to get stuck in the tape loop of "Woe is me," "Why, did this happen to me?" Malachite is here for you to break free.

Physically malachite encourages clear communication with the third and fourth light wheels and can be very helpful for food disorders or addictions that are often stimulated by heartbreak or grief. It opens cellular communications, and the sodium potassium gateways, allowing for nourishing microminerals and electrolytes to go in and out of the cell. After a heart injury, like a stroke, malachite will help restore strength and vitality to the cells and the DNA. Malachite also assists with copper deficiencies by revitalizing absorption and assimilation of copper when worn around the wrists and fingers.

MINOR ARCHETYPES

∞ Rose Quartz

Rose quartz connects to the emotional body and releases suppressed emotions, in wave patterns, slowly lightening up the heart center. It helps nourish and soften emotions in a very soothing and loving way, gently. Rose quartz is also a very powerful crystal and can be used to softly bring to the surface emotions that have long been buried because they are too painful to discuss or relate to. Repressed emotions cause disease and rose quartz frees the body from this attachment.

Rose quartz is also crucial when experiencing times of stress. Stress immeasurably impacts the function of the heart and cardiovascular system. This stone soothes the emotional body, wrapping you in a loving embrace and facilitating the movement of connection to your higher self.

∞ Peridot

Peridot warms and nourishes the heart like beaming wildflowers in a meadow full of sun. This crystal acts like a beacon directly into the heart center, turning up the volume of your deepest desires. It also encourages the release of past regrets, and waters the seeds of self-encouragement and desires. Peridot removes all blockages to receiving love, not only self-love but love from those around us nourishing and cherishing the child within.

Peridot helps strengthen any heart and blood related illnesses. It increases the release of red blood cells from the spleen, increases hemoglobin, and increases oxygen in the body.

CRYSTAL ADDITIONS

∞ Rhodochrosite
∞ Watermelon Tourmaline

NOURISH THE HEART CRYSTAL GRID

Pick an area of the body where you feel stagnant or blocked energy. This is the area of where you will focus on sending nourishing healing. Lie down on your back on the floor. Place a salmon colored cloth over your entire body on top of the stone grid. Relax for 30-60 minutes. By lying in the full moon for this healing session you will receive the most benefits. Drink a glass of malachite charged water after this attunement. Immediately after the treatment cleanse the crystals and stones.
(See Appendix C)

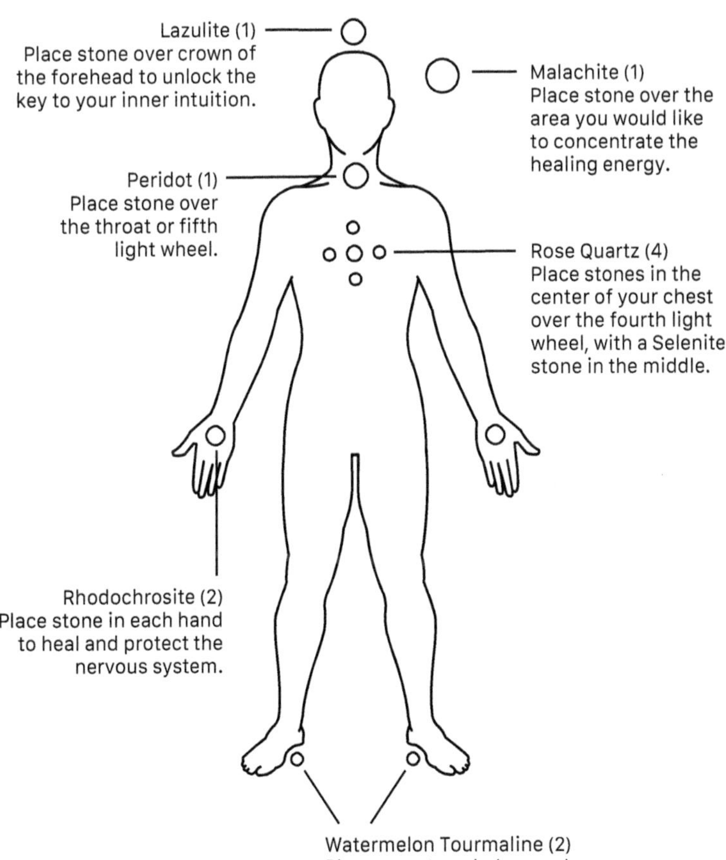

NOURISH THE HEART – ENERGETIC AND VIBRATIONAL TECHNIQUES

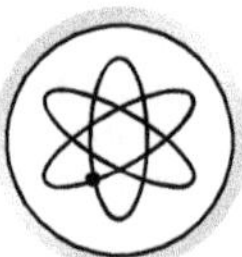

MAJOR ARCHETYPE

HEART NOURISH HYDROTHERAPY

- ∞ 118 ml Rose floral water or hydrosol
- ∞ 118 ml Neroli hydrosol
- ∞ 59 ml Gardenia monoi
- ∞ 2 drops of Jasmine absolute (Jasminum grandiflorum)

Luxuriate in a warm water bath for at least 20 minutes and enjoy the beautiful sense of nourishment from your skin through to your soul.

MINOR ARCHETYPES

Nourish the Heart EOBT

Place one drop of neroli essential oil between the first two fingertips of the right hand, inhale deeply and tap meridian point Pericardium-8 (P8), Palace of Weariness for 30 seconds with the intention of filling your heart and all cells in your body with unconditional love.

Location: In the deepest part of the well of the palm when the hand is gently cupped.

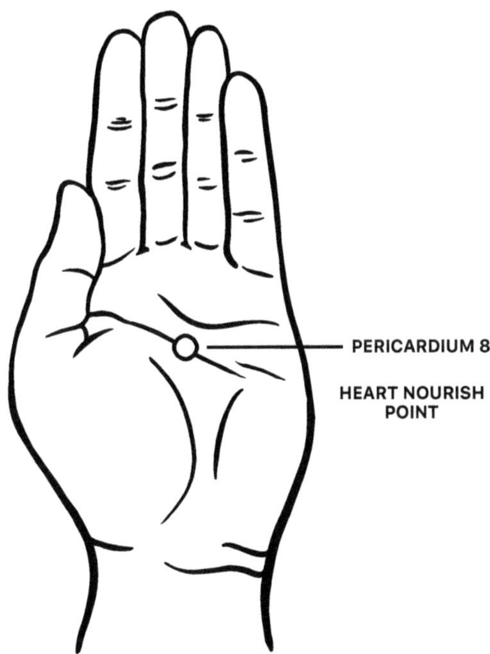

Nourish the Heart Water Ceremony

This form of vibrational alchemy imprints the vibration, life force, and specific healing energy of the crystal into one of the most nourishing and restorative elements, water. Taken on an empty stomach in the morning, it allows for a rapid cellular response and often a tangible feeling of shift of emotional energy and awareness.

Take your cleansed and programmed crystal and add it to a glass or pitcher of fresh clean water. Wrap your hand around the vessel and align your intention to infuse water molecules with the consciousness of love, gratitude, and the desire to lovingly nourish your heart and being on every level.

To enhance the alchemy of the intervention, infuse with a salmon-colored light. After 20 minutes, remove the crystal, thank it for sharing its vibration and drink the water as desired. Note: Remember to strain the crystal prior to drinking and enjoy with the intention of allowing the spectrum of vibration to permeate and heal at the cellular level. Needed:

- ∞ 1 piece of Malachite
- ∞ 1 vessel of water

Infuse as instructed above and drink throughout the day. Refrigerate unused portions for later use.

NOURISH THE HEART – FLOWER AND GEM ESSENCES

FLOWER ESSENCES

MAJOR ARCHETYPE

PINK LOTUS

AW Pink lotus is a flower of awakening. I encountered the potent alchemy of the lotus on my first aromatic journey to India some twenty years ago. Our gracious hosts paddled out into a smallish body of water at dawn to pick the pink, blue and white lotus flowers just before they began to open and greet the day. I can still vividly recall the sweet, otherworldly aroma and the sensation of the subtle movements of the pink lotus as it opened in my hands. It was expansive and transportive, awakening and opening my heart in new ways. This lotus reminds us of the beauty of our sacred human heart and how the Divine is expressed everywhere around us. This flower essence assists in opening the crown and pineal glands in conjunction with the heart. Past life influences stored in the cells are opened and rise to the surface for clearing. This essence vibrates the resonance of divine love and joy and assists in allowing the heart to receive love with greater trust and innocence.

MINOR ARCHETYPES

Peony

Peony reminds us of the sweetness and beauty of life. It activates the purity and innocence in the emotional and astral bodies and awakens the same within our cellular consciousness. This essence stirs the playful nature of the child within, reminding us to view the challenges of life with an open and light heart.

Bleeding Heart

Bleeding heart balances the heart center and assists in stabilizing the emotions of grief and despondency relating to loss of loved ones. It nourishes the parts of our heart that hold conflict with another by bringing compassionate release to relationships that are no longer congruent with our authentic self. This essence activates the thymus gland and expands the soul seat light wheel above the heart to access the longings of the soul for the current incarnation.

FLOWER ESSENCE ADDITIONS

- ∞ California poppy
- ∞ Peach

GEM ESSENCES

MAJOR ARCHETYPE

BLUE TOPAZ

Blue topaz assists you to open to the frequency of clairaudience (being able to hear on an intuitive level). It elicits a sense of unconditional love, of safety, joyfulness, and youthful energy regardless of age. This essence invigorates our youthful nature and is excellent as an antiaging remedy. This essence rejuvenates the etheric level of the auric field and invigorates the emotional and physical body. Blue topaz opens your spiritual connection and is a wonderful essence to use in meditation to deepen your practice. Alleviating tensions connected to the heart; this essence helps you to open yourself to intimate connection with another.

NOURISH THE HEART – INTENTIONS

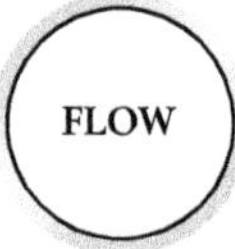

MAJOR ARCHETYPE

FLOW

MINOR ARCHETYPES

- ∞ I am loved, I am love, I am loving
- ∞ I trust in my ability to lead with my heart
- ∞ In my sacred human heart, I give and receive my love

ADDITIONAL INTENTIONS

- ∞ I invite and allow harmonious relationships into my life
- ∞ I am one with all humanity
- ∞ I live in peace
- ∞ I love myself when I hate myself and cause my own suffering

NOURISH THE HEART – MEDITATION MUDRA

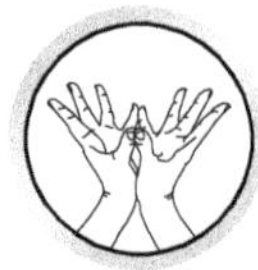

Padma Mudra

Flowing on the river of bliss,
my heart opens to the nourishing waves of love and compassion.

The Padma mudra is a symbolic gesture of the lotus flower and nourishes the heart center and heals all aspects or areas you may feel are "shattered or fragmented", limiting your ability to fully love. This mudra also opens the connection between the lower chakras of the physical body and Earth to the upper physical and atmospheric chakras. This mudra allows an endless healing of memories and trauma letting them surface and flow out easily from the conscious and subconscious thought field. This beautiful flower mudra opens the heart, granting access to emotional healing with an awakened feeling of self-compassion and acceptance.

Padma Mudra Alignment

1. Place your hands in front of your heart center and face the palms together with the fingertips pointing upward.
2. While keeping the bottom of the hands, pinkies, and thumbs together, open and unfold your hands like a blossoming lotus flower.
3. Take a deep breath, let your body relax.
4. You may now either do the meditation below or 10 minutes of *Wave Breathing* (to access the wave breathing please go to www.zenergy-medicinals.com).
5. You may also use this mudra at any time you are feeling you are out of alignment with your heart, passion, and sense of purpose. This mudra also sustains cardiovascular health and stimulates the thymus gland and can be used alternating with the thymus tapping to strengthen immune response.

∞ To access the heart mudra meditation please go to www.zenergy medicinals.com

∞ Take a deep breath in, inhaling the sweet aroma of your essential oil, inviting the aromatic molecules to come into your cellular consciousness.
∞ Form the Padma mudra with your hands and take several breaths to open and align to the flow of love. Feel the openness created with the lotus flower as this feeling permeates every cell of your body. Visualize you are lying in the middle of a lightly flowing river and this water cleanses your body releasing any stagnant energy as you feel lighter with each breath.
∞ Take another deep breath in, envisioning an emerald, green light, a sphere of light right in front of your heart. A golden light begins to swirl with it. Golden emerald light encircling you.
∞ A pathway appears in front of you. As you see yourself, place the first step upon this soft green mossy pathway. You experience a gentle warm

and sweet breeze, fragranced gently with aromas of pine, earth, and moss. And each step that you place forward, you feel yourself sinking a little bit more deeply into the safety and protection of Mother Earth.

- ∞ A light appears from a clearing within the woods. The light of the sun emanating to the very center … surrounded by tall trees … oak, pine, creating a sense of solidness, protection, safety, and nurturing.
- ∞ In the very center of the circle, you see where the light is beaming clearly down upon a bench. Move forward and take a seat on this bench that fits perfectly to your body.
- ∞ You begin to relax and let go of all the fear, the anxiety, the uncertainty. All of that which is unclear, letting go in this moment. Feeling your body, your being, being filled with this golden light, your attention comes back to your heart, where that golden emerald light is still pulsating.
- ∞ Breathe in deeply to this space, into the very center of your heart. Freeing yourself from everything that feels limited, limiting, constrictive. Feeling a tremendous resounding sense of being safe, protected, connected, clear, open.
- ∞ With each breath, feel the loving embrace of the emerald light. Repeat the intention three times either silently or aloud: "Flowing on the river of bliss, my heart opens to the nourishing waves of love and compassion."
- ∞ Open to the greater truths of your being. You can get up from the bench and walk back towards the opening in the wood, back down the path, feeling lighter, revitalized, clear.

NOURISH THE HEART – SACRED GEOMETRY

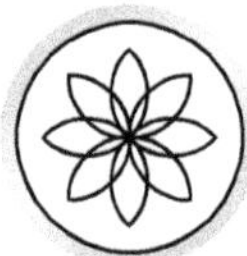

MAJOR ARCHETYPE

NOURISH THE HEART SACRED GEOMETRY

Our intentional and original depiction of Nourish the Heart sacred geometry depicts an eight petaled flower. The number eight is also associated with the infinity symbol and the limitless healing capacity of love. This form of sacred geometry vibrates the energy of wholeness, uniting fragmented aspects of the heart and soul back into cohesion.

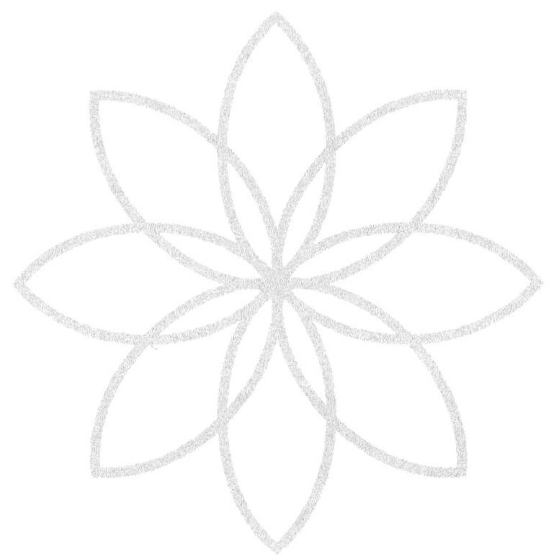

NOURISH THE HEART – NUTRITION

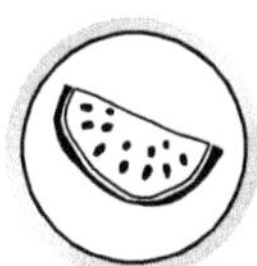

MAJOR ARCHETYPE

WATERMELON

Ahhh, watermelon, just thinking about the sweetness of this fruit makes your mouth water, and there's a reason. It's made up of 92 percent water and is one of the most hydrating fruits. It also is rich in lycopene, which lowers blood pressure, reduces the thickness of the arterial walls, and decreases cholesterol. It also contains the amino acid citrulline which increases nitric oxide levels in the body, helping to generate and repair DNA that has been damaged by free radicals. It also contains vitamins A, B6, and C, magnesium, and potassium, promoting a healthy functioning heart (Massa et al., 2016).

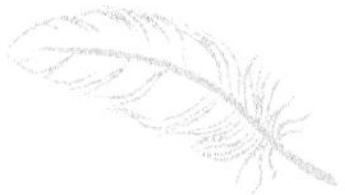

Try juicing watermelon, adding a pinch of sea salt, chili pepper, and some fresh lime juice, and serve over ice for a refreshing summer cooler.

MINOR ARCHETYPES

Strawberries

Strawberries contain many plant compounds for supporting the heart. Ellagic acid is a polyphenol antioxidant removing toxins from the intercellular fluid and protecting the DNA from free radical damage. They also contain procyanidins, another form of antioxidants, that protect the heart by blocking nitrosamines from forming (Basu, Rhone, & Lyons, 2010).

Dark Chocolate

Dark chocolate is not only delicious but rich in flavanols, reducing blood pressure, insulin sensitivity, and cholesterol. It's also packed with two under-consumed minerals, iron and magnesium, both important for cardiac function and red blood cell production. And, yes, we are saying to eat more dark chocolate – yippee! (Rull et al., 2015).

NUTRITIONAL ADDITIONS

- ∞ Cacao
- ∞ Lobster
- ∞ Dates
- ∞ Cranberry
- ∞ Adzuki bean
- ∞ Liver
- ∞ Quince
- ∞ Vanilla bean

NOURISH THE HEART – DISCOVERY DIVE – HEALING A BROKEN HEART

As sensitive as our sacred human heart can be, it is also incredibly resilient. When our hearts are open, we can feel the joy of life and the depths of love and connection that simply is not possible when our hearts are closed. We are born open, free, pure, and innocent. Life imprints our experience upon us in a myriad of ways.

Our early childhood family dynamics model our first experiences of love and what it means to connect with our hearts to another. We then spend our lives furthering this dance back and forth with an open and closed heart and then witness how it affects our future interrelational dynamics. We pay a heavy price by operating from a broken, closed heart, and not just with our relationships. Every decision we make in how we care for ourselves and others, every choice in business or career dealings and, as importantly if not more so, how we view the world and greater universe around us from a point of expectation. Belief system and expectation run hand in hand. Expectation filters our perception of reality and when this comes from a place of brokenness, we can prove again and again how painful life is.

Are you ready to craft a new story of creation in your life? To heal the deep places of dysfunction, loss, and struggle and set yourself free to experience the fullness and beauty of what it means to meet yourself first and then another with a pure, open, and innocent heart of your youth? Even if you are not 100 percent all in yet, dive into this self-discovery to clear the pathway.

What was the first major loss you experienced in your life? Was it a person, a relative? A pet? What were the circumstances?

What was the greatest "gift" or "teaching" you received from this being or circumstance?

How and where in your body do you feel that loss today? Take a moment to close your eyes, take a deep breath and feel where this emotion is in your body.

When did you experience heartache for the first time? In your family? In a relationship? Have you ever felt enslaved or abused, and if so, how? Do you still feel this emotion in your heart and chest?

Are you ready and willing to receive love NOW? What would this new relationship look like? Describe this new relationship in as much detail as you can. Dream your heart's biggest desire!

NOURISH THE HEART – DISCOVERY DIVE – CULTIVATING A PRACTICE OF GRATITUDE

Cultivating a consistent practice of gratitude is powerful. It offers us greater openness, joy, resilience, and the ability to create new, healthy neural pathways. Creating your gratitude practice before bed allows you to focus on positive experiences from the day to weave a heart centered, peaceful sleep journey into the higher dimensions when resting.

We have outlined a few different areas of life and encourage you to create your own system and style, naming at least three items, simple or otherwise for each.

In my body (health), I AM grateful for:

In my home, I AM grateful for:

In my work, I AM grateful for:

In my primary relationship, I AM grateful for:

In my family, I AM grateful for:

In my work relationships, I AM grateful for:

In my community, I AM grateful for:

FREEDOM PHOTON WHEEL™

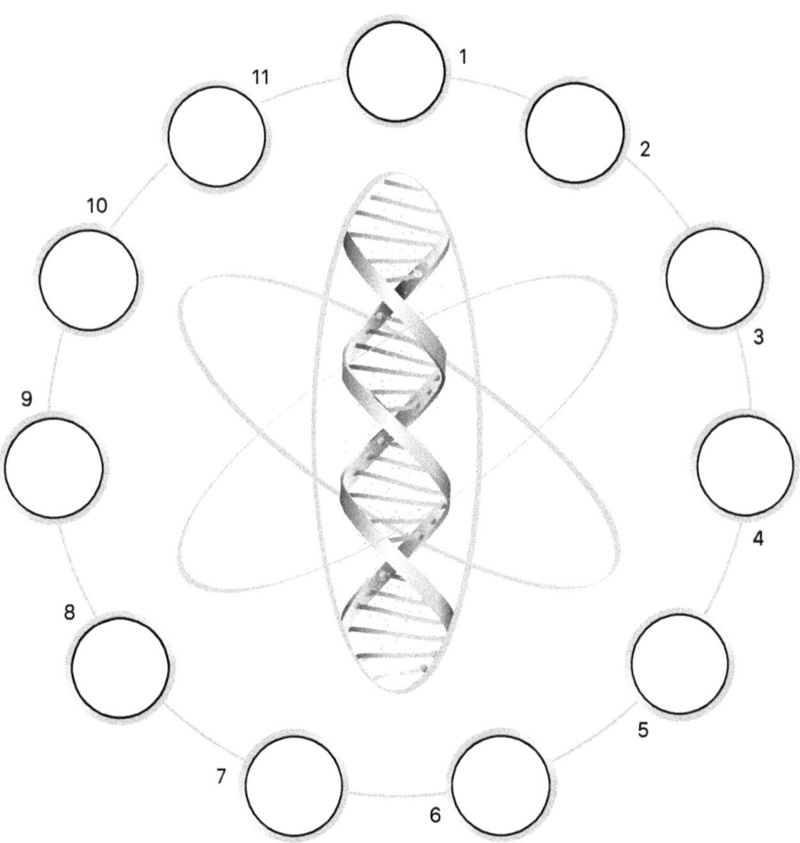

NOURISH THE HEART
YOUR PERSONAL FREEDOM PHOTON WHEEL RITUAL

Moon Phase

Perform your ritual during any moon cycle.

Intention

"I give and receive my love. My love nourishes every part of my being down to the DNA level and through my genetic lineage."

Select, Align, and Activate

Select your interventions according to the instructions in Chapter Five. Inhale and apply your chosen essential oil for 30–45 seconds. Use your botanical tincture or tea as directed. You may also listen to the meditation and use the mudra from this chapter while attuning your FPW.

Affirm

"Divine consciousness assists me in allowing the vibration of unconditional love to permeate my cells, particles, and all structures of my body, physical and nonphysical and all that I have carried through my lineage, my mother and father bloodline. I am anointed with the fullest experience of giving and receiving love."

ACTIVATE THE HEART

Once we have gone through the layers of letting go and cultivating a loving place, we are ready to live from and lead with our hearts. Unifying Heaven above and Earth below, our hearts are open and ready to activate and evolve into portals of creation. Holding the concentric point of the center of the infinity symbol, we activate the heart on every level down to the DNA to access the zero-point field, the dimension of limitless potential. It is from here that we begin to see and experience what is possible when we let go of the past and assimilate the wisdom for our future.

Activating the heart allows us to shift from a linear, mentally focused, and limited dimensional reality to come into a new center of being. We can source new levels of balance, connection, and expansion in nature and be lit by the vibration of love. From the perspective of your superhero self, think of it as activating a brand-new GPS system: this is the full-on high-tech version. In addition to guiding your course via your own true north, it also discerns what relationships, career choices, manners of authentic communion, communication, and intimacy serve your highest good. That is the beauty of living and leading with a heart fully open and activated.

Physically activating the heart is about flow. Turning on or igniting the fiery engine within. ALL SYSTEMS ON! When the heart is physiologically functioning smoothly you can feel this surge running through your body. Yes, this is subtle, but as you learn to listen more attentively with your inner source or spirit you will begin to feel the shift of the heart activation. We like to think of it like the lava flowing under the Earth's crust. Moving through all the nooks and crannies. Igniting your DNA and cells with a fire of passion and love.

HEART ACTIVATE FREEDOM PHOTON WHEEL

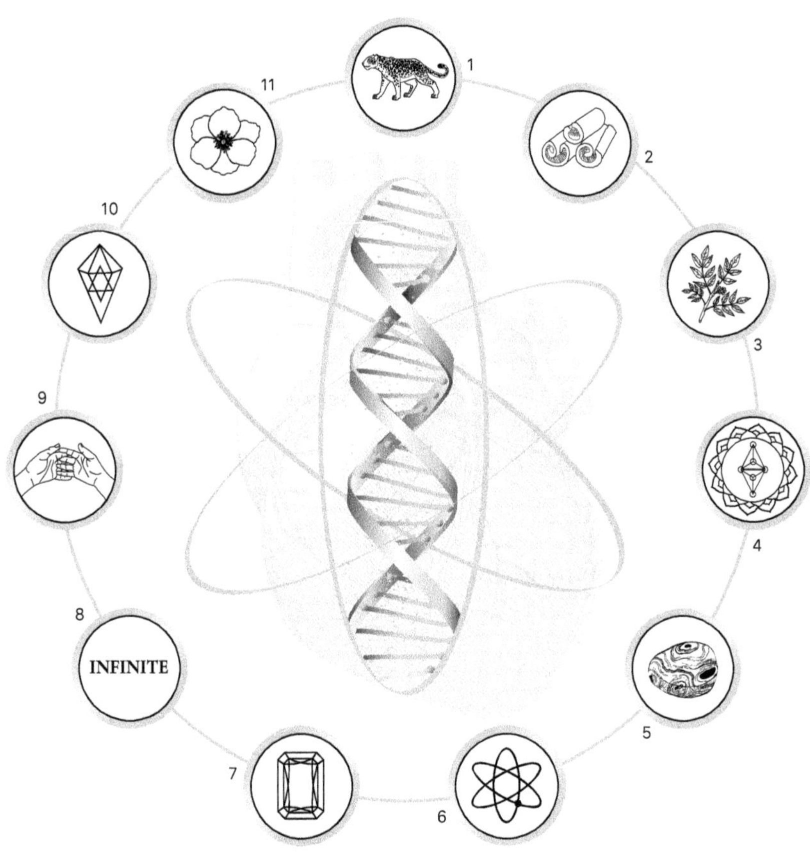

1 Alchemy Animal: Leopard
2 Aromatherapy: Cinnamon
3 Botanical: Prickly Ash
4 Light Wheel: Hridaya-agni
5 Crystal: Alantisite
6 Photon Vibration
7 Flower or Gem Essence: Emerald
8 Intention: Infinite
9 Meditation Mudra: Ushas
10 Sacred Geometry
11 Nutrition: Rosehip

HEART ACTIVATE
INFINITY INFLUENCERS

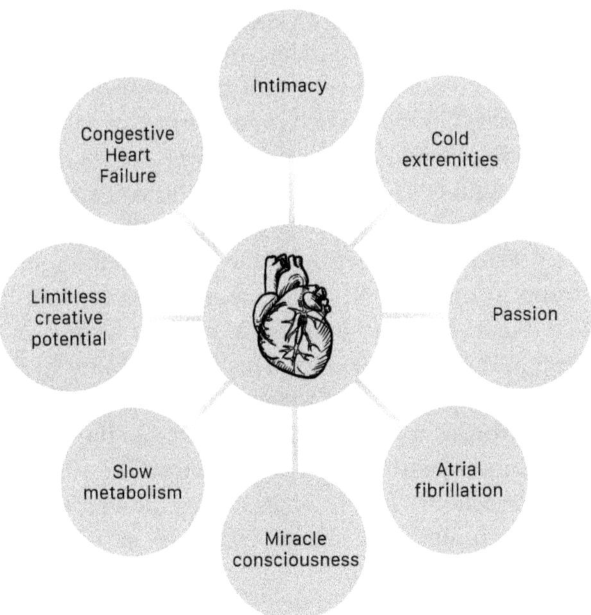

ACTIVATE THE HEART – ALCHEMY ANIMALS

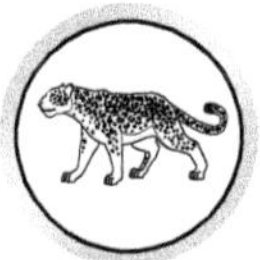

The activate alchemy animals of the heart embrace the fire element and light the flame of our limitless love within. As you will see these animals are fierce, in the most loving way, and their magic and power is infinite. You may connect or attune to this power when you want to embody clarity, radiance, metamorphosis, and fire.

MAJOR ARCHETYPE

LEOPARD

The leopard is often connected to a vision quest where you are searching deep within for your own power. The leopard encourages you to search and ask within, "What is the source of my power and how can I tap into its limitlessness?" Often when on a journey of self-discovery and testing the boundless waters of our power we can rock the boat of those around us. You might be challenged about who you are becoming. Stay strong, dear leopards, for your power is your truth.

The leopard teaches us to rekindle the power within our hearts and to stand strong in our beliefs and seize all opportunities to embrace this renewed vigor. Imagine you are a leopard hiding in the grass, poised to leap and seize your prey. This is the vitality of the leopard. Fierce, powerful, playful, and at times a little sneaky but always with the mindset of "This is my truth." This is not from the ego. This power comes from the inner heart saying, "I deserve it."

Creature Connection: "I fully embrace my power. I believe in me. I seize all opportunities of self-growth and expansion with love and light."

MINOR ARCHETYPES

Phoenix

The magnificent phoenix is a mythical and magical alchemy animal symbolizing transformation through death and rebirth by flame. This strength or flame within the phoenix never dies and connects us to aspects of longevity and the hidden wisdom of knowing what is always best.

When you are drawn to this sun guardian, hold on because you are going to need the strength for what lies ahead. All aspects of your life that are no longer serving your true purpose will be released. You will burn them in the sacred flame. We even suggest a fire ceremony. Write down all things in your life not inspiring you or holding you back, light a fire, and toss them in. Watch those old beliefs burn up in flames.

Creature Connection: "I release all belief systems holding me back from my truest desires. I rise from the ashes on the wings of the phoenix renewed and transformed."

Scorpion

The scorpion is an alchemy animal of isolation and intense passion. When you are drawn to this archetype, it's time to take a day or even a few days of alone time. When was the last time you had time with just you and only you? Book a weekend retreat and rediscover who you are.

The scorpion also symbolizes the need for passion, sex, and some much-needed loving. Let's get real here. When was the last time you had an orgasm or pleasured yourself? Make a date in your calendar, right now, for some sex. We are not talking about a regular quickie with your sweetie but a full-on night of passion. Let loose and embrace your inner scorpion – dominate the bedroom tonight. We approve!

Creature Connection: "I fulfill all my sexual desires and arousals. I am magnetic. I am charismatic. I drink the love potion of life and rediscover me."

ANIMAL ADDITIONS

∞ Hummingbird
∞ Seal
∞ Fire ant
∞ Ladybug

ACTIVATE THE HEART – AROMATHERAPY

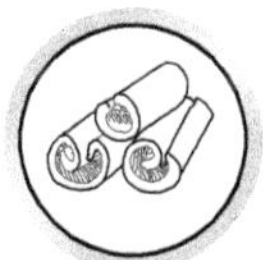

MAJOR ARCHETYPE

CINNAMON – *Cinnamomum cassia*

Part Extracted: Bark or leaves

Core Properties: antioxidant, antimicrobial, antifungal, antidiabetic, antiseptic, antiviral
Safety: Skin and mucous membrane irritant, dilute prior to use

Warming and stimulating aromatically, the medicine of cinnamon brings strength to the heart, the will, and the emotions. Ruled by the sun and the element of fire, cinnamon assists in restoring vital life force, and passion for life and love. It is a renowned aphrodisiac and awakens or reinvigorates sexual fire between two people. It breathes spirit back into the body, the mind, and the soul.

Cinnamon is an oil of encouragement, reminding us that it is possible to bounce back from illness, loss, heartbreak, and soul ache to source that deep reservoir of resilience that is intrinsic to human nature. This oil is indicated to dissolve an inability to move forward, lift, and expand out of the depths of darkness and any places where a sense of weakness presents itself in the nooks and crannies of the shadow self.

Ancient civilizations revered, traded, and relied on cinnamon for the potent medicinal effect of preventing infections and limiting the contagious nature of disease. Cinnamon was so highly revered that it was coveted during the time of the Black Death in Europe in the mid 1300s. The highly antiseptic nature of cinnamon indicates use for colds and flus, particularly with a strong antiviral action; this oil should be a staple in every medicine chest, particularly as the planet continues to shift and different bacterial and viral strains challenge humanity.

Special Notation: Cinnamon is produced from the leaf as well as the bark of the plant. The oil from the bark has a high rate of dermal toxicity and should not be used on the skin. Cinnamon leaf should be used at dilution rates well under 1 percent.

Activate the Heart – Cinnamon Boudoir Mist to Invigorate Passion

∞ 3 drops of Cinnamon essential oil (*Cinnamomum cassia*)
∞ 1 drop Clove essential oil (*Syzygium aromaticum*)
∞ 2 drops Ginger essential oil (*Zingiber officinale)*
∞ 2 drops Ylang Ylang essential oil (*Cananga odorata superior extra*)
∞ 5 drops Patchouli essential oil (*Pogostemon cablin*)
∞ 8 drops Geranium essential oil (*Pelargonium graveolens*)
∞ 1 drop Rose absolute (*Rosa damascena*)

Blend into a 60 ml bottle of distilled water and shake well. Infuse with your intention to ignite passion. Mist bedroom and linens as desired. Not for direct use on skin.

MINOR ARCHETYPES

Hyssop – *Hyssop officinalis*

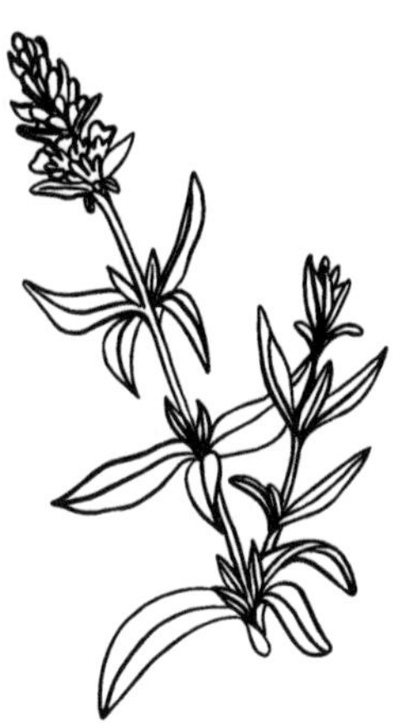

Part Extracted: Flowering tops

Core Properties: antibacterial, anticatarrhal, antifungal, anti-infectious, antirheumatic, antiviral, decongestant, expectorant, febrifuge, immune tonic, insect repellent, rubefacient
Safety: Due to the high ketone content in hyssop, those with high blood pressure, or who are epileptic or pregnant or breastfeeding should avoid it. Use sparingly at low dilution rates under a standard therapeutic dilution of 2.5 percent.

AW I was first introduced to hyssop in the form of a medicinal herb. As a child I had experienced chronic bronchitis as a result of allergies. Every year, in spring and fall, I would have such a severe bout of bronchitis that I would be in bed, sick for a week. After leaving home at nineteen and settling in Cape Cod, MA I found myself sick, without health insurance, and with very little money in the bank. Somewhere I heard the mention of herbal medicine. I went out, purchased a book and five herbs and went home and made a medicinal tea. I was amazed by how quickly I healed and without the use of harsh pharmaceuticals that I had been prescribed in the past. Since then, I have not experienced bronchitis. From that moment on, I made teas, tinctures, and other remedies for all my friends and family to heal by. Not long after, I found essential oils and I knew they would be my lifelong passion.

Hyssop essential oil brings expansion to the heart energetically, increasing emotional intelligence regarding relationships. The sweetly herbaceous aroma connotes ancient roots. There is a potent virility that comes through the aromatic molecules and this oil assists in restoring vital life force and the innate healing force within each of us. Where there is cold in the body or emotions, hyssop warms and strengthens, including the spirit and our individual will. This biblical oil was often called upon for purification and protection and referred to by its Hebrew name "holy herb." It can guide us to find the holy temple within our hearts where we connect with our own divine light and then from there, we can invite another to enter this sacred space. It helps to purify our emotions, especially those surrounding the heart, and strengthen our ability to discern the truth and to protect from unhealthy and unsupportive people and relationships that do not nurture and honor our true nature.

Hyssop also activates the third eye with focus and insight and helps to realign the hara line, the line of effortless intention, with solid strength and clarity. This oil is also indicated for colds, respiratory complaints, immune support, and to balance circulation.

Activate the Heart – Hyssop Bronchial Herbal Tea

- ∞ 1 part Hyssop – *Hyssopus officinalis*
- ∞ 1 part Thyme – *Thymus vulgaris*
- ∞ ½ part Licorice root – *Glycyrrhiza glabra*
- ∞ 1 part Eucalyptus leaf – *Eucalyptus globulus*
- ∞ 3 large slices fresh Ginger root – *Zingiber officinale*

Add ginger to 473 ml of water. Bring to a boil, then add loose herbs, stir, and turn off heat. Steep for 10 minutes and strain. Sweeten as desired and drink two cups a day for three days. If pregnant, asthmatic, or you have high blood pressure, consult your healthcare practitioner before use.

Ylang Ylang – *Cananga odorata*

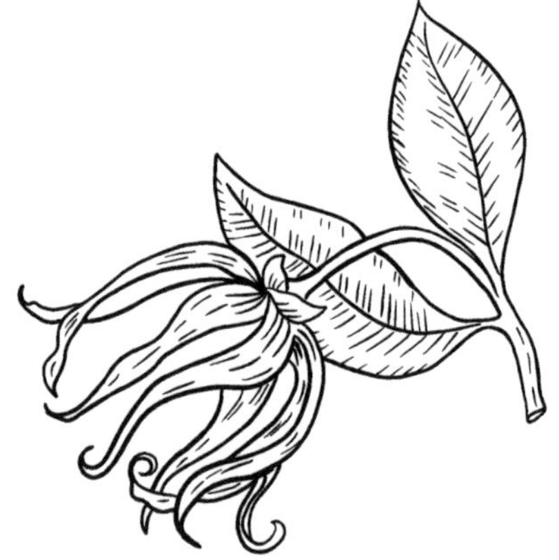

Part Extracted: Flower

Core Properties: antiseptic, antibacterial, antidepressant, anti-inflammatory, antiparasitic, aphrodisiac, hypotensive
Safety: nontoxic, nonirritant

Known as the Queen of Flowers, ylang ylang is one of the most potent aromatics for emotional release. Through inhalation, it has an immediate action of engaging the heart. The deeply penetrating aroma is rich, sweet, and heady.

Hypnotically captivating, ylang ylang permeates the heart, accesses the very center, and expands outward creating ripple effects of openness and desire for true connection.

Ylang ylang, through its aromatic alchemy, brings the light of healing the relationship with our mother, whether it is an unhealthy adult dependence on approval, acceptance, or an emotional imbalance resulting from a cold mother withholding her love and nurturance. This oil brings its healing energy through our mother bloodline to restore the divine feminine principle within. This oil assists in releasing emotions of an extreme nature, especially anger, jealousy, frustration, and disappointment, allowing the higher aspects of the feminine to emerge with compassion, wisdom, and open heartedness.

Ylang ylang has the unique ability to calm and clear emotions from the heart and energetically through the DNA as well as to activate the creative nature and depths of intimate bonding with another. Ylang ylang stimulates inner beauty through connecting the heart with the soul. Aphrodisiac in nature, ylang ylang helps us connect to our sensual nature and align our sexuality to our hearts, opening for deeper connection at the soul level through sexual union. Ylang ylang activates our desire for deep sensual connection, and is beneficial for frigidity, impotence, and other sexual dysfunctions. It is also helpful for clearing trauma of a sexual orientation through the bloodline.

Ylang ylang sings of the voluptuous nature of life. Its medicine reminds us not to become rigid in our thinking, but to stay fluid, open, and consistently invite in the grandest, most expansive experience of life. With its deeply feminine aroma, ylang ylang invites us to embrace our emotions, freeing ourselves to feel and release versus stuffing, compacting, and limiting the life force within us.

This oil helps to activate the female creative mind and support creation from a place of effortless intention. Ylang ylang medicine also heals the split of the feminine archetype, bringing light into the places of betrayal, competition, and ego to bring unification through the feminine aspects to the collective consciousness.

Ylang ylang produces up to five grades of essential oils, with the loveliest aromatically as well as energetically termed, ylang ylang superior extra. The uplifting nature of ylang ylang reminds us of the joy of being alive. This oil is tremendously helpful to alleviate anxiety of a heart-based nature.

Activate the Heart – Ylang Ylang Perfume to Awaken Joie de Vie

- ∞ 11 drops Ylang Ylang essentials oil (*Cananga odorata superior extra*)
- ∞ 4 drops Blood Orange essential oil (*Citrus aurantium*)
- ∞ 4 drops Wild Orange essential oil (*Citrus sinensis*)
- ∞ 1 drop Black Pepper essential oil (*Piper nigrum*)
- ∞ 5 drops Bergamot essential oil (*Citrus bergamia*)
- ∞ 1 drop Carrot Seed essential oil (*Daucus carota*)

Blend into 5 ml jojoba or coconut oil. Infuse with the intention to awaken joy and apply as you would a perfume on pulse points and to the heart.

Additional Essential Oil

- ∞ Ambrette Seed *Abelmoschus moschatus*

HEART ACTIVATE AROMATHERAPY
DNA BLUEPRINT BENEFITS

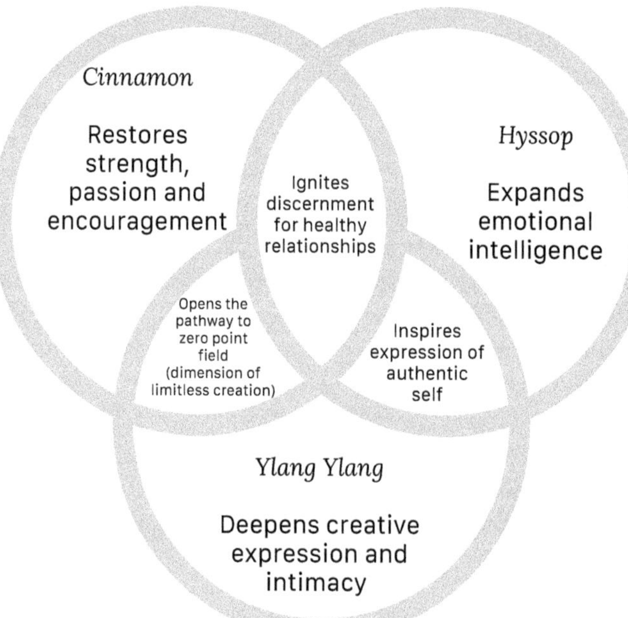

ACTIVATE THE HEART – BOTANICAL MEDICINE

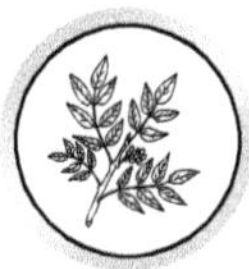

MAJOR ARCHETYPE

PRICKLY ASH – *Zanthoxylum americanum*

Parts Used: Bark and berries

Prickly ash is a stimulating herb activating cardiac circulation. It promotes blood flow out from the heart to the peripheral tissues, warming the skin, organs, and joints. It's useful for any sign of poor circulation including rheumatic conditions or a lack of skin tone. Prickly ash is useful for fragile states of health where blood flow is stagnant and no longer moving through the tissues due to a narrowing of the arteries.

It is nicknamed the toothache tree as it was a Native North American remedy for toothache and is still used today for many painful conditions. Externally it can be used as a stimulating ointment for pain relief.

Emotionally prickly ash is like a gentle pin cushion. When the heart has been emotionally stagnant or locked up without the key for a long period of time, to open the floodgates all at once can be traumatic. Prickly ash does this in a subtle way. It stimulates and activates the energetic aspect of the heart to start pulsing waves of love and joy into the heart center.

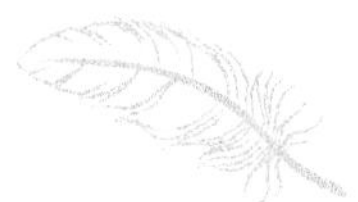

Place a small sachet of dried bark and berries under your mattress or pillow to activate the heart center "love wave." Add crystals from the Activate the Heart section to enhance this process.

Activate the Heart – Prickly Ash Physical Uses

Activate: Circulation of blood flow, alterative, activates DNA synthesis
Cardiovascular: Sluggish circulation, antispasmodic, slow and a weak heart.
Nervous System: Rejuvenating tonic
Adrenals System: Stimulates sluggish adrenals – activates the fire within of the frail and ill
Immune System: Antimicrobial, antiviral, and lymph stimulant
Musculoskeletal: Chronic rheumatism
Digestive System: Poor digestion, flatulence, abdominal cramps, and bitter stimulant
Reproductive: Uterine cramps

Activate the Heart – Prickly Ash Emotional Uses

Releases fear of never finding love
Releases anxiety of chronic health conditions
Activates the twin flame

Activate the Heart – Prickly Ash Energetic Uses

When taken before bed, it stimulates positive dreams and prevents repeating nightmares
Used in fire initiation ceremonies for activation
Use in FPW sacred ceremony for love activation

Activate the Heart – Prickly Ash Dosage

Decoction: 1 tablespoon of Prickly Ash berries with 354 ml cups of water. Drink 1 cup 2x/day
See Appendix B on how to make a decoction
Tincture: 0.5–1 ml 3x/day
Topical: Can be used externally for rheumatic pains as a poultice or oil.

Activate the Heart – Prickly Ash Cautions and Contraindications

Low dose herb – follow dosage guidelines
Pregnancy

Activate the Heart – Prickly Ash Freedom to Circulate Oil

Ingredients:
2 parts Prickly Ash bark – *Zanthoxylum americanum*
2 parts Cleavers – *Galium aparine*
1 part Poke root – *Phytolacca spp.*
1 part Red root – *Ceanothus americanus*
½–1 teaspoon Cayenne powder

Directions: See Appendix B for directions on how to make an infused oil
Application: Apply 3–4 times per day over thearea to promote circulation.
Note: avoid open wounds and sensitive areas

MINOR ARCHETYPES

Nettle Leaf – *Urtica dioica*

Parts Used: Leaf and root

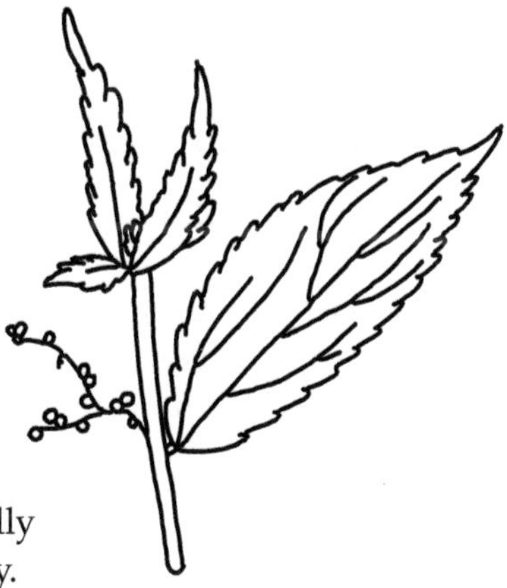

You might be familiar with this common plant, nettle, used most often for detoxing the system as a diuretic, but the genetic and ancient DNA of this plant is for heart activation. Just by being in the presence of this intense ally you can feel the activation of your body. Now is the time many of the plants are being activated for their true purpose in helping heal and evolve the planet. Nettle is one of these botanicals. If this ally grows near you, we would like you to please take the time to connect with the new DNA activating within this plant and your cells. Note: this plant has formic acid so please don't touch this plant unless you have gloves, or it will sting you.

Nettles activate the electrical conduction of the heart dispelling many underlying heart conditions due to misfiring. Think of nettles as the spark plug activating the genetic code within the cardiovascular system.

Activate the Heart – Nettle Physical Uses

Activate: Electrical system of the heart, DNA expression
Cardiovascular: Swelling, conduction disorders (heart block), congestive heart failure, hypertension, and anemia
Nervous System: Clears a foggy mind
Adrenal System: Rebuilds stamina (via nutrients)
Urinary System: Increases urine and eliminates waste
Musculoskeletal System: Arthritis, gout, swollen joints, joint pain, and muscle pain.
Male Reproductive System: Benign Prostatic Hyperplasia
Female Reproductive System: Heavy bleeding
Integumentary System: Nervous eczema
Respiratory System: Hay fever and allergies
Nutrition: Rich in minerals – Calcium, potassium, and iron

Activate the Heart – Nettle Emotional Uses

Limitless possibilities – you begin to see complicated situations with clarity
Attracts new supportive relationships
Stings you into to action
Emotional strength – activates your inner warrior

Activate the Heart – Nettle Energetic Uses

Place in a sachet on your altar for protection from unwanted energy and relationships
Place a bouquet of flowers in the room to accelerate recovery from illness
Used in ceremony as a rite of passage and transformation

Activate the Heart – Nettle Dosage

Infusion: 1 tablespoon per cup of water. 3x/day
Tincture: 1 ml 3x/day

Activate the Heart – Nettle Cautions and Contraindications

Pregnancy – Overnight infusion for minerals may be allowed – consult your physician

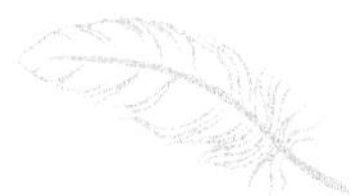

Activate the Heart – Free Your Inner Warrior Tea

14 g Nettle leaf – *Urtica dioica*
14 g Dandelion leaf – *Taraxacum officinale*
7 g Hawthorn berries – *Crataegus monogyna*
2.5 g dried Ginger root – *Zingiber officinale*

Combine herbs and steep in for 709 ml for 8 minutes. Drink 3 cups per day.
See Appendix B for how to make an infusion

Cinnamon – *Cinnamomum zeylanicum*

Parts Used: Bark

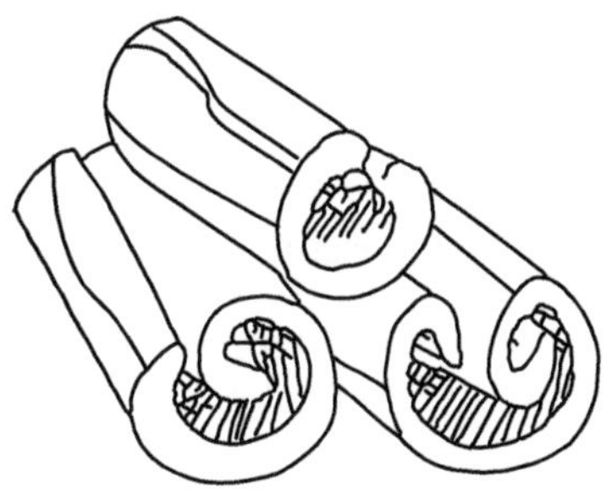

Physically cinnamon is a warming herb strengthening the circulatory and digestive systems. It activates the fire and power of the heart in conditions of a slow and sluggish nature. It's especially useful in conditions of physical debilitation. Cinnamon is also a wonderful herb for the digestive system and soothes an irritable bowel system and aids the pancreas in insulin regulation. If you have a history of eating disorders, cinnamon is the botanical ally to turn to for letting go of these past cellular deteriorations. If you are having difficulties losing weight, cinnamon can help break down the "safety" wall we build as a trauma protection mechanism and replace it with a gentle loving embrace.

The sweetness of cinnamon melts a hardened heart and soothes the cravings of the sugar beast. It brings joy and warmth into cells allowing them the ability to repair DNA more quickly in a relaxed state.

Activate the Heart – Cinnamon Physical Uses

Activates: Heat – the fire within, physical debilitation, DNA repair
Cardiovascular: Hypertension, increases circulation
Nervous System: Stress and tension
Adrenal System: Balances cortisol
Respiratory System: Bronchial spasm
Female Reproductive: Menstrual cramps
Digestive: Diarrhea, spastic colon, constipation, and candida
Immune System: antibacterial, antifungal, antiviral
Endocrine System: Diabetes, blood sugar balancing
Μυσχυλοσκελεταλ Σψστεμ: Pain relief

Activate the Heart – Cinnamon Emotional Uses

Intimacy – positive self-sexual image
Harmony and honesty for troubled relationships
Allows vulnerability for healing

Activate the Heart – Cinnamon Energetic Uses

Sprinkle cinnamon on your altar to attract love and empower your sacred intentions
Childhood trauma healing
Develop intuition opening to the divine inspiration
Releasing cellular patterning of eating disorders

Activate the Heart – Cinnamon Dosage

Infusion: 1 teaspoon per 236 ml of water. Drink 236 ml 3x/day
Tincture: 10–15 drops 3x/day

Activate the Heart – Cinnamon Cautions and Contraindications

Pregnancy

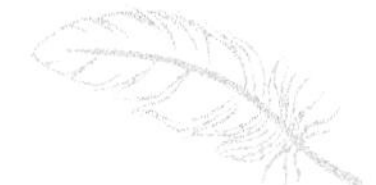

Activate the Heart – Cinnamon Freedom from the Flu Hot Toddy

Feeling under the weather? Cinnamon to the rescue!

Combine in a small saucepan:
8 g Cinnamon chips – *Cinnamomum zeylanicum*
4 g Ginger root – *Zingiber officinale*
Juice of 1 lemon
236 ml water
4 g sweetener
Heat till combined and drink hot.

Dosage: 3 cups/day until symptoms resolve

BOTANICAL ADDITIONS

∞ Licorice – *Glycyrrhiza glabra*
∞ American Ginseng – *Panax quinquefolius*
∞ Passionflower – *Passiflora incarnata*

HEART ACTIVATE BOTANICAL MEDICINE
DNA BLUEPRINT BENEFITS

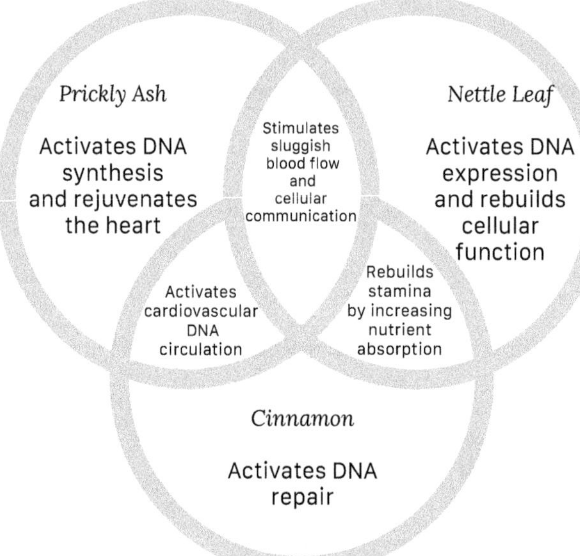

ACTIVATE THE HEART – LIGHT WHEELS

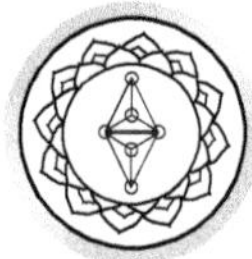

MAJOR ARCHETYPE

THE 148th LIGHT WHEEL, HRIDAYA-AGNI

Hridaya-agni translated means heart-fire or flaming heart. This light wheel activates the fire within and harmonizes the beat of your heart with the beat of the universe. Hridaya-agni is devotion. Devotion to finding true love, not of others but of yourself. We are most often the hardest on ourselves and this light wheel beckons you to hear the call of true love within. It directs you to find peace within by calling forth the guidance of the universe, tapping into the many, many beings in the universe which have not yet been actualized in our plane or in this universe. There is such a great labyrinth of knowledge swimming around us, all we must do is listen, turn up the volume, and tune into the station.

MINOR ARCHETYPE

∞ The 32nd light wheel, Dvaatrimshat

Dvaatrimshat is part of the past life light wheel clusters. This cluster holds all of your past life trauma and experiences at the higher realm and akashic records. Dvaatrimshat is your life's path and any negative karma or hurt you have picked up in this lifetime or another one is stored here for access. By access, this means that during meditation and activation this karma can be released by a simple change of vibration. Activate this change by using the mudra and sound archetypes from activating the heart for eight days. You might not feel a profound change but a more subtle change over the next week. We suggest using a journal and keeping notes of any changes in your vibration or energy field that might occur over the next week.

COLORS

MAJOR ARCHETYPE

MAGENTA

Magenta activates the heart through self-expression and emotional vulnerability. When this color is activated, trust your intuitive heart and lead with your heart instead of your head with all upcoming decisions. Magenta also encourages you to speak the true feelings of your heart and not to be afraid to wear your emotions on your sleeve.

SOUND

∞ Alta

Alta stimulates the energy of expansion, connection, and flow of unity consciousness, an ancient knowing and wisdom extending beyond the planet. It also expands the heart to receive greater love, connection, and nurturance. It aligns the heart with the alta major light wheel, which sits at the base of the skull at C1 – Atlas, the point of initiation for transmission from your higher self.

ACTIVATE THE HEART – CRYSTALS AND STONES

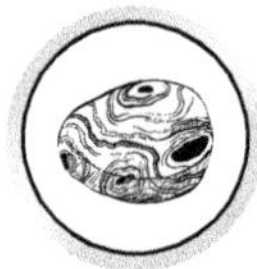

MAJOR ARCHETYPE

ATLANTISITE

Atlantisite carries the vibration of love. This powerful crystal ignites the kundalini, life force, within guiding you to a path of unlimited potential. Atlantisite connects to the power of the ancient lost times in history and their magic alchemy including the Egyptians and the Lemurians. It is also a stone of great compassion aiding in forgiving yourself and others from emotional pain.

Atlantisite is also a great stone of manifestation and abundance, and if you are guided to use this stone in your sacred intentions know that your dreams are becoming a reality. It draws in the energy of the higher light wheels, clearing and activating them and pouring a healing vibrational energy into your light body.

Atlantisite increases the strength of your red blood cells helping with blood disorders as well as other heart deficient conditions. It activates the red blood cells facilitating nutrients to travel through the cells energizing the mitochondria of the cells. Atlantisite is a stone of mineral absorption and by activating water overnight with this stone and then drinking it the next day you will help your body absorb necessary minerals.

MINOR ARCHETYPES

∞ Ruby

Ruby is another master healing stone that assists in reigniting the heart. Ruby stimulates all aspects of the heart and thymus creating spiritual and emotional balance, stability and openness. It activates healing with our masculine nature, clearing energy through the father bloodline. Ruby amplifies thought and facilitates inspiration in leadership. Ruby also has regenerative action physically, stimulating optimum charge in the cellular structures and nadis and is recommended for any cardio-vascular imbalances.

∞ Gaia Stone

The gaia stone connects you to the goddess energy of Gaia and connects to the heart of Earth. Gaia heals the emotional wounding of humanity and of the Earth bringing harmony to all the planetary chakras. This stone protects the heart from abuse and violence, clearing past and future karmic relationships of heart wounding. It is also helpful when the heart center is overactivated and you are experiencing disturbed or restless sleep. Place the stone under your pillow to sleep soundlessly through the night.

Physically the gaia stone activates circulation and clears excess heat from the heart and the head. The gaia stone frees the body from ailments of heat such as headaches, hot flashes, and irregular body temperature.

ACTIVATE THE HEART CRYSTAL GRID

Set the intention for your healing attunement of awakening to new ideas and supportive relationships. Place a black cloth, cotton or silk is best, on the floor. Place a white cloth over your entire body on top of the stone grid. Relax for 30-60 minutes. You may listen to healing music such as the sound of Alta Major. Drink a glass of Atlantisite charged water throughout the day after this attunement. Immediately after the treatment cleanse the crystals and stones. (See Appendix C)

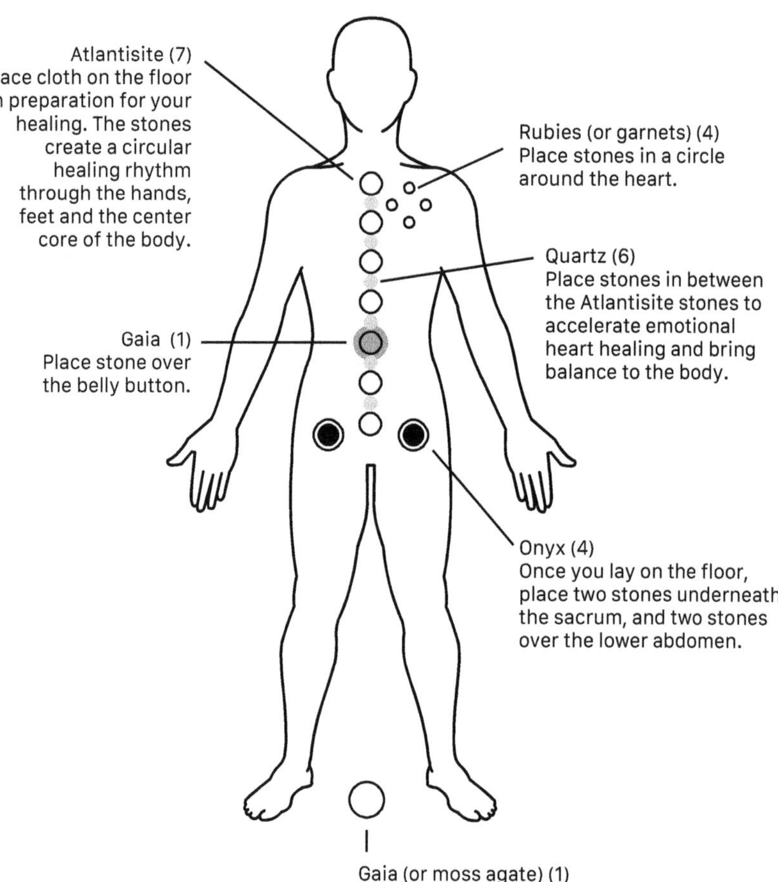

ACTIVATE THE HEART – ENERGETIC AND VIBRATIONAL TECHNIQUES

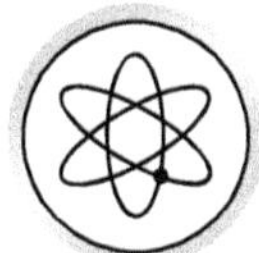

MAJOR ARCHETYPE

HEART ACTIVATE HYDROTHERAPY

- ∞ 4 drops Ylang Ylang essential oil (*Cananga odorata superior extra*)
- ∞ 1 drop Ambrette Seed CO_2 extract (*Hibiscus abelmoschus*)
- ∞ 2 drops Cistus essential oil (*Cistus ladaniferus*)
- ∞ 10 drops of Passionflower essence
- ∞ 10 drops Diamond gem Essence
- ∞ 8 ounces of brewed Cinnamon herb tea

Add all ingredients to the bath and soak for at least 20 minutes. If you have sensitive skin, you may want to skip the cinnamon tea.

MINOR ARCHETYPES

Heart Activation Visualization

Close your eyes and visualize a diamond shaped symbol entering the very center of your heart. This symbol is filled with light that fluctuates between a pulsating magenta to a pulsating golden light. As this light begins to fill your heart, the diamond in the center of your heart expands until it surrounds your entire energy field with this diamond light. Now invite in the intentions for all that you want to create in your life and allow the diamond frequency to energize those intentions until you can see, feel, or experience them as being fully actualized.

Activate the Heart EOBT

Place one drop of ylang ylang essential oil between the two fingertips of the right hand, inhale deeply and tap Heart-1, Utmost Source, Entry to Heart Meridian for 30 seconds with the intention to fully open, activate, and unify the physical and cosmic heart.

Location: In the deepest part of the well in the center of the armpit.

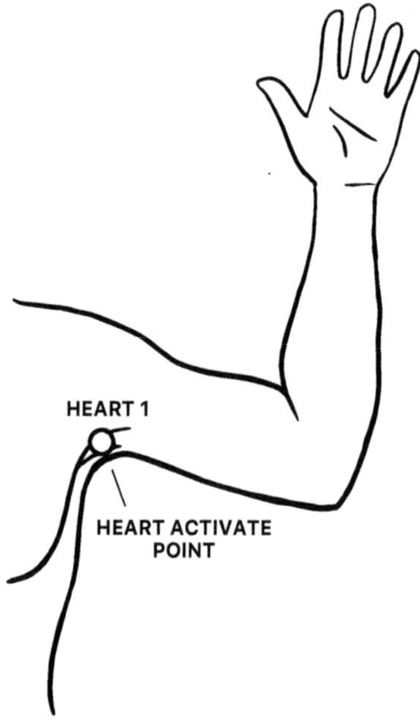

ACTIVATE THE HEART – FLOWER AND GEM ESSENCES

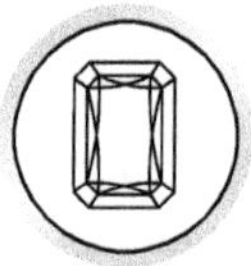

FLOWER ESSENCES

MAJOR ARCHETYPE

APPLE BLOSSOM

Apple flower essence holds the energetic imprint and energy of the apple blossom. The blossoms for this essence are best collected before dawn in the presence of the new moon. It carries the energy of the dawn, new beginnings, and expansion as well as the teeming void of possibilities of the new moon.

Apple blossom brings balance to conflicting thoughts and emotions. It is an essence of relationship, bringing balance to codependency, and fosters long lasting relationships; it enhances trust and the ability to give and receive in a healthy way. All encourages heart expansion and transformation at the core level. Apple blossom supports fertility on all levels. It invites you to be calmly active and actively calm.

MINOR ARCHETYPES

Pecan

Pecan bolsters self-confidence and inner strength. This essence supports realignment of the hara, the line of effortless intention. Using this essence for six months will support the hara to elongate and strengthen encouraging the discovery of your life or soul purpose. Pecan essence also offers an aphrodisiac quality and is beneficial for couples that are looking to restore their sensual chemistry. This essence can also be used to enhance magnetism and awaken new levels of confidence regarding inner beauty.

Passionflower

Passionflower bridges the human heart and auric field with that of divine consciousness, opening the spiritual body to greater levels of awareness. It assists in the understanding of universal truths and the interconnectedness of all realities, past, present, and those still unfolding. It opens the heart to divine love and unity. If you have yet to experience the vast beauty and sacred geometry of the passionflower, invite the intention to do so. It is truly exquisite, articulating both the complexity and magnificence of creation. This essence can be used to inspire creativity for new projects and to bring unmanifest concepts into form.

GEM ESSENCE

MAJOR ARCHETYPE

EMERALD

Emerald essence with its grand affinity for the heart, opens, expands, and aligns the physical heart with the cosmic heart. It invites the personality aspects to open to a universal understanding of self at the soul level. Emerald opens the soul seat center, where all the longings for this incarnation are held, attracting people and circumstances that are in alignment with the soul's high purpose. Emerald aligns the meridian points and energy centers, or light wheels with the cosmic consciousness of Mahatma, the source of unconditional love.

ACTIVATE THE HEART – INTENTIONS

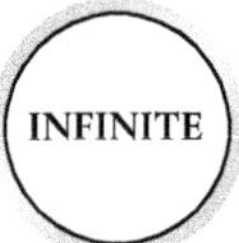

MAJOR ARCHETYPE

INFINITE

MINOR ARCHETYPES

∞ I charge and ignite my heart, all the cells and the blood vessels
∞ I live, love, and lead from the deep wisdom of my heart
∞ I have everything I need within me to flourish in all areas of my life

ADDITIONAL INTENTIONS

∞ My infinite love heals all
∞ My heart holds the potential for all creation
∞ The light within my heart illuminates my highest path

ACTIVATE THE HEART – MEDITATION MUDRA

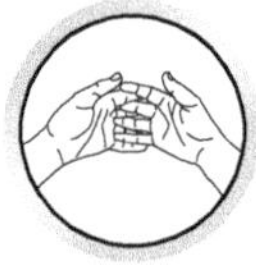

Ushas Mudra

I assimilate the infinite light rays of the universe,
embracing and living my highest joy, passion, and purpose.

Ushas mudra connects the cells and DNA of the heart with the infinite light rays of healing and illuminates a path of expansion and openness. Take a moment to imagine you are sitting on the beach watching the sunrise. When you feel the first ray of sun upon your face, this is the feeling of Uṣhas, of unending lightness. With the Ushas mudra, you will open to the infinite possibilities of not only self-love but of loving all those around you with compassion and without judgement. This mudra activates your "soul dream" and aligns with your heart's truest vision of love and intention.

Ushas Mudra Alignment

1. Place your hands in front of your heart center and face the palms together with the fingertips pointing upward.
2. Interweave your fingertips together and with the little finger closest to your heart center.
3. Lightly touch your thumbs together. If this position becomes tiresome you may rest your hands upon your lap.
4. Take a deep breath, let your body relax.
5. You may now either do the meditation below or 10 minutes of *Cellular Breathing* (to access the cellular breathing technique please go to www.zenergymedicinals.com).
6. You may also use the mudra any time you want to invoke clarity and intention regarding health conditions or alignment with your inner being and purpose.

Activate the Heart Meditation

∞ To access the meditation please go to www.zenergymedicinals.com

∞ Take a deep breath in, inhaling your single note or essential oil formula for 30–45 seconds.
∞ On your next breath in, see, feel, allow, imagine an opalescent cocoon surrounding your physical body. Imagine it created from filaments of every spectrum of light. Open, relax, and sink into the nurturing protection of this chrysalis.
∞ Hold the Ushas mudra and take several breaths to align and awaken your inner heart. With each breath, feel the openness of your heart,

chest, and lungs, allowing a feeling of peace, calmness, and clarity to envelope your being.

- ∞ And on your next breath envision a rose-colored light in the shape of a sphere emanating and pulsating right in front of your heart. This light begins to penetrate and permeate your heart space deep into the very center.
- ∞ This rose-colored light fills the entire chrysalis cocoon around you and then becomes more salmon in color, pulsating at the center of the heart, breathing in the intention "I love myself. I love myself when I hate myself and I cause my own suffering."
- ∞ Feel yourself relax even more deeply into this vibration of compassion of self love and acceptance. This is the pathway of true knowing and transformation of you as the glorious butterfly, allowing the illumination of divine uniqueness that speaks many volumes of your truth and gifts.
- ∞ On the next breath in, you begin to hear faintly a song that is most familiar to your heart. It is the very song that reverberates to the core of your being and back through the entirety of the cosmos. It is the song of the One.
- ∞ See, feel, allow, imagine the melody to fill your being with great comfort, through loving and accepting yourself wherever you are on the journey. Wherever you are in your own healing spiral, back to your core, your quintessence, you are worthy of love in all forms, in all places within your being.
- ∞ With each wave of healing, the doorway of limitless opportunity opens wider and wider, and you feel a greater sense of freedom. Repeat the intention three times either silently or aloud: "I assimilate the infinite light rays of the universe. Embracing and living with passion and purpose."
- ∞ Filled with nourishing love, offer a prayer of love and gratitude in your heart for the healing within your being, your lineage, and through that to the collective consciousness of the planet, of humanity, all kingdoms of life animals upon it. In great gratitude. So be it.

ACTIVATE THE HEART – SACRED GEOMETRY

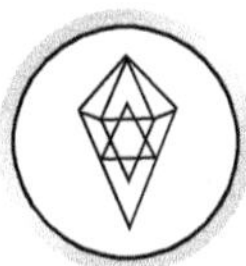

MAJOR ARCHETYPE

ACTIVATE THE HEART SACRED GEOMETRY

This intentional and original depiction of sacred geometry encompasses both the pyramid and diamond configurations. The diamond has a laser focus activation quality to access the very core of the heart, to the dimension of the zero-point field. It expands with great clarity the sacred alchemical chamber or temple of cocreation with the Divine for the evolution and advancement of the individual soul as well as the individual's' ability to create benevolence for the planet.

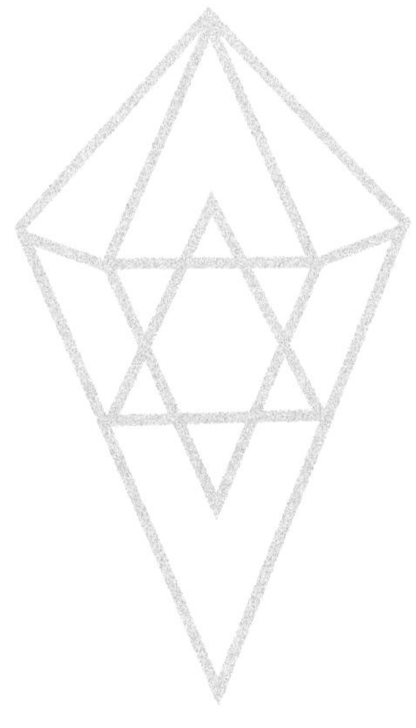

ACTIVATE THE HEART – NUTRITION

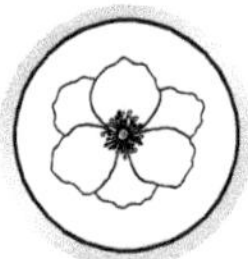

MAJOR ARCHETYPE

ROSEHIPS

Rosehips are abounding in nutrients and cardiovascular disease fighting properties. They are brimming with antioxidants such as quercetin, vitamin C, ellagic acid, and catechins. Rosehips protect and activate the heart by lowering blood pressure and cholesterol levels. They are also anti-inflammatory as the key constituents combat oxidative DNA damage and cease further cellular and telomere damage. Fabulous for antiaging (Andersson et al., 2012).

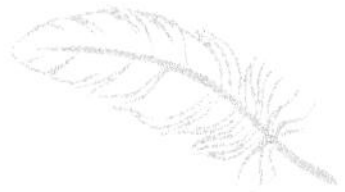

Activate the Heart – Rosehips Tea

Ingredients
- ∞ 950 ml filtered water
- ∞ 200 g dried Rosehips – *Rosa canina*
- ∞ 4 g dried Ginger root – *Zingiber officinale*
- ∞ 2 g Cinnamon chips – *Cinnamomum zeylanicum*
- ∞ Sweetener of choice to taste.

Boil 475 ml of the water, remove from heat, add the rosehips, ginger, and cinnamon. Cover and steep for 20 minutes. Strain and discard herbs. Add the sweetener and remaining 475 ml water. Chill and serve over ice with a slice of lime.

MINOR ARCHETYPES

Cacao

Cacao comes from the pod-like fruit of the *Theobroma cacao* tree and is one of the richest sources of the antioxidant, polyphenol, and is abundant in flavonols (a class of flavonoids) as well. Flavanols protect the integrity of the blood vessels increasing circulation through the arterial system and the heart (De Araujo et al., 2016).

Goji Berries

Goji berries are an antioxidant superfood. High in antioxidants, they protect the DNA and the mitochondria from damage and instigate the mitochondria to increase replication resulting in increased energy. Gojis are little nuggets of energy, increasing stamina, focus, protecting the heart, and lowering blood pressure. They come in a dried form, like raisins, and can be hydrated and added to foods or soaked in water and ingested in smoothies and as a tonic.

NUTRITIONAL ADDITIONS

∞ Beet
∞ Red pepper
∞ Acai
∞ Pomegranate seeds
∞ Apple
∞ Garlic

ACTIVATE THE HEART – DISCOVERY DIVE – CALLING IN LOVE, JOY, AND PASSION

Challenging all old patterns and belief systems around love and happiness is the first step to shattering the glass ceilings and walls you have built around you. Imagine living in the mansion of your dreams, and instead of enjoying each room of your beautiful home, you close off all but the smallest of rooms and that becomes all you can see.

Many of us have grown up on stories and fairy tales that set the stage for either the rescued or the rescuer, victim or perpetrator, non-emotional and emotional hysteria, caretaker and dependent, and so on. We've grown up with specific beliefs of what it means to be loved and taken care of by another and more importantly by ourselves. In the previous exercises, you have been clearing old patterns and beliefs of grief, disappointment, sadness, anger, betrayal, pain, struggle, and loss with the knowledge that until these emotions are allowed, embraced, and integrated fully as the wisdom of life teachings that they are designed to be, they will continue to perpetuate the patterning in the DNA and with that our external and internal environments as well as creations.

In the previous chapters, you have learned that when you are triggered by a certain belief system and pattern, you have the ability in the moment of emotional reaction to bring yourself back to presence.

You can witness your experience in the moment. It takes practice, yet it is highly rewarding. You are either in pattern or in presence. When we are in presence the old paradigms of how we relate to ourselves and therefore each other can be transformed to new levels of health and harmony.

Instead of closing our hearts, shutting down and pushing love and others away, further reinforcing separation and the distorted belief system when triggered, we can create a new way of being. Through presence, we can energetically move through the pain of the past and open to experience love, joy, and bliss as we are designed to from the perspective of divined consciousness.

As you prepare to initiate your Heart Activate Freedom Photon Ritual please invite these questions deep into your heart: What if your old story of love, happiness, and fulfillment simply didn't exist anymore? What would your life look like from the perspective of your biggest dream?

Let's consider for a moment that calling in this BIG VISION and all the support, help, guidance, needed to cocreate it was as easy as picking up the phone to call your best friend? Let's use that term for spiritual teachers, guides, guardians, avatars, and angels. We like to call them "My team of Divine Light."

As you begin to contemplate these next BIG questions, ask yourself, "What does my heart long to create?"

What would your optimum experience of self-care be? How much would you rest? What would you eat? How would you exercise? Would you get regular therapy, massage, energy work?

What would your dream relationship look like with your spouse or partner? Where would you live? How would you love each other, make love to each other? How deeply would you communicate with them? What would you create together? Would you travel, where to, and how often?

What would this feel like in your heart, your body, and in your cells? How would your emotions respond? This step is tremendously important! Spend the next few minutes allowing yourself to have these feelings and then jot them down here! You will come back to this as you activate your Freedom Photon Ritual.

FREEDOM PHOTON WHEEL™

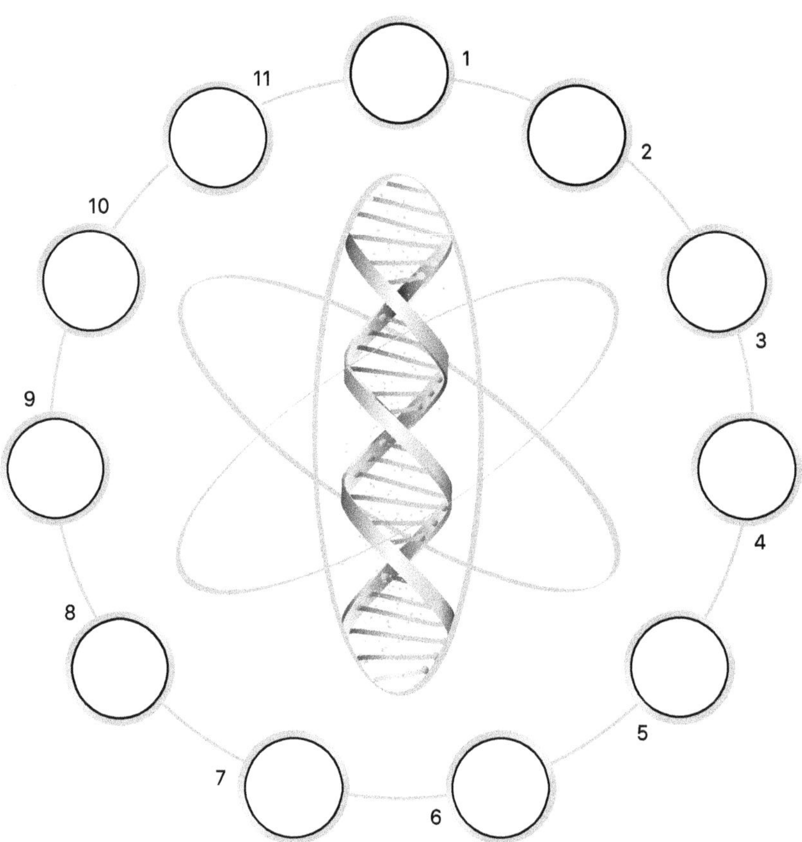

ACTIVATE THE HEART
YOUR PERSONAL FREEDOM PHOTON RITUAL

Moon Phase

It is best to perform your ritual when the moon is waxing from the new moon to the full moon, to align with the phase. However, the power of your intention and momentum is key so if you are inspired at another time, go for it.

Intention

"I call forth, activate, and allow the full DNA sequence for INFINITE love and unity through every level of my being and genetic lineage."

Select, Align, and Activate

Select your interventions according to the instructions in Chapter Five. Inhale and apply your chosen essential oil for 30–45 seconds. Use your botanical tincture or tea as directed. You may also listen to the meditation and use the mudra from this chapter while attuning your FPW.

Affirm

"Divine consciousness, assist me in allowing the highest experience of INFINITE love, joy, and bliss through my lineage and my mother and father bloodlines so that I may emanate and embody the full spectrum of love and compassion."

CHAPTER 7

Unlocking Your Unlimited Energy – The Adrenals

When was the last time you jumped out of bed with vim and vigor to greet the day and all the miracles held therein? The adrenal system is unique as it is governed by two elements, fire and water. Both are required, in balance, for this system to fully heal and engage. All trauma through the mother and father bloodlines of your heritage are contained within the two precious adrenal glands. The imprint of fear and anxiety of being fully alive, entirely safe, in physical form, on the Earth is held here. Chronic stress over time depletes the energy here and diminishes connection to the core of the Earth, which offers an unending supply of energy, life force, and vital connection.

The adrenal system represents our relationship with the past experiences in our DNA from our lineage as well as the past experiences of life on this planet. War, violence, and dominance of power through slavery and abuse of all varieties held within your bloodline and that of the collective consciousness of the Earth is stamped on the adrenal system of every human being, which is why after the age of seven, every person experiences some degree of adrenal fatigue.

This is also a reminder of the great importance and personal responsibility we have for our own healing, holographically, from the microcosm to the macrocosm. From our individuated human perspective, our cells and DNA are microcosms of the macrocosm of our spirit, soul, auric field, and the vastness of our "quintessence." From a unified perspective, every human being contributes to the collective consciousness. Therefore, as we heal the pains of the past held within our DNA as a representation of the totality of who we are, we heal the macrocosm of humanity, allowing our greater evolution as a unified human race.

Bringing the focus of healing to the adrenal system allows for us to elevate through the "Soul Purpose Triad" from living a life of surviving to a life of thriving. When we perpetuate a cycle of survival, we are in a constant state of dis-ease. This can manifest as chronic exhaustion, illness, emotional imbalance, dysfunctional relationship patterns, financial scarcity, and so on.

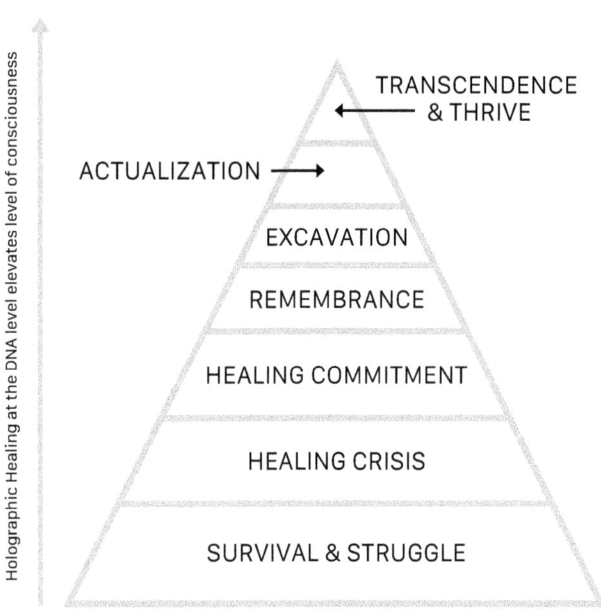

When struggle is constant, dis-ease is constant.

Thriving is the new paradigm of opportunity for human existence and engagement. Moving into a deeper state of trust in yourself, the Earth beneath you for support, the universe all around you to co-create beauty, magic and miracles, health, vibrancy, and intimate relationships. A life of thriving offers a state of abundance and resources, of vital life force and connection. It is this invitation we offer to you as you explore and excavate a deeper understanding of yourself and your relationship with freedom, sovereignty, and the ability to renew your commitment to this life in all its glory.

THE INNER WORKINGS OF THE ADRENAL SYSTEM

∞ To access the meditation please go to www.zenergymedicinals.com

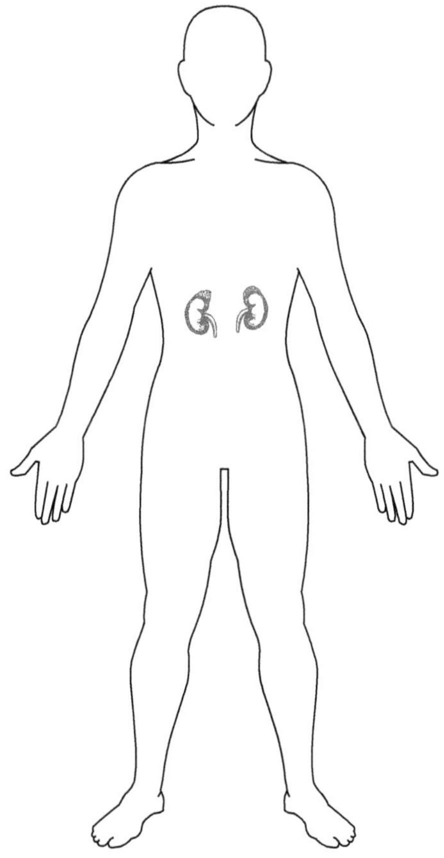

ENDOCRINE SYSTEM

The endocrine system includes all the glands of the body and the hormones produced by those glands. The glands are controlled directly by stimulation from the nervous system as well as by chemical receptors in the blood and hormones produced by other glands. By regulating the functions of organs in the body, these glands help to maintain the body's homeostasis. Cellular metabolism, reproduction, sexual development, sugar and mineral homeostasis, heart rate, and digestion are among the many processes regulated by the actions of hormones.

ADRENAL GLANDS

The adrenal glands are a pair of triangular glands found immediately superior to the kidneys in the back side of the body. The adrenal glands are each made of two distinct layers, each with their own unique functions: the outer adrenal cortex and inner adrenal medulla.

ADRENAL CORTEX

The adrenal cortex produces many cortical hormones in three classes: glucocorticoids, mineralocorticoids, and androgens.

- Mineralocorticoids, as their name suggests, are a group of hormones that help to regulate the concentration of mineral ions in the body.
- Glucocorticoids have many diverse functions, including the breakdown of proteins and lipids to produce glucose. Glucocorticoids also function to reduce inflammation and immune response.
- Androgens, such as testosterone, are produced at low levels in the adrenal cortex to regulate the growth and activity of cells that are receptive to male hormones. In adult males, the number of androgens produced by the testes is many times greater than the amount produced by the adrenal cortex, leading to the appearance of male secondary sex characteristics.

ADRENAL MEDULLA

The adrenal medulla produces the hormones epinephrine and norepinephrine under stimulation by the sympathetic division of the autonomic nervous system. Both hormones help to increase the flow of blood to the brain and muscles to improve the "fight or flight" response to stress. These hormones also work to increase heart rate, breathing rate, and blood pressure while decreasing the flow of blood to and function of organs that are not involved in responding to emergencies during the "rest and digest" time.

PSYCHO-SPIRITUAL ASPECTS OF THE ADRENALS

ADRENALS PSYCHO-SPIRITUAL PATHWAY

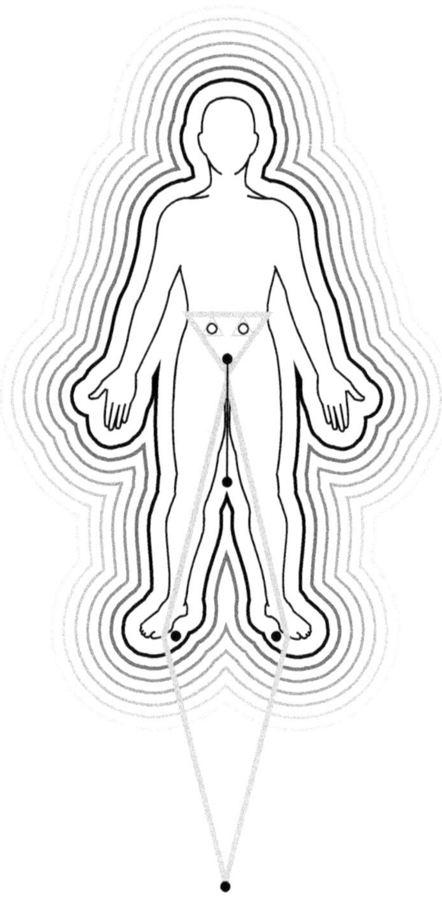

The adrenal glands are held in etheric pyramid temples of golden amber light, both individually and together. They receive the vital life force from the core of the Earth, up through the soles of the feet as well as through the root light wheel, uniting and co-mingling at the dantian point. The health and vitality of the Earth connection and resultant nature of the lifeforce received by the individual directly relates to the subconscious beliefs, thoughts and emotions connected to this incarnation. The dantian then nourishes the adrenal glands with this healing light and regenerative resource.

As discussed in our introduction, the adrenal system is a key receiver and transmitter of life force. The adrenals are deeply connected to the root chakra or Muladhara light wheel. Yes, we realize chakra is an overused randomized word these days, yet that does not diminish the fact that its origins date back to 1500–500 BC in some of the oldest texts known as the Vedas. Looking more closely at the power of the adrenal system we can liken it to the root structure of our "tree of life," receiving the nutrients as energy to feed our system. The adrenal system can only take in as much of this planetary life force, or nourishment, as our system allows based on both our level of openness in the root chakra and the degree of trauma, we have experienced in our life to date.

On a primary level, through the connection to the root chakra, the adrenal system is deeply connected to our will to live and our sense of belonging – belonging in our bodies, in our family of origin, and being fully on the planet. Because the adrenal system is responsible for our fight or flight response, this system holds all areas of trauma around feeling safe.

Furthermore, it is the experience of strong emotion such as fear, anger, sadness, and other acute or chronic stress related pressures by which we further tax the adrenal system, creating dark colored bands of heavy energy around the adrenals. The levels of stress caused from traumatic experiences may be actual or perceived to still pose a threat to the system at large. The level of health of our adrenal system is a key indicator of how our bodies have been able to adapt to stress and deal with traumatic experiences.

When our adrenal system is balanced and strong, we feel a sense of connectedness to the Earth, ourselves, and the world around us. We also experience physical vitality, groundedness, renewable energy, and the abundance of life.

When out of balance, we can experience low levels of energy, high levels of fatigue, mood swings, addictions, and a sense of being disconnected and isolated.

DETOX THE ADRENAL GLANDS

Welcome to detoxing the adrenal glands! Are you ready to feel energized? To feel the energy coursing through this system we first must open the channels that are hindering energy and create flow. Imagine a flowing river of energy through your body as you work through this next DNA section.

DETOXING THE ADRENALS – THE PHYSICAL PERSPECTIVE

Most of you know what it feels like to be tired and drained of energy as if the life source has been sucked out of you. The adrenal glands communicate with our body through many different levels of fatigue. Hans Seyle developed the theory of three stages of stress or adrenal fatigue called the GAS or general adaptation syndrome.

1. The alarm or reaction stage – this is the normal fight or flight response to stress.
2. The resistance stage – this is the stage when your body is experiencing stress for long periods of time and continually must manage the stress. You might experience irritability, frustration, and poor concentration. This stage leads to stage three.
3. The exhaustion stage – this stage is for chronic stress when your body gives up. You may experience fatigue, burnout, depression, anxiety, and decreased stress tolerance.

In the detox phase of the adrenal system, you will be working with the archetypes to discharge or release the cells that have been overworked and are still in a state of stasis in the system. Your body will begin to return to a parasympathetic state and rest before moving into the nourish and activate stages of healing.

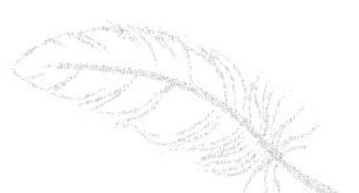

We suggest getting out your journal and to start making a list of messages your body is sending you in relation to adrenal fatigue and detoxification. What stage do you think you are in? What level of fatigue are you currently experiencing?

DETOXING THE ADRENAL GLANDS – THE PSYCHO-SPIRITUAL PERSPECTIVE

Detoxing the adrenal system is crucial for us to fully take back our sovereign life force. We most often hear of the adrenals in relation to adrenal fatigue and chronic stress related exhaustion. The following pages are rich with adaptogenic plant and vibrational medicine to restore vibrancy. Less discussed and just as critical for our full vitality to flourish is the exploration and intention for healing the past. Unwinding patterns around self-sabotage, self-abuse, and addiction is key to healing through the DNA and family lineage. Memories of slavery are a perspective which also drains life from the adrenal glands. It is important to note that slavery comes in many forms and is not wholly tied to race: there are caste systems aplenty outside of Eastern philosophy. Gradations of intimidation and violence with or without mandates can include human trafficking, forced and imbalanced marriage or labor, imbalance in business partnerships, and more. Any time there is intention followed with action to "have power over" another, imbalance ensues. The shame and guilt connecting to having less abundance, less energy juxtaposed with having more resources than another depletes our energy and connection.

Detoxing the adrenal glands allows us to unwind the memories both in the cells and in the auric field that keep us frozen in fear: fear of the past, not only our own but all memories of being unsafe and brutalized in our DNA, mother and father bloodlines. Where there is sexual trauma in the past, and particularly that which runs along the family lineage, is bound here, depleting life force energy as well as the will to live. The adrenal system invites us to let go of any beliefs of limitation and struggle. Limitation in this regard can relate to energy and vitality, prosperity and resources, or even the limitation of being in the container of human form vs. the limitless expansive nature of spirit.

Trauma Held in Adrenal System – Stella

Stella uncovered memories of sexual abuse later in life. It was not until her early forties that she began to have flashbacks. Small snippets of memory that seemed disjointed but evoked intense feelings of panic and despair that seemed to suck all the air from the room around her. She spoke of living most of her adult life with a nagging feeling that she could not quite put her finger on. As we explored her history, she talked of her sister's multiple experience of sexual abuse and how she found out that her mother had also experienced abuse as a young adult. Stella experienced chronic exhaustion. She had a strong desire and positive intention to heal and stop the pattern from being passed on down her line to her own daughter. This perspective is important to acknowledge the power of healing at the DNA level to put an end to distorted patterns in the mother and father bloodlines. It only takes the courage of one to dive into their spiral of healing, to bring the light of healing through the layers and through the lineage, to transform the future by healing the past just as we are doing here throughout these pages and dimensions of possibility that are opened herein as we find a way to source our inner personal power and benevolence.

ADRENAL DETOX FREEDOM PHOTON WHEEL

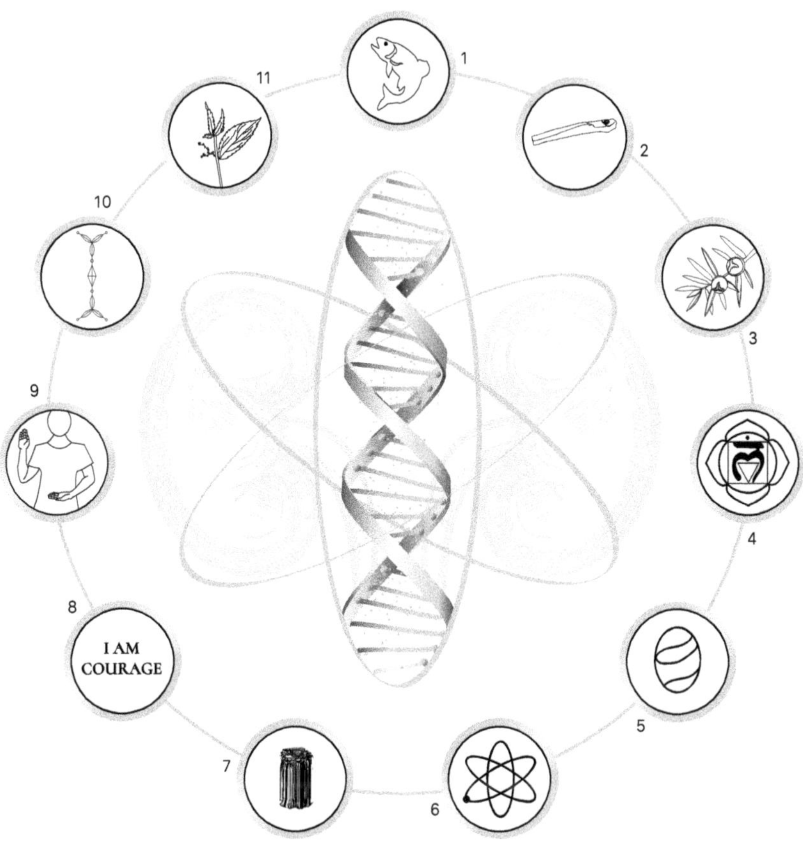

1 Alchemy Animal: Salmon
2 Aromatherapy: Palo Santo
3 Botanical: Juniper
4 Light Wheel: Muladhara
5 Crystal: Opalight
6 Photon Vibration
7 Flower or Gem Essence: Black Tourmaline
8 Intention: I Am Courage
9 Meditation Mudra: Abhaya Varada
10 Sacred Geometry
11 Nutrition: Nettle

ADRENAL DETOX
INFINITY INFLUENCERS

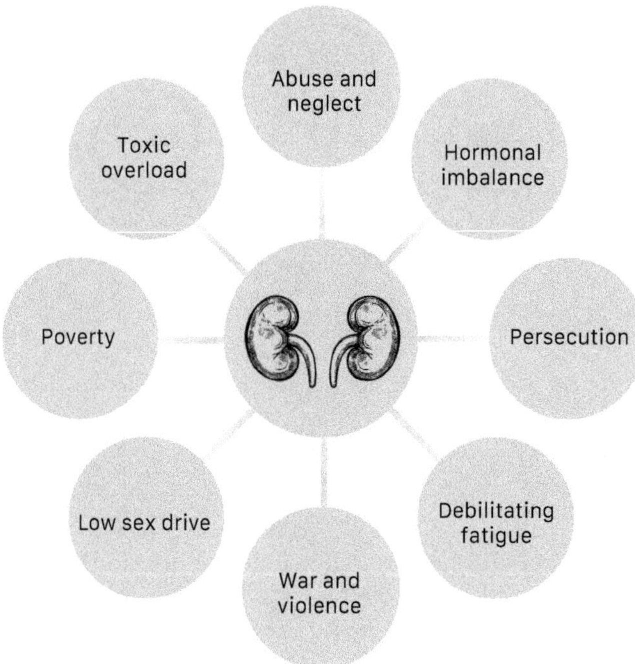

DETOX THE ADRENALS – ALCHEMY ANIMALS

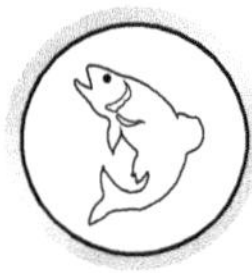

The detox alchemy animals of the adrenals embrace the water element and assist with filtration. Filter from a physical perspective engaging the adrenals and the kidneys to release toxins but also from the emotional viewpoint liberating from fear.

MAJOR ARCHETYPE

SALMON

The salmon alchemy animal exemplifies freedom and happiness. Imagine, for a moment, you are a salmon in the river fighting to swim upstream with the other salmon. The salmon fights for its dreams and has the strength and drive to never give up. If this archetype is appearing for you, it is time to gather guidance and face your fears. Fear is an emotion. The adrenals are intensely connected to fear and fear holds you back from living your dreams – really living your life to its fullest potential.

The vibrant salmon, with a similar shape to the adrenal glands, is about rebirth. The rebirth of your energy. Giving you the strength of a thousand salmon swimming together towards happiness. The salmon connects you to the eternal spring of life which has a never-ending wave of power. Tune in to the energy of the salmon when you are meeting a challenge head on and you need the courage to face your greatest fears.

Creature Connection: "I swim with the courage of the salmon. Submerging myself completely in the waters of renewal and rebirth. I call upon my guides and ancestors for support and guidance on this new river of dreams."

MINOR ARCHETYPES

Skink

The skink alchemy animal signals it's time to take an internal audit at what's zapping your energy and what's ruling your energy center? It's easy to get caught up in day-to-day life and not take time out for self-care. The skink reminds you it's time to take a break, lay out on the sunny deck, read a book, walk on the beach, anything to break your routine of depletion.

The skink is able to regenerate anything they have lost so take this to heart. Are you regenerating new energy from your vital core or are you recreating the same illness repeatedly in a different way? It's easy to rename a problem. The skink offers its alchemy to transform this old impression and create a new one.

Creature Connection: "I slow down the momentum of my daily life. I relax. Like the skink, I lay in the sun enjoying each moment to the fullest."

Octopus

The octopus alchemy animal is an animal adept at camouflage and signifies you are pretending to be someone you are not. It's time to be honest with yourself and your intentions progressing onward on this healing path. Ask yourself "What's really holding me back from unlimited energy?" Get out your journal on this one!

The octopus is extremely agile and will guide you quickly through any fear barriers, helping you to adapt and adjust to these new aspects of yourself. Now is not the time to get up to the wall and break through it with a sledgehammer. Now is the time to leap over the wall and glide easily to the next day.

Creature Connection: "I glide easily through the storms of the sea adapting to each new wave of motion with a renewed sense of life and exploration."

ANIMAL ADDITIONS

∞ Catfish
∞ Shark

DETOX THE ADRENALS – AROMATHERAPY

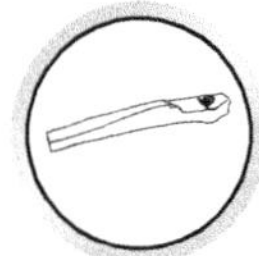

MAJOR ARCHETYPE

PALO SANTO – *Bursera graveolens*

Part extracted: Wood

Core properties: antiseptic, anti-inflammatory, and antibacterial
Safety: nontoxic, nonirritant, over harvested

Many are familiar with palo santo wood for the sacred purification and energy cleansing practice through burning. Its aroma is deep, earthly, and woodsy. This South American "holy wood" produces an essential oil with such potent depth it easily transcends space and time. The spirit of palo santo, although rooted at the very core of the Earth, also expands to the template of purity within cosmic consciousness. This lends it the ability to heal through the mother and father bloodline at core patterns that have been passed through the lineage and held within the subconscious. Like how burning the wood dissolves negative energy, the essential oils support the unwinding of energy connections that constrict the life force in the adrenals.

Palo santo can take us into the deepest, darkest places within and bring the immutable strength and power of the light to transform. It invites this healing energy into the most entrenched blocks or calcifications of energy with the invitation to shift, to be set free, and to release the quintessence or life force that is held within the distorted configurations in our shadow self.

The adrenals hold life force, and all distorted energy and belief systems around being alive tend to accumulate here. This creates energetic bands that constrict the life force in the adrenal area, limiting life force, limiting vitality. This makes palo santo an excellent choice for detoxifying the adrenal glands, physically, emotionally, and spiritually through the DNA.

The vibration of palo santo palo has a very powerful ability to clear our masculine side and come through and bring healing light to our male bloodline in the DNA. Particularly when there has been energy around rigidity in thinking and sexuality from the male perspective, domination, control, and templates around things being hard ... that life must be hard, work must be hard. All these belief systems that are held within the adrenals can benefit from palo santo, bringing with it the intention to heal the father bloodline and the relationship to the divine masculine within.

Detox the Adrenals – Palo Santo Massage Oil

- ∞ 7 drops Palo Santo essential oil (*Bursera graveolens*)
- ∞ 3 drops of Carrot Seed essential oil (*Daucus carota*)
- ∞ 2 drops of Juniper essential oil (*Juniperus communis*)
- ∞ 3 drops Grapefruit essential oil (*Citrus paradisi*)

Blend these oils together in 30 ml of your carrier oil, and then infuse it by holding it in your hands with the intention to cleanse and purify the adrenals. Massage a 5 ml size amount into the lower back, in the kidney/adrenal area.

MINOR ARCHETYPES

Juniper – *Juniperus communis*

Part extracted: Berries

Core properties: antiseptic, antirheumatic, astringent, antispasmodic, analgesic, diuretic, and tonic
Safety: nontoxic, nonirritant

The rich aroma, fresh, crisp, and green of juniper berry connotes clarity. Produced from the female seed cones of juniper, it, has a very cleansing effect on all levels. In the auric field, it helps to dissolve energy accumulations or blocks, and particularly in the emotional body where there's' an excess imbalance of feelings or emotions.

Its bright and clean aroma lifts the spirits and brings an expansive new potential into thought processes and the mental body. It also helps to breathe new life into existing projects or relationships that become lackluster, invigorating them with fresh, clear energy for creativity and passion.

Juniper also has a regulating effect on the endocrine system, balancing hormone production that is currently excessive or lacking. There is both a lightness and a sense of power that juniper berry offers, which make it an excellent choice for clearing the adrenal glands from the heaviness associated with exhaustion, overwhelm, and chronic overuse of the will.

When we generate life force from our will center and chronic patterns of push force, overwork, overdoing, or over giving, we become disconnected from our renewable resource of Earth, energy, and vital life force connected therein. And because of that, we disconnect from the potential of creation by effortless intention.

Juniper helps to clear excess energy in multiple natures; excessive pent-up anger from excessive frenetic energy that is masculine nature, excessive talking, or obsessive thought patterns.

Detox the Adrenals – Juniper Room Clearing Spray

- ∞ 12 drops of Juniper Berry essential oil (*Juniperus communis*)
- ∞ 4 drops of Lemon essential oil (*Citrus limonum*)
- ∞ 6 drops of Grapefruit essential oil (*Citrus paradisi*)
- ∞ 4 drops of Rosemary essential oil (*Rosmarinus officinalis*)
- ∞ 4 drops of Pine essential oil (*Pinus pinaster*)

Blend your essential oils in 60 ml of distilled water, shake well before use. Infuse with your intention to cleanse and purify the energy in your home, office, and personal space.

Grapefruit – *Citrus paradisi*

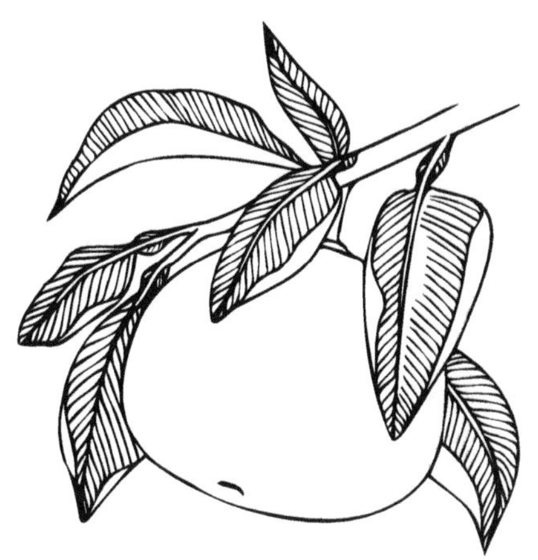

Part extracted: Peel

Core properties: antidepressant, antiseptic, aperitif, diuretic, disinfectant, lymphatic stimulant, tonic, and anti-infectious
Safety: nontoxic, potential irritant and sensitizer, photo toxic

Bright and clear, grapefruit's refreshing aroma is uplifting and invigorating. It generates a vortex of bright light in the auric field and lifts dross or density with an upward swirling action. Grapefruit has a similar effect on the adrenal system by penetrating the cellular level and clearing layers of depressed energy as well as emotion.

One of the best oils for self judgement, grapefruit breaks down energy blocks in the auric field, particularly the mental and emotional body. In the mental body, grapefruit helps to clear negative thought forms and patterns of negative self-talk. From the emotional perspective, grapefruit helps to release pent-up frustration, anger, and resentment. It also helps to clear energetic debris picked up from other people and places.

Grapefruit's ability to break down energetic accumulations also applies to the breaking down of fats in the body and stimulating digestion and lymphatic drainage, which make it an excellent choice for weight loss.

Note this oil is phototoxic and potentially sensitizing. A dear friend applied grapefruit directly to the skin without diluting it and then went into the hot Bermuda sun for a prolonged period. She burned severely and broke out in a rash of small, white bumps. Twenty years later, she still cannot go into the sun without breaking out in that same rash. Sensitization can have lifelong effects. Remember, just because something is natural doesn't mean it is always safe.

Educate. Explore. Discern.

Detox the Adrenals – Grapefruit Lymph Circulation Body Oil

∞ 5 drops of Carrot Seed essential oil (*Daucus carota*)
∞ 7 drops of Juniper essential oil (*Juniperus communis*)
∞ 3 drops of Fennel essential oil (*Foeniculum vulgare*)
∞ 10 drops of Grapefruit essential oil (*Citrus paradisi*)
∞ 6 drops of Cypress essential oil (*Cupressus sempervirens*)

Blend into 60 ml organic jojoba and massage a 5 ml amount onto legs, belly, neck, and armpits to increase circulation and toxin release.

ESSENTIAL OIL ADDITIONS

∞ Myrrh – *Commiphora myrrha*

ADRENAL DETOX AROMATHERAPY
DNA BLUEPRINT BENEFITS

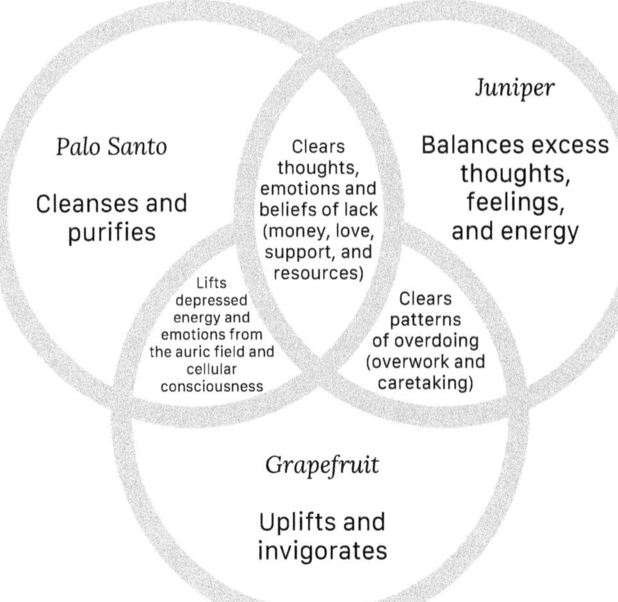

DETOX THE ADRENALS – BOTANICAL MEDICINE

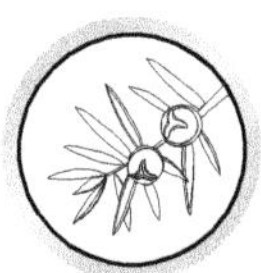

MAJOR ARCHETYPE

JUNIPER BERRY – *Juniperus communis*

Parts Used: Berry

Juniper is a tonic herb as it tonifies the adrenals and kidney through stimulation. Juniper is most indicated in chronic congestive states of the adrenal system. It regulates hormonal balance and increases production of both corticosteroids and catecholamines of the adrenal glands. This is important for re-establishing energy or an energy baseline for improvement. Quite often when the adrenal detox herbs are needed the system is so depleted it has used up all the reserves. Juniper enables the adrenals to slowly build back up the reserves to establish stability and groundedness to the Earth.

Juniper is also used in arthritis and rheumatism because of its anti-inflammatory and diuretic properties. It can be applied topically as an analgesic for painful joints, sprains, and bruises.

One major benefit of juniper berries is they are rich in antioxidants. Antioxidants help your body to prevent and fight disease because they relieve oxidative stress caused by excess free radicals in your system. Juniper berries contain three extremely important antioxidants for phase two liver detoxification: superoxide dismutase (SOD), catalase, and glutathione peroxidase.

Juniper is another one of our ancient botanical allies carrying the genetic information of the ancient Egyptians and Greeks. They considered juniper a purifying and protective herb and used it for sacred ceremonial and medicine. Take a deep breath in and connect to the magnificence of Juniper and channel, the unbounding energy of the Earth and of our ancestors.

Detox the Adrenals – Juniper Physical Uses

Detox: Releases fluids and eliminates toxins, expels damaged cells and DNA, and restores vitality

Adrenal System: Regulates and increases production of corticosteroids and catecholamines

Cardiovascular System: High blood pressure, normalizes electrolyte balance

Nervous System: Insomnia

Urinary System: Diuretic – increases urinary output, flushes out bladder infections

Musculoskeletal System: Arthritis, joint pain and swelling

Digestive System: Digestive bitter – gas, bloating, digestive upset

Immune System: Antiseptic, antibacterial, antifungal

Integumentary System: Eczema, psoriasis, heals scars, prevents wrinkles, and breaks down cellulite

Detox the Adrenals – Juniper Emotional Uses

Strengthens will power
Provides clarity in confused states
Protection from fear

Detox the Adrenals – Juniper Energetic Uses

Cleansing and protection – hang above altar for doorway
Actualize your full potential
Release sexual blockages and cellular imprints

Detox the Adrenals – Juniper Dosage

Decoction: Steep 1 T of crushed berries in 8 oz. of hot water for 20 minutes – drink one cup 3x/day
Tincture: 30 drops 3x/day

Detox the Adrenals – Juniper Cautions and Contraindications

Pregnancy, kidney disease, and kidney infections

Detox the Adrenals – Juniper Freedom to Flow

This formula aids the body in releasing excess fluids and cellular toxic DNA fragments.

Ingredients:
15 ml Juniper – *Juniperus communis* liquid extract
15 ml Nettle leaf – *Urtica dioica* liquid extract
10 ml Lemon balm – *Melissa officinalis* liquid extract
10 ml Sarsaparilla – *Smilax ornata* liquid extract

Directions: Combine the liquid extracts into one small bottle.

Dosage: 3 dropperfuls 3x/day for 1–3 weeks

MINOR ARCHETYPES

Dong Quai – *Angelica sinensis*

Part used: Dried root

Dong quai is a beautiful lighthearted herb in the umbelliferae family with small disc shaped flowers arranged in an umbel like fashion. We love the airiness of this plant reminding us to not take life so seriously. It is all going to work itself out – if we just let go.

The root of this plant is where we draw its healing properties. It allows the adrenals and kidneys to filter more efficiently, establishing a clearer hormonal path of communication. The adrenal medulla and cortex are then able to produce cells of higher function and stability, providing a foundation of energy, blood sugar balancing, blood pressure regulation, and immune cell activation.

Detox the Adrenals – Dong Quai Physical Uses

Detox: Clears cellular debris from the extracellular space and matrix. Reconfigures DNA into correct formation and code
Adrenal System: Promotes recirculation of the adrenal hormones – Improving energy and sleep
Cardiovascular System: Cardio-protective, reduces arterial plaque, invigorates the blood
Nervous System: Sedative
Urinary System: Urinary tonic
Reproductive System: Amenorrhea, dysmenorrhea, PMS, endometriosis, tones the uterus, estrogenic, menopause and infertility
Digestive System: Decrease inflammation, IBS, and relieves constipation
Liver: Hepatoprotective
Immune System: Immunostimulant
Musculoskeletal: Arthritis

Detox the Adrenals – Dong Quai Emotional Uses

Purify the emotions – clear old emotionally draining baggage
Release patterns of failure – inspire new creative dreams
Courage to open to new experiences

Detox the Adrenals – Dong Quai Energetic Uses

Open the mind to your soul purpose – vision quest
Absolution of family bloodline karma
Lightness for astral travel

Detox the Adrenals – Dong Quai Dosage

Decoction: Steep 1 tablespoon in 236 ml of hot water for 20 minutes – drink one cup 3x/day
Tincture: 30 drops 2–3x/day

Detox the Adrenals – Dong Quai Cautions and Contraindications

Pregnancy, acute hemorrhagic conditions and diarrhea
Contraindicated if taking prescription blood thinners

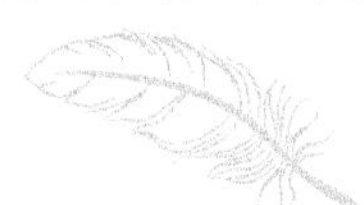

Detox the Adrenals – Dong Quai Freedom to Conceive Sitz Bath

Decoct: ¼ cup of Dong Quai with 946 ml of water for 20 minutes. Add to the sitz bath. Do the sitz bath every other day for 3 weeks. Break for a month and repeat if necessary.
Note: The 1 week off per month for women is during menstruation. For men, the bath water should not be more than body temperature. See Appendix B for Sitz Bath Instructions.

Sarsaparilla – *Smilax rotundifolia*

Parts Used: Root

You might be familiar with this sweet root, famous for its original use in flavoring root beer. We are not using the herb in that format here, but we do want you to think about the sweetness of life and whether you are nurturing your adrenal glands or energy? Sarsaparilla was historically used as a revitalizing tonic in the spring to perk up the body and metabolism after a long hibernating winter. This is the strength we draw upon from sarsaparilla.

Revitalize. Rejuvenate. Replenish

Sarsaparilla is also a superstar as a hormonal herb, engaging the second light wheel. It is helpful for hormonal imbalance and sexual dysfunction and boosts libido. It supports the DNA by pulling out disruptive endotoxins from the bloodstream. An endotoxin is a toxin that is present inside a bacterial cell and is released when the cell disintegrates. When the adrenal glands are detoxing, it's important to use an herb to help pull out the toxic residue otherwise you may be worse – more fatigued and more depleted. Not good!

Energetically sarsaparilla works on the family lineage of sexual trauma and sexually transmitted disease. It was used historically to treat syphilis and today we use it to clear these genetic imprints. Remember when we talked previously about how you carry the history of your family and your lifetime family through every part of your DNA? It's just as important to clear the DNA imprint from past dysfunction as it is the present. We usually see patients improve 50 percent faster when they clear the past genetic deterioration from their cells.

Detox the Adrenals – Sarsaparilla Physical Uses

Detox: Releases endotoxins and wastes from the blood and the imprint from the DNA
Adrenal System: Alterative returning vitality and tonic
Cardiovascular System: Reduces swelling and edema
Nervous System: Hormonal depression
Endocrine System: Metabolic stimulant, pituitary stimulant
Urinary System: Diuretic and diaphoretic
Reproductive System: Hormonal tonic for males and females, aphrodisiac, testosteronic, progesteronic, menopause, and libido
Digestive System: Toxic gut with poor absorption
Immune System: Immuno-stimulant, antibiotic, autoimmune disease
Musculoskeletal System: Anti-inflammatory, antirheumatic. and gout
Integumentary System: Antiseptic, itchy rashes, psoriasis, and wound healing

Detox the Adrenals – Sarsaparilla Emotional Uses

Releases thought patterns, loops, and manifests new loops
"I have energy for sex and intimacy" – Aphrodisiac
"I have energy to live my dreams"
"I let go of all relationships that are zapping my energy"

Detox the Adrenals – Sarsaparilla Energetic Uses

Connection to the healing powers of the Inca Empire and the Sun God, Inti
Release family STD and sexual abuse from the DNA
Spiritual cleansing of the second light wheel – energize

Detox the Adrenals – Sarsaparilla Dosage

Decoction: Steep 2 teaspoons Sarsaparilla in 236 ml of hot water for 15 minutes – drink one cup 3x/day
Tincture: 30 drops 2x/day

Detox the Adrenals – Sarsaparilla Cautions and Contraindications

Pregnancy

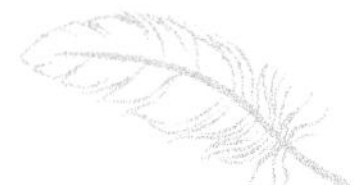

Detox the Adrenals – Sarsaparilla Essence Freedom from Sexually Transmitted Diseases

This tonic assists the body in detoxing the DNA imprint of STDs. **Note:** See your practitioner if an STD is suspected for proper care and treatment.

Ingredients:
28 g dried Sarsaparilla root – *Smilax rotundifolia*
28 g Lemon balm – *Melissa officinalis*
Alcohol of choice
Water
Glycerine
44 drops of Mariposa Lily Flower Essence
Follow the instructions for making the 2 extracts, let mature for 4–6 weeks, strain and add the flower essence
Dosage: 3 dropperfuls 2x/day for 1 month, rest for one month and repeat as needed
See Appendix B on how to make a tincture.

BOTANICAL ADDITIONS

- ∞ Lemon Balm – *Melissa officinalis*
- ∞ Lemon – *Citrus limon*
- ∞ Spikenard – *Aralia racemosa*
- ∞ Nettles – *Urtica dioica*

ADRENAL DETOX BOTANICAL MEDICINE
DNA BLUEPRINT BENEFITS

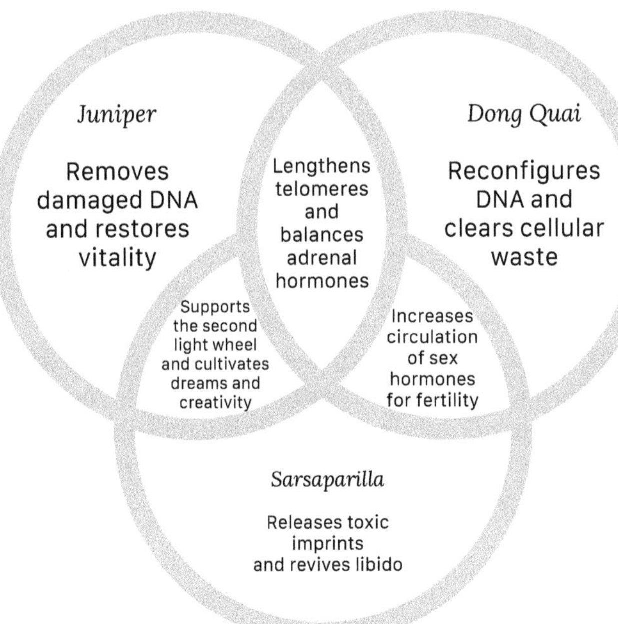

DETOX THE ADRENALS – LIGHT WHEELS

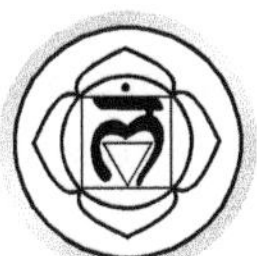

The light wheels of the detox adrenal system connect the body to the magnetic force of the Earth. You will discover heightened stamina, spirit, and strength as the planetary light wheels are activated within the core of the Earth and transmitted into your light wheels.

MAJOR ARCHETYPE

THE 1st LIGHT WHEEL, MULADHARA

The first light wheel is known as the root light wheel and is the connection to the Earth and the planetary light wheel, the earth star (the Earth's chakra). It is connected to the power of the Earth, stabilizing and grounding your energy during times of depletion. Muladhara connects the endocrine system and the adrenal system clearing stagnant sex hormones.

Muladhara is considered the great recycling bin of the light wheel system. It processes accumulated energy as well as unused energy and recycles it through the system for appropriate usage. Have you ever had the thought, "If only I could tap into the energy of the Earth?" This light wheel is the intermediary of this life force.

Physically muladhara relates to sexual dysfunctions such as endocrine disorders and hormonal imbalances. This light wheel is linked to safety and our sense of survival. When this light wheel is imbalanced, eating disorders may develop due to the fear of not having basic needs met and feeling threatened.

MINOR ARCHETYPE

∞ The 5th light wheel, Vishuddha

Vishuddha is the bridge connecting the adrenals to the center of the throat through communication. You will experience freedom of self-expression and liberation as this light wheel is activated releasing feelings of depression and depletion of sexual endurance. This light wheel is a place of truth where you can vocalize your authentic sexual needs and desires.

COLORS

MAJOR ARCHETYPE

AMBER

Amber is the color of self-expression and unreserved personality. It is an energizing color both physically and mentally and can be worn or placed in the environment for tapping into this life force especially when you are feeling worn out.

It can be very helpful for stimulating the appetite when managing anorexia and cachexia due to cancer related illness.

SOUND

Khei

∞ Khei elicits a soothing and balancing energy to the adrenal glands, like bathing them in a water bath. There is a peaceful quality that is induced through this sound, particularly beneficial to balance feelings of overwhelm.

DETOX THE ADRENALS – CRYSTALS AND STONES

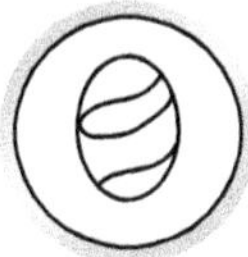

MAJOR ARCHETYPE

OPALIGHT

Opalight is a powerful crystal of resolution. Patterns of physical and emotional depletion are often linked with a karmic tie. No matter what modalities have been employed previously without releasing this karmic tie from the trauma timeline the life force remains stagnant.

Opalight helps to realign karmic or old belief patterns that are ingrained within the DNA and to reorganize the patterns to ones of harmony and synchronicity. This stone can shine the light on areas of your life that are stuck and where the energy for moving forward has become stagnant.

Opalight works on the DNA of the cell releasing genetic damage carried down through past generations and realigning the DNA for present and future generations. It can be very useful for healing and discovering root causes of disease or dysfunction that are deeply intertwined within the body and DNA.

Opalight functions most efficiently at night to resolve karmic ties in the dream state where the physical and emotional body are less active. It also quells insomnia resulting from an overactive adrenal gland and cortisol imbalance and practicing the crystal attunement before bed will be the most effective.

MINOR ARCHETYPES

∞ Carnelian

Carnelian activates the creative life force of the adrenal glands. It helps boost confidence and gives courage when you have lost the passion to pursue your life's purpose. This is the stone of action. We lovingly have nicknamed this stone the "couch potato." Why is this you might be asking? This stone kicks you off the couch and lights a fire under your butt – so, get moving!

Physically carnelian strengthens and reinforces vitality. It is especially useful for detoxifying addictive substances that have damaged the energy such as caffeine, alcohol, pharmaceuticals, or other drugs. It also aids females transitioning off toxic birth control and oral contraceptives that have changed the natural rhythm of the sex hormones.

∞ Diamond

The diamond is an timeless crystal holding the DNA or genetic memory of the ancient rulers connecting them to the divine source above. Diamonds are powerfully energetic stones. The diamond is like the previously discussed onyx, but the diamond is clear and connects the upper light wheels with a clear and pure white light. It clears and dispels all stagnant energy from the adrenal glands and sex organs encouraging precise energetic flow through the systems.

Note: You can use the rough or raw form of diamond for healing which is more cost effective; just please make sure to buy from a reputable source and purchase diamonds that are conflict free.

CRYSTAL ADDITIONS

∞ Emerald

DETOX THE ADRENALS CRYSTAL GRID

Do this crystal attunement grid 30-60 minutes before bed for better sleep and to facilitate DNA detox during the night. You may listen to healing music such as the sound of the ocean or rain. Immediately after the treatment cleanse the crystals and stones. Add the cleaned Opalight stones to a glass of water. Let sit overnight and then drink in the morning when you wake up. (See Appendix C)

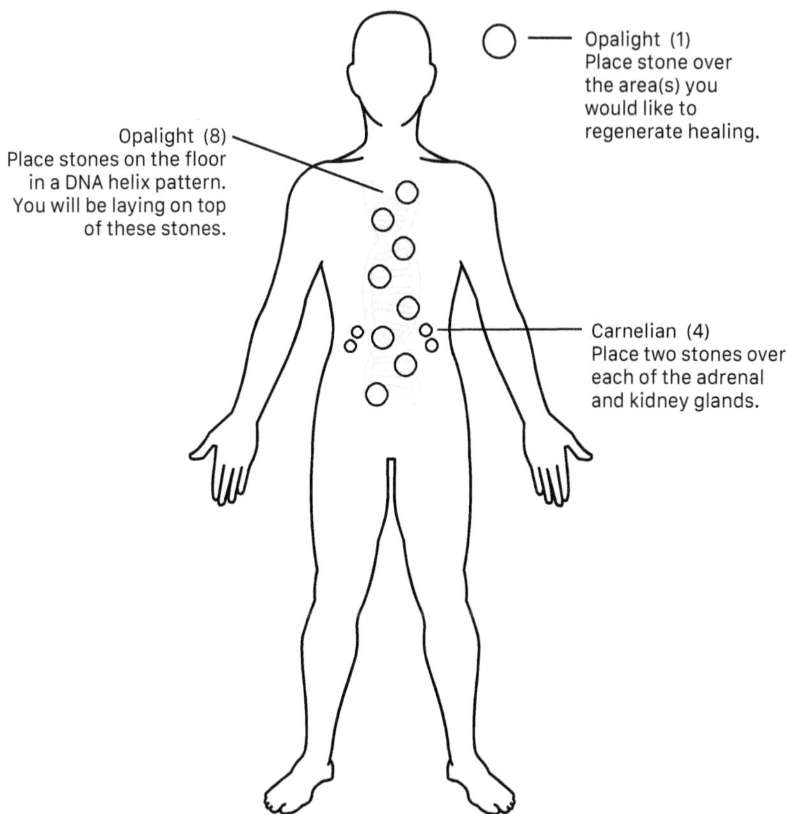

DETOX THE ADRENALS – ENERGETIC AND VIBRATIONAL TECHNIQUES

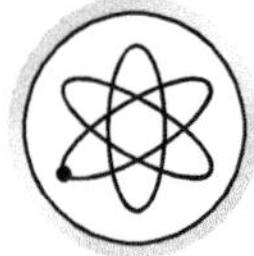

MAJOR ARCHETYPE

ADRENAL DETOX HYDROTHERAPY

- ∞ 453 g of Epsom salts
- ∞ 226 g Celtic sea salt
- ∞ 56 g of Seaweed – kelp powder
- ∞ 4 drops of Palo Santo essential oil (*Bursera graveolens*)
- ∞ 3 drops Juniper essential oil (*Juniperus communis*)
- ∞ 4 drops Lavender essential oil (*Lavendula angustifolia*)

Add all ingredients to a bath of warm water and soak for 20 minutes.

MINOR ARCHETYPE

Detox the Adrenals – Dantian – Visualization

Take a deep breath into your dantian point, approximately one inch below your navel. This is the one single note that holds you in physical form, with a tone and vibration unique to you. See, feel, allow, imagine this point expanding and pulsating golden light. Now envision your dantian forming a pyramid with your adrenal glands. The dantian is the lower point or apex that is connecting deep down into the Earth. Now invite your intention for your adrenals to flush out all the toxins and energetic debris down to the cellular and molecular level. The energy being released is flushing down to the point of the pyramid and then downward, returning to the Earth and dissolving. On your next breath in, see, feel, allow, imagine your adrenal glands to be renewed and revitalized.

Detox the Adrenals EOBT

Place one drop of palo santo essential oil between the first two fingertips of the right hand, inhale and tap the Kidney-5, Xi-Cleft point and tap thirty seconds with the intention of letting go of all fears, constrictions, and karmic entanglements.

Water Spring, K-5 (Xi-Cleft) point of the Kidney Meridian-Location: On the inside (medial aspect) of the ankle in the valley formed between the Achilles tendon and the prominence of bone that is the medial malleolus, inferior to the malleolus on the edge of the heel bone (calcaneus).

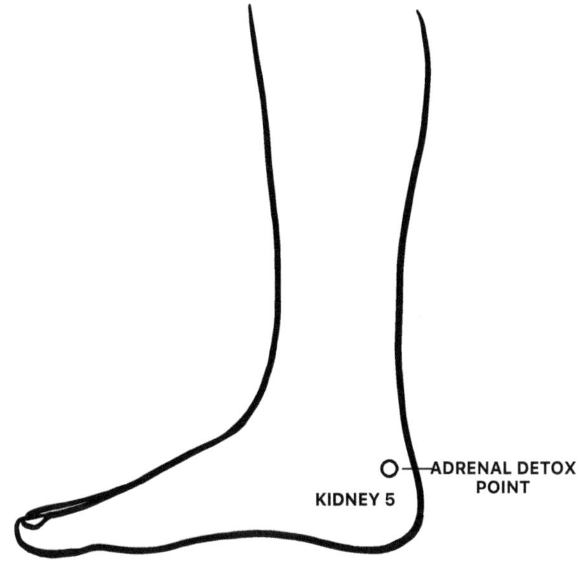

DETOX THE ADRENALS – FLOWER AND GEM ESSENCES

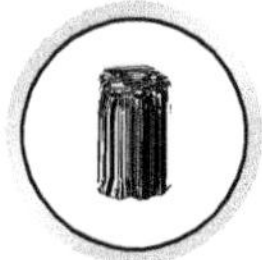

FLOWER ESSENCES

MAJOR ARCHETYPE

LEMON BALM

Lemon balm is the "great balancer" of energy, and emotions bringing a wave of peace through to the nervous system. This essence is helpful for those with back injuries and helps to clear the energy of the injury from the spine. Calming and balancing to emotions of an extreme nature, this essence is helpful to alleviate deep levels of exhaustion as well as frustration, reminding us to connect with the joyful vitality of life. Lemon balm is also good for lessening the depression associated with incarnating and experiencing life from a limited perspective in human form, reminding us that life within form and on this planet is a gift of creation, given to create magnificence.

MINOR ARCHETYPE

Thuja

Thuja clears deep miasma of core dis-ease in cells. This essence is a powerhouse of purification and helps to clear the auric field of heavy energy and past life blockages that are hindering current energy flow. Thuja's power to clear out the old is particularly helpful for the adrenals and breaking up energy accumulations around the adrenal glands that constrict life force. This essence is also good for clearing the Manipura light wheel in the solar plexus which is often damaged from power struggles and energetic cords that drain life force.

Birch

Birch is an essence of liberation. Infused with the template of purity, it helps to clear energetic connections to vows and contracts with dark energies through mother and father bloodlines. This sacred essence helps to heal tribal energies of violence, greed, and slavery held in the adrenal glands.

FLOWER ESSENCE ADDITIONS

∞ Sarsaparilla

GEM ESSENCES

MAJOR ARCHETYPE

BLACK TOURMALINE

Black tourmaline deeply connects us to the strength and grounding force of the Earth, imperative for the adrenals to be able to both release the density of energy that comes from physical day to day life and to receive a regenerative flow of life force from the Earth. This essence protects you from negative energy and projection from others. It unifies the male and female aspects of your triad and is one of the most potent remedies for healing and balancing the adrenal glands.

DETOX THE ADRENALS – INTENTIONS

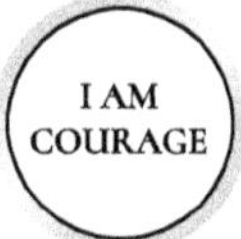

MAJOR ARCHETYPE

I AM COURAGE

MINOR ARCHETYPES

∞ I release all karma and entanglements holding me back from freedom
∞ I embrace and release my inner fears with the courage of a tiger
∞ I am fierce

ADDITIONAL INTENTIONS

∞ I release fear
∞ I am fearless
∞ My past is a springboard for the dynamic, powerful person I am today

DETOX THE ADRENALS – MEDITATION MUDRA

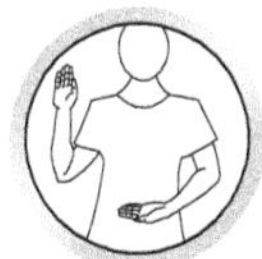

Abhaya Varada Mudra

I am a free sovereign being of light.
My energy is fully my own.

Abhaya Varada mudra invokes a feeling of safety by releasing any fears holding you back from your fullest potential and by grounding and connecting deep into the crystalline grid of the Earth. When the sympathetic nervous system is rampant, running from the bear, the emotion and feeling of insecurity consumes every aspect of the DNA. Ultimately this results in a zapping of all energy reserves. The Abhaya Varada mudra instills a sense of confidence and centeredness by releasing fear and anxiety and opening the first and second chakras.

Abhaya Varada Mudra Alignment

1. Hold your right hand at the level of the right shoulder, with the palm facing forward.
2. Hold the left hand directly below the belly button, palm facing upward, with the little finger resting gently on the stomach.
3. Take a deep breath, let your body relax.
4. You may now either do the meditation below or ten minutes of *Gaia Breath* (to access the Gaia Breath technique please go to www.zenergymedicinals.com).
5. You may also use this mudra at any time you are feeling anxious or fearful about a current illness or life changing circumstance.

∞ To access the mudra meditation please go to www.zenergymedicinals.com

∞ Breathe in your essential oil synergy for 30–45 seconds.
∞ Hold the Abhaya Varada mudra and take several breaths to align and attune to your inner adrenal glands. With each breath, feel the connection to the core crystalline grid of the Earth as all tension and stress melt away.
∞ Connect and breathe in the nourishment, abundance, strength, vitality of Mother Gaia, of planet Earth.
∞ This connection is imperative for the physical form to thrive and with that all personality aspects: the: the male, the female, and the child within.
∞ Observe the state of your adrenals currently. Do they look plump and vital? Thriving with life force? Does the life force seem to circulate and become electric and then static? Pop in and out of frequency and disconnection? Do they appear hydrated? The adrenal system

gives us the great opportunity to thrive. And every belief that is held within our system regarding being alive in this body on this planet at this juncture of time and space is felt and held here. Take another moment to invite your adrenal system to show you through imagery, visual signs, or symbols, any wisdom. Any information and intelligence that's' held here. It is all within your DNA.

∞ Now invite in the clearing, the letting go, the detoxification of all patterns, images, and beliefs around survival, struggle ... perceived or actual through this current life and then down through your family lineage on both the male and female lines. All experiences, struggles, strife, battle. All the battles won or lost. Letting go of the patterns of stress, fatigue, and deep exhaustion seep out from the adrenal system, allowing it to be transmuted by the elements and your sacred geometry.

∞ Allow that nourishment to come into the adrenal system in golden light for deep rejuvenation, allowing the adrenals to fully activate with the purity and power of the life force at the core of Mother Earth. Letting this golden amber light ignite in the center of each adrenal and move outward spherically in waves, waves that ebb and flow and continue to pulsate activations by the life force into the very core of your DNA.

∞ With each breath, feel yourself being supported and connected to Gaia, Mother Earth. Feel the safety and warmth of her dear embrace. Repeat the intention three times either silently or aloud: "I am a free soveriegn being of light. My energy is fully my own."

∞ From this moment forward. Seven generations forward, seven generations back. Purity and power are yours.

DETOX THE ADRENALS – SACRED GEOMETRY

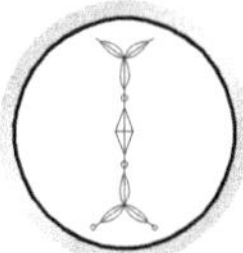

MAJOR ARCHETYPE

DETOX THE ADRENALS SACRED GEOMETRY

This intentional and original sacred geometric design depicts the adrenal glands connected by a tri-petaled flower and central connecting diamond, allowing the glands to release the energetic and cellular density and debris to open a flow of amber light and life force from the Earth.

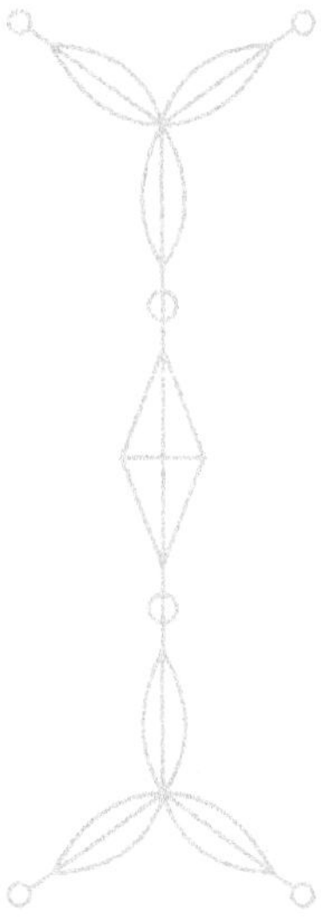

DETOX THE ADRENALS – NUTRITION

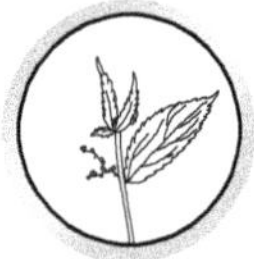

MAJOR ARCHETYPE

NETTLES

Nettles are so prolific they are often considered a weed; good thing we love and support this nutritious green ally and we hope you will grow to love it too. This plant is so packed with essential nutrients that consuming half a cup of fresh nettles per day will meet many of the daily vitamin requirements: vitamins A, C, and K, calcium, magnesium, iron, and more.

Nettles also are diuretic and extremely beneficial for detoxing the adrenals and kidneys, increasing urine production and eliminating toxic cellular debris and other waste (Tahri et al., 2000). We recommend making a hot or cold infusion of the leaves and drinking one cup three times per day. See Appendix B for instructions on how to make the infusion.

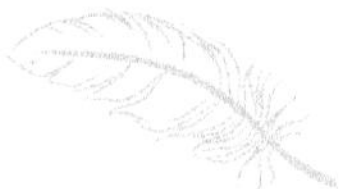

Harvest a fresh bunch of spring nettles, making sure to wear gloves, and add them into your favorite soup in the place of spinach or kale, for the detox and diuretic properties.

MINOR ARCHETYPES

Dandelion

Dandelion greens are another nutritious and lovely weed loaded with fiber, minerals, and vitamins. Dandelion's diuretic properties will decrease excess fluid in the body enhancing detoxification and weight loss. This potassium rich plant stimulates the adrenals and kidneys to remove toxins via urinary output and is especially helpful for ridding the body of environmental toxin exposure (Clare, Conroy, & Spelman, 2009).

Marsh

Marsh samphire is a succulent saltwater plant in the parsley family high in vitamins, minerals, and antioxidants. Its potent diuretic nature stimulates toxic release from the adrenal system, regulates blood pressure, and decreases systemic inflammation. It's a tasty asparagus cousin and can be eaten raw or lightly steamed with salt, pepper, and lemon.

DETOX THE ADRENALS – DISCOVERY DIVE – DETOXING FEAR

This Discovery Dive will assist you in releasing genetic fears held within your DNA to free you to fully experience and express your life force in the myriad of manners that your heart, soul, and spirit long to in this lifetime. Oftentimes, we do not realize we are frozen in certain ways, whether it is from having the fullness of health, the depth of relationships and intimacy, the profession we have always dreamt of, and so on. Our systems become so complacent and comfortable in the status quo that we start to believe that is all there is. And yet, somewhere there is and has always been a voice within you, no matter how vociferous or quiet, that knows there is more.

Your adrenal organs have held the remembrance of fear, anxiety, violence, scarcity, slavery, limitation, desperation, isolation, extremes in all manifestations of the human experience: hot, cold, control, constriction, addiction, movement, overwork, and stress and trauma in all other forms ... AND this system is also your superhero power pack to an infinite amount of life force and vitality, freedom, and strength. You are unlocking the vitality in each moment of this journey together.

So, let's dive in!

We invite you to settle into your sacred space and the altar you created for your journey of transformation. Choose an element or two from the Freedom Photon Wheel, in particular an essential oil or crystal to anchor and deepen the process. Invite your intention for the highest level of graceful release of what no longer serves you to free your being, your life force, and your light.

Do I feel safe? Do I belong here?

On this planet? In this body? In my family of origin?

Do I feel fully free? How and how not?

Do I show up fully for myself? Or do I show up more fully for others? How so?

What stops me from living the most dynamic life possible?

Do I feel enslaved? To what or who? My spouse, children, parents, employer, government, the Divine? All are possible. And often, at the core level we experience some combination therein, even to the Divine. When we offer our lives to service of the greater god, that too can also feel constrictive and unfulfilling if we are not in balance.

Does it feel safe to consistently live fully empowered? Or is it more comfortable to stay quiet, small, and sick? If it is the latter, who in my family of origin or current circle feels threatened if I shine as brightly and beautifully as I can?

Here's a big one!! Do I breathe fully and from my lower belly or do I take shallow breaths from my upper chest? When we breathe fully and deeply, we cannot be anxious or afraid!

Do I feel safe in my body? Is there any place that feels more vulnerable than another in your body? How and why?

What were my parents or grandparents most afraid of? What am I REALLY afraid of? What fears am I ready to fully let go of?

What would it be to live a life free from exhaustion? What would my life look like if I did not feel pulled by those in my family, work, or other relationships? What would my life look like if I put my own needs first and foremost? What would it be like to live my life feeling FULLY FREE and ALIVE?

Take the time to sketch or jot down any descriptive words or thoughts as they come to you … THIS is a crucial step in creating the runway for your new self to launch from!

FREEDOM PHOTON WHEEL™

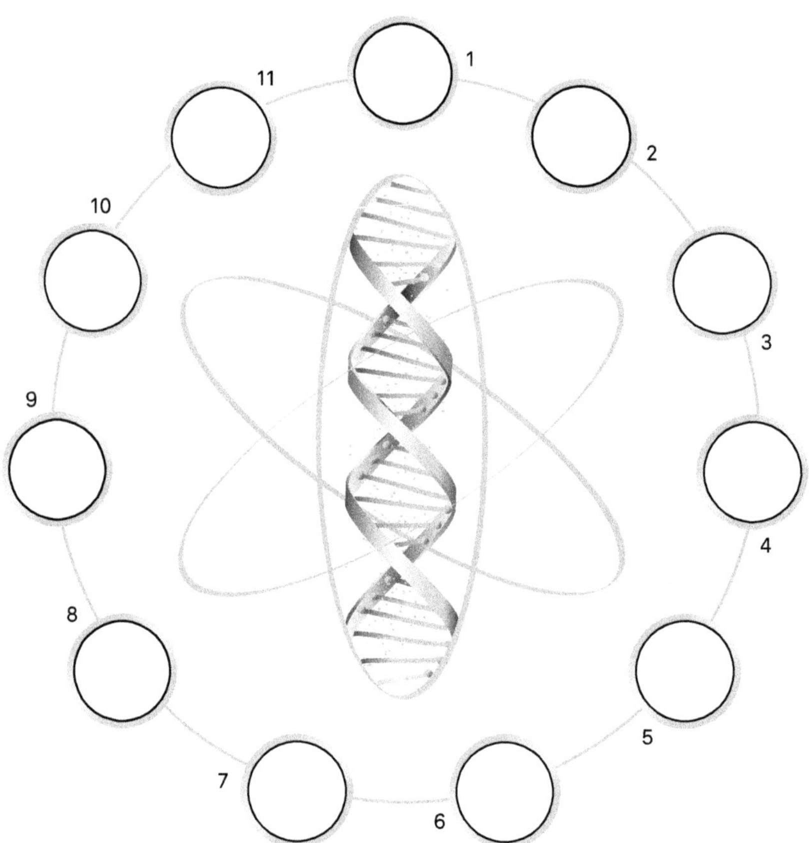

DETOX THE ADRENALS
YOUR PERSONAL FREEDOM PHOTON RITUAL

Moon Phase

It is best to perform your ritual when the moon is waning from the full moon to the new moon, to align with the phase. However, the power of your intention and momentum is key so if you are inspired at another time, go for it.

Intention

"I release all energy of constriction and limitation through my genetic lineage that binds any level of my essence and life force from experiencing full sovereignty as a divine being of light. "

Select, Align, and Activate

Select your interventions according to the instructions in Chapter Five. Inhale and apply your chosen essential oil for 30–45 seconds. Use your botanical tincture or tea as directed. You may also listen to the meditation and use the mudra from this chapter while attuning your FPW.

Affirm

Divine Consciousness, assist me in releasing and dissolving (see below) of all that I have carried through my lineage, my mother and father bloodline, so that I allow the fullest experience of my own life force, sustainable energy, and vitality.

Release

Exhaustion. Overdoing. Struggle. Scarcity. Limitation. Slavery. Abuse (of self and others). Fear. Anxiety.

NOURISH THE ADRENALS

The adrenal system, like all others, craves a deep amount of nourishment. We are quickly reminded when self-care in this regard is neglected. This system is one of the most sensitive and can dip back into previous patterns easily if we slip our consistent healthy habits. Conversely the adrenal system can access unlimited resources of energy and power.

This speaks to elements of fire and water that infuse the adrenals with the needed energy for balance and optimization. This potential can be accessed by cultivating a habitual practice of intentional "earthing" – connecting with the life force of the Earth to bathe the adrenals with the amber light restoring their golden essence and vitality. Just as we are constantly shifting and changing on our own journey of healing, Mother Earth is constantly changing, upgrading her frequency during this time of great shift. By inviting this practice in daily you can continuously nourish the adrenals to invigorate and recalibrate your energy.

The adrenal system holds all the collective "fight or flight" based trauma from time immemorial. This often-forgotten system of the body is key to transform personal and planetary consciousness related to war, persecution, abuse, and slavery. It is only through the practice of loving ourselves unconditionally and honoring our commitment and connection to the Earth and each other, that we will sustainably heal and transform our lives to our grandest vision. We must also acknowledge the primary conflict held in the adrenals, to live or to die. To live fully, we need to learn to love our bodies, our home of Mother Earth, and that we incarnated into our families of origin for a very specific environment and purpose for the growth of our soul.

ADRENAL NOURISH FREEDOM PHOTON WHEEL

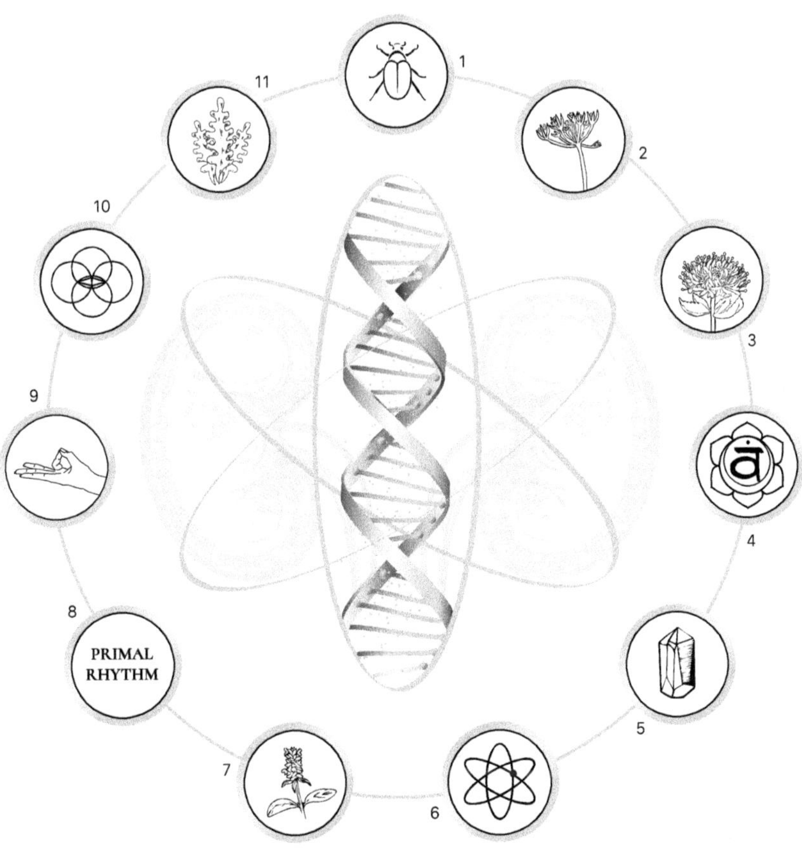

1 Alchemy Animal: Scarab Beetle
2 Aromatherapy: Carrot Seed
3 Botanical: Rhodiola
4 Light Wheel: Svadhisthana
5 Crystal: Fluorite
6 Photon Vibration
7 Flower or Gem Essence: Self Heal
8 Intention: Primal Rhythm
9 Meditation Mudra: Jala
10 Sacred Geometry
11 Nutrition: Sea Lettuce

ADRENAL NOURISH INFINITY INFLUENCERS

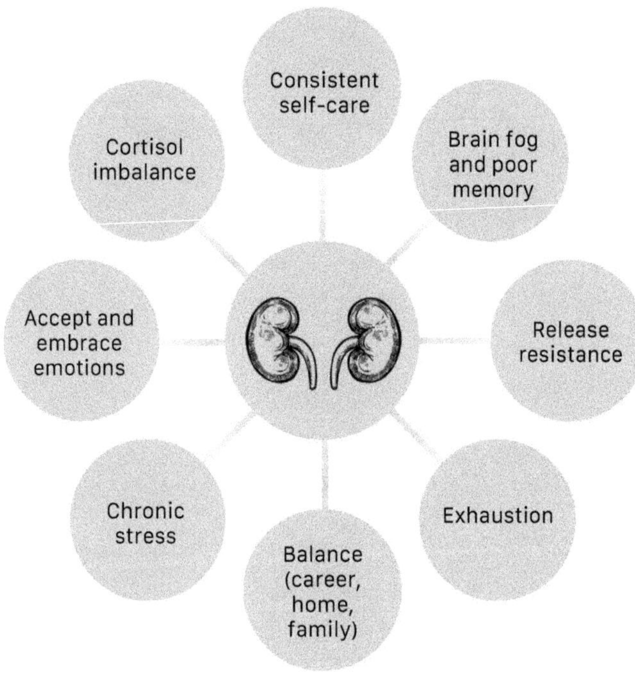

NOURISH THE ADRENALS – ALCHEMY ANIMALS

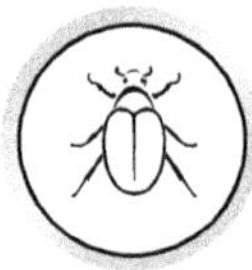

The nourish alchemy animals of the adrenals are your connection to the mystical realm. They help you to embrace and infuse the healing alchemy of the magical and supernatural: mystery, metaphysics, imagination, spirituality, and power.

MAJOR ARCHETYPE

SCARAB BEETLE

The ancient scarab beetle is well known as an insect or creature of metamorphosis and transformation. The scarab empowers and nourishes the adrenal gland with determination and resilience fueling the body and the spirit. Did you know that the scarabs beetle has super strength and can lift to 600 times its weight? Amazing! This is the energy you want to envision and take to the core of your being during your meditations and to your sacred altar. The unlimited strength of the scarab combines both elements of the Earth, grounding you, and the element of Air connecting to the spiritual realm.

Physically the scarab allows you to hone or tune with a keen sense into what your body needs. You can sense more easily when the cells and the DNA are out of alignment with your body and its life force, facilitating renewal.

Creature Connection: "Magic lives in me and vibrates through every cell of my being."

MINOR ARCHETYPES

Manatee

The manatee is a wonderful water creature aligning the adrenals deeper to your etheric body, human energy field, or aura. In stages of fatigue the etheric body is often depleted. The manatee's message is to slow down and swim through the waters of life with ease. Allow any emotions or feelings that have been affecting your etheric body to "wash off your back." It's now time to leave all the stagnant energy you have been carrying around in your old suitcase at the front door and start your new life adventure with trust and ease.

Creature Connection: "I sail through the waters of life with ease. I call out to you, Manatee, to carry away my burdens and refill each layer of my body with spirit."

Luna Moth

The luna moth is one of the most mystical alchemy animals, with the reminder to live each day to the fullest, enjoy each second. It has a very short life span and only lives as a winged adult for ten days. The moth message is to let go of the past, to stand grounded in the present moment, and to have your eyes open to the unknown future ahead. Feel the freedom of this journey towards the light of your futures with a new sense of determination. Stay true and strong on the continued quest to fulfill your dreams with a renewed vigor.

Creature Connection: "I call upon the winged beauty of the luna moth to surround my body with the light. I am free to live in the present. I embrace fully with excitement the future and the unknown."

NOURISH THE ADRENALS – AROMATHERAPY

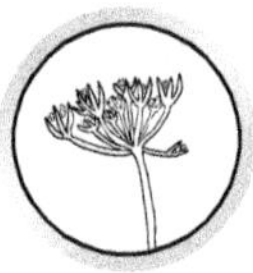

MAJOR ARCHETYPE

CARROT SEED – *DAUCUS CAROTA*

Part extracted: Seed

Core properties: antiseptic, carminative, cytophylactic, depurative, diuretic, emmenagogue, hepatic, stimulant, tonic, and vermifuge
Safety: nontoxic, nonirritant

Carrot seed medicine nourishes on multiple levels. It warms, fills, soothes, stimulates, and is regenerative to our physical, mental, emotional, and spiritual aspects. It assists us to open our Earth connection and receive the richness of energy, life force, and abundance that's held there. It activates the meridian points and energy chakras or light wheels to receive more energy and more light. It vibrates at golden frequency to support, stabilize, and regenerate organ and glandular function. Carrot seed has a fiery strength, and yet fluidity about it, which makes it a unique and excellent choice for filling the adrenal system with much needed energy. Its expansive aroma and energy can permeate some of the deepest places of fatigue within. This type of exhaustion is more than physical, and even emotional, but a soul level weariness that many beings are currently experiencing. Carrot seed medicine weaves its potent alchemy through all aspects of our existence to restore, reunite, and revitalize.

It stimulates liver cells and skin cells and fills the adrenals with comfort, strength, and hydration. Its rich, earthy, and voluminous aroma opens the heart, the sacral center, while expanding the Earth connection to reconnect to our center. It supports the alignment of the hara to the Earth connection, recalibrating the lower chakras.

A wondrous beauty oil, carrot is deeply nutritive. It enriches the skin and hair and adds moisture, connecting us to our infinite source of beauty from the inside out.

Nourish the Adrenals – Carrot Seed Beauty Serum

∞ 3 drops Carrot Seed essential oil (*Daucus carota*)
∞ 2 drops Geranium essential oil (*Pelargonium graveolens*)
∞ 3 drops of Sandalwood essential oil (*Santalum austrocaledonicum*)
∞ 2 drops Rose otto essential oil (*Rosa damascena*)
∞ 2 drops Neroli essential oil (*Citrus aurantium var. amara*)
∞ 15 ml Rosehip seed oil
∞ 15 ml Apricot seed oil

Essential oils and plant oils derived from the seed offer deeply nutritive plant medicine in the form of vitamins, minerals, bioflavonoids. Blend all ingredients together, shake and infuse with your intention for your inner beauty to shine. Add this to your morning and evening skincare routine. After cleansing while your skin is still warm and your cells are open, apply a few drops of the serum before you add your face cream.

MINOR ARCHETYPES

Bergamot – *Citrus bergamia*

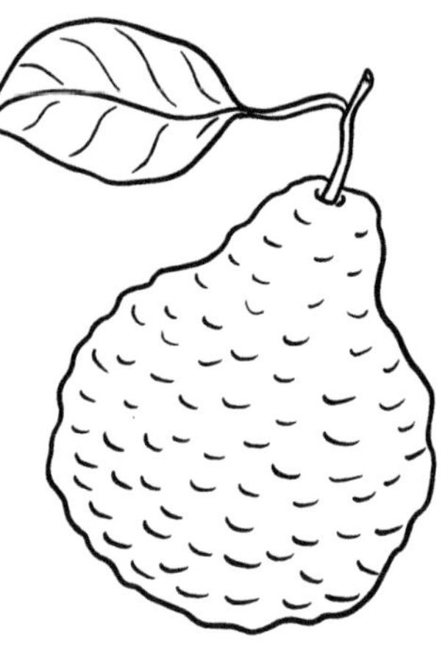

Part extracted: Peel

Core Properties: Calmative, antispasmodic, carminative, and digestive stimulant, antidepressive, soporific, anti-inflammatory, antiseptic
Safety: nontoxic, potential irritant and sensitizer, phototoxic

Ruled by the sun, the aroma of bergamot is bright and citrus spicy. Its medicine lifts, opens, and expands the spirit with a zest for life. Bergamot brings this energy through the cells and the bloodlines where there is patterning of a depressive nature. The spirit of bergamot beckons you to wake up, knowing there are many levels of sleeping.

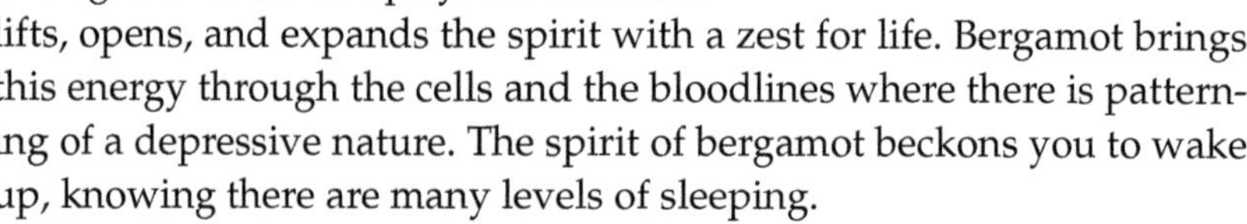

This oil gently coaxes the places of resistance within to let go and let the breath of spirit within. It infuses a playful and free nature into those that feel they must constantly be in the trenches and hardness of life.

Bergamot connects the adrenal glands with the joy and ease that life can offer, lifting and transmuting the heavy energy of overdoing, overwhelm, and releasing the strain of chronic stress through the cellular consciousness and DNA.

Bergamot can bring ease to a heavy heart and mind, replacing it with ripples of pleasure and laughter. This bright oil is an excellent choice for those affected by SAD (seasonal affective disorder) because of its close link to the sun. From a cosmic perspective, it links us with the Great Central Sun, opening us to greater universal and cosmic consciousness, helping us to evolve our understanding of the vastness of light and creation that we hold at our fingertips.

Detox the Adrenals – Bergamot Bright Energy Mist

- ∞ 8 drops of Bergamot essential oil (*Citrus bergamia*)
- ∞ 4 drops of Mandarin essential oil (*Citrus reticulata*)
- ∞ 2 drops Carrot Seed essential oil (*Daucus carota*)
- ∞ 2 drops organic Ylang Ylang essential oil (*Cananga odorata superior extra*)

Blend into 30 ml distilled water and shake well before use. Mist your home or other personal space to lift and brighten the energy and your outlook on life.

Myrrh – *Commiphora myrrha*

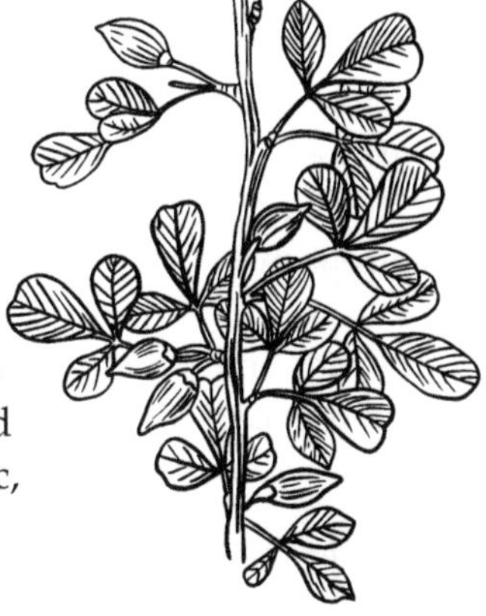

Part extracted: Resin

Core properties: anti-catarrhal, anti-inflammatory, antimicrobial, antiphlogistic, antiseptic, astringent, balsamic, carminative, cicatrisant, emmenagogue, expectorant, fungicidal, sedative, digestive and pulmonary stimulant, stomachic, tonic, vulnerary
Safety: nontoxic, nonirritant

Myrrh whispers the memory of ancient Earth and healing arts. The essential oil distilled from the resin of the plant with its mystical aroma seeps into places of trauma, held in the subconscious, surrounding them, with its universal understanding of pain. Pain from the human perspective, helping us to break up the energetic patterns and calcified energy in the trauma or energy blocks. It helps to clear this distortion and separation.

Myrrh connects and communes with us through this deep acceptance for all that we have experienced on our journey. Bringing this through the DNA and our mother and father bloodlines, enveloping the places of deep sadness, loss, pain, and grief with the loving embrace of universal compassion, transforming some of the darkest places of loss held in the collective consciousness of humanity.

With an affinity for healing on multiple levels, myrrh is beneficial for gum disease, skin afflictions, bronchial conditions, and has the nature of bringing peace to all areas of inflammation in our bodies and spirits. Quelling past disappointment, loss, and the pain of moving forward without those loved ones we have lost along our way.

Myrrh medicine is an oil that honors birth and death and the spiritual transformation that involves both. Myrrh gently and powerfully encourages the adrenal system to let go of the memories of loss, pain, guilt, shame, betrayal, and violence as well as constriction. It brings understanding that the past has been an evolutionary process of transcendence. Myrrh medicine invites us to dissolve the old to birth the new.

Rooted in religion and spiritual tradition through millennia, myrrh offers an expansive energy of tranquility and acceptance of the self through the trials and tribulations of life.

Nourish the Adrenals – Myrrh Rebirthing Oil

∞ 7 drops of Myrrh essential oil (*Commiphora myrrha*)
∞ 3 drops of Frankincense essential oil (*Boswellia carterii*)
∞ 2 drops of Spikenard essential oil (*Nardostachys jatamansi*)
∞ 3 drops of Vetiver essential oil (*Vetiveria zizanioides*)

Blend into one tablespoon of coconut oil and anoint as you would a perfume as part of your intention to let go and rebirth anew.

ESSENTIAL OIL ADDITIONS

∞ Cedarwood – *Cedrus atlantica*

ADRENAL NOURISH AROMATHERAPY
DNA BLUEPRINT BENEFITS

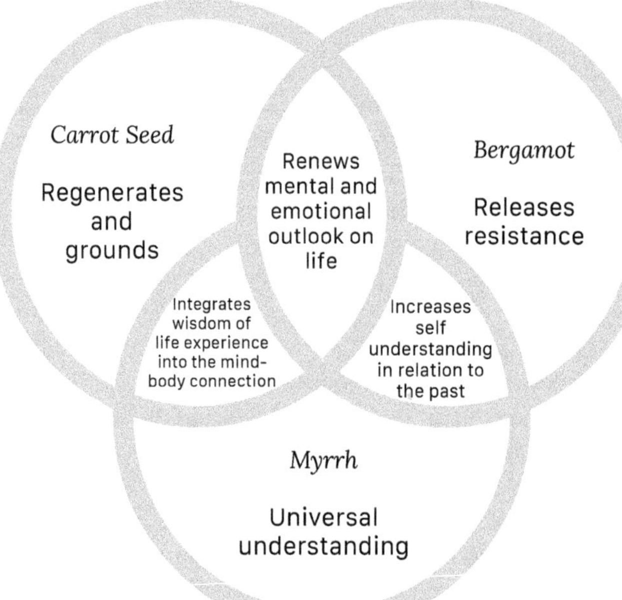

NOURISH THE ADRENALS – BOTANICAL MEDICINE

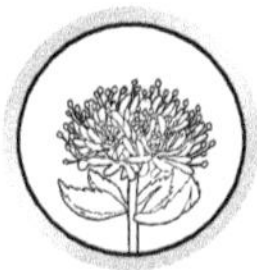

MAJOR ARCHETYPE

RHODIOLA – *Rhodiola rosea*

Part used: Root

Have you been feeling burned out? Rhodiola is the botanical for you. This adaptogen nourishes the adrenals, resisting stress, increasing energy, and decreasing brain fog or mental fatigue. If you have been working at a desk job, studying or sitting for long periods of time, rhodiola will get you up and functioning efficiently again. Rhodiola works in conjunction with the nervous system providing a protective effect for neurotransmitters (especially dopamine and serotonin) enhancing both short term and long-term memory. This powerful antioxidant is also cardioprotective and has been studied for its use with stress induced cardiac events.

Stress has been linked to many inflammatory cellular dysfunctions: depression, neurodegenerative diseases, peripheral inflammation, autoimmune diseases, and is anticarcinogenic. Rhodiola reduces the inflammatory marker, C-reactive protein, known for increasing oxidative stress and inducing DNA damage. We like to think of rhodiola as the "queen stress protector" providing a defensive barrier against harmful cells and other inflammatory agents.

The dazzling yellow flower of rhodiola shouts out, "I am happy and filled with energy." It nourishes the second and third light wheels providing energy as well as personal power. Use this herb anytime you are needing support physically, cleaning the house, or running a race, or are emotionally under periods of undue stress. Let the rhodiola botanical diva support and nourish every mitochondrial cell with full power.

Nourish the Adrenals – Rhodiola Physical Uses

Nourish: Harmonizes mitochondrial DNA – improving energy
Adrenal System: Lowers cortisol, increases energy, and improves body's resistance to stress
Cardiovascular System: Antioxidant and cardioprotective
Nervous System: Depression, improves cognitive function, reduces mental fatigue, and protects neurotransmitters
Musculoskeletal System: Headaches
Immune System: Improves thymus function and T cells
Endocrine: Improves thyroid function, supports metabolism, weight loss, and burns fat
Reproductive: Fertility and stamina

Nourish the Adrenals – Rhodiola Emotional Uses

Embracing pleasure and relaxation
Discharging worry and troubled thoughts
Strength for tragic situations in states of panic and fear

Nourish the Adrenals – Rhodiola Energetic Uses

Releases DNA family lineage of mental disorders
Reconnects the body and spirit in union after trauma
Cradles the energy of the sun for energy strength

Nourish the Adrenals – Rhodiola Dosage

Decoction: Steep 1 tablespoon Rhodiola in 236 ml of hot water for 15 minutes – drink one cup 3–6x/day
Tincture: 60 drops 3x/day

Nourish the Adrenals – Rhodiola Cautions and Contraindications

None known

Nourish the Adrenals – Rhodiola Freedom to Soar Honey

Ingredients:
28 g Rhodiola – *Rhodiola rosea*
28 g Schisandra – *Schisandra chinensis*
8 g Ginger root – *Zingiber officinale*

Honey Dosage: 1 tablespoon 3x/day
See Appendix B on how to make a medicinal honey

MINOR ARCHETYPES

Devil's Club – *Oplopanax horridus*

Parts Used: Root and lower stem bark

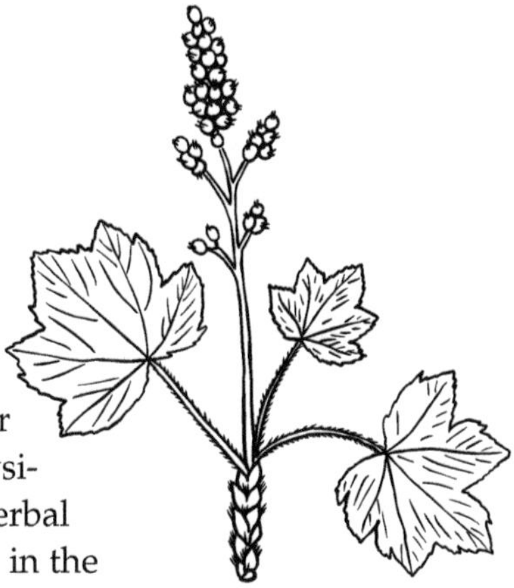

Devil's club is a powerful adrenal nourishing botanical used for exhaustion and is especially useful for debilitating fatigue from a painful physical or emotional illness. Turn to this herbal adaptogenic ally when your vitality is in the toilet, so low you can barely get out of bed in the morning. It's also a dynamic herb to add to immune boosting formulas for both acute and chronic illnesses.

If you have ever harvested or seen devil's club in the forest, you'll know it has large thorns, and caution as well as gloves must be used when harvesting. So, what do these spikes symbolize? These spikes summon your inner and ancient tribal warrior providing a coat of armor for protection. Invoke oplopanax when you need to learn new energetic skills to protect yourself in challenging and oppressive situations.

The genetic history of devil's club is very diverse and has been used by indigenous cultures spiritually and medicinally. When using or harvesting this plant call upon your elders and the ancient wisdom of magic within your DNA for strength and healing. Call upon the power of this ally for telomere lengthening and rejuvenation of the DNA.

Nourish the Adrenals – Devil's Club Physical Uses

Nourish: Antiaging, telomere elongation, and adrenal burnout
Adrenal System: Mental and physical exhaustion
Cardiovascular System: Blood purification and cardiovascular disease
Nervous System: Mental health – loss of reality
Endocrine System: Appetite stimulant, diabetes
Reproductive System: Fertility
Digestive System: Bitter digestive – constipation
Gallbladder: Gallstones
Immune System: Colds and flu respiratory support, Anticarcinogenic, and autoimmune conditions
Musculoskeletal System: Anti-inflammatory and analgesic
Integumentary System: Acne and dandruff – topical wash

Nourish the Adrenals – Devil's Club Emotional Uses

The strength of a warrior to accomplish anything
Lift the weight of the world off your back
Provides support and comfort during stress

Nourish the Adrenals – Devil's Club Energetic Uses

Purification ceremonies – add to an amulet or fire
Travel into the transcendent realms
Heal the world form karmic war and destruction

Nourish the Adrenals – Devil's Club Dosage

Infusion: 1 tablespoon of Devil's Club per cup of water, infused for 22 minutes. Drink 1–3 cups/day
Tincture: 44 drops 2x/day
Topical: Steam bath, poultice for inflammation and pain

Nourish the Adrenals – Devil's Club Cautions

Berries are poisonous
Pregnancy
Monitor with blood sugar conditions

Nourish the Adrenals – Devil's Club Elixir Freedom of the Warrior

1 part Devil's Club – *Oplopanax horridus*
½ part Hawthorn berries – *Crataegus monogyna*
½ part Motherwort – *Leonurus cardiaca*
¼ Red Raspberry leaf – *Rubus idaeus*
¼ part Rose Petals – *Rosa damascena*
Honey or Glycerite
Alcohol of choice
Combine all ingredients
Dosage: 1T 3x/day
See Appendix B on how to make an elixir.

Tulsi – *Ocimum tenuiflorum*

Parts Used: Leaf and flower

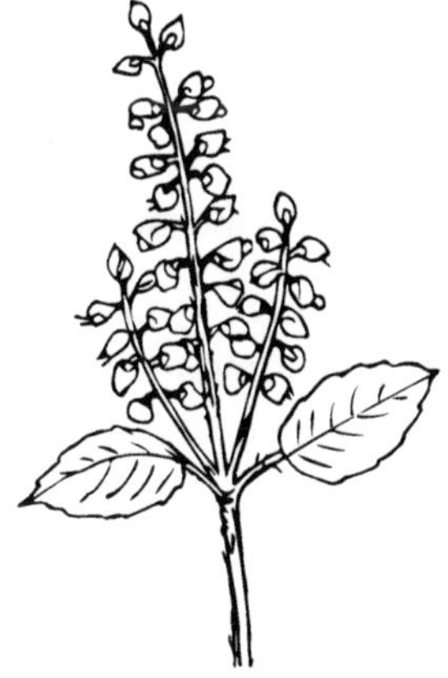

Tulsi, holy basil, is a majestic ayurvedic botanical and symbol of Hinduism. It's most used for calming and soothing the nervous system due to its high flavonoid content, benefiting the body during times of chronic stress. Tulsi is the champion adaptogen helping the body to deal with all levels of stress and adrenal fatigue. Tulsi has a positive physical effect on the body both physically and mentally.

Tulsi is also an environmental protectant assisting the body in detoxing pollutants and heavy metals, decreasing the overall toxic load. This botanical ally releases mental stress built upon the fears and anxiety by which environmental toxins could be affecting the body, often called MCS, multiple chemical sensitivity.

Emotionally tulsi opens the heart and mind encouraging gratitude for life and living things. It encourages us to appreciate the little things in life like a child seeing a butterfly for the first time: awe, love, excitement, and appreciation. It also creates space in your life to live without attachments and to live each moment with both feet in the present.

Nourish the Adrenals – Tulsi Physical Uses

Nourish: Reduces adrenal stress and balances cortisol
Adrenal System: Alterative, exhaustion, lowers stress
Cardiovascular System: Cardiotonic
Nervous System: Depression, anxiety, memory
Endocrine System: Diabetes and blood sugar balancing
Reproductive System: Balances hormones
Respiratory System: Congestion, stuffy nose, and sinus pressure
Digestive System: Carminative, demulcent
Immune System: Antiviral, antifungal, immunomodulator cancer prevention, diaphoretic, and natural antibiotic
Musculoskeletal System: Headaches and migraines, analgesic
Integumentary System: Acne and skin infections

Nourish the Adrenals – Tulsi Emotional Uses

Calming in times of emotional distress
Grounding to the Earth when emotionally distanced
Harmony and balance, clearing stuck emotions

Nourish the Adrenals – Tulsi Energetic Uses

Balances the electromagnetic forces of the light wheels
Prosperity and abundance abounds
Devotion and gratitude to spirit and the planet

Nourish the Adrenals – Tulsi Dosage

Infusion: Steep 7 g dried Tulsi in 1 liter of water. Steep for 30 minutes to 6 hours. The longer steeped, the more potent the medicine will be. Strain and drink at room temperature or slowly reheat without boiling.
Can be stored in the refrigerator for 24–48 hours.
Tincture: 60 drops 3x/day

Nourish the Adrenals – Tulsi Cautions and Contraindications

Pregnancy

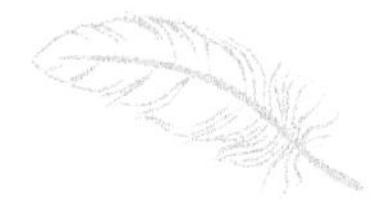

Nourish the Adrenals – Tulsi Mocktail Freedom to Dance like a Diva

Ingredients:
15 ml Tulsi – *Ocimum tenuiflorum* liquid extract
8 oz. Sparkling Mineral Water
Dash of sweetener – optional
Mix all ingredients together and have a dance party to celebrate life!
Let your inner Diva shine!

BOTANICAL ADDITIONS

- ∞ Goji Berry – *Lycium barbarum*
- ∞ Lion's Mane – *Hericium erinaceus*
- ∞ Calendula – *Calendula officinalis*

ADRENAL NOURISH BOTANICAL MEDICINE
DNA BLUEPRINT BENEFITS

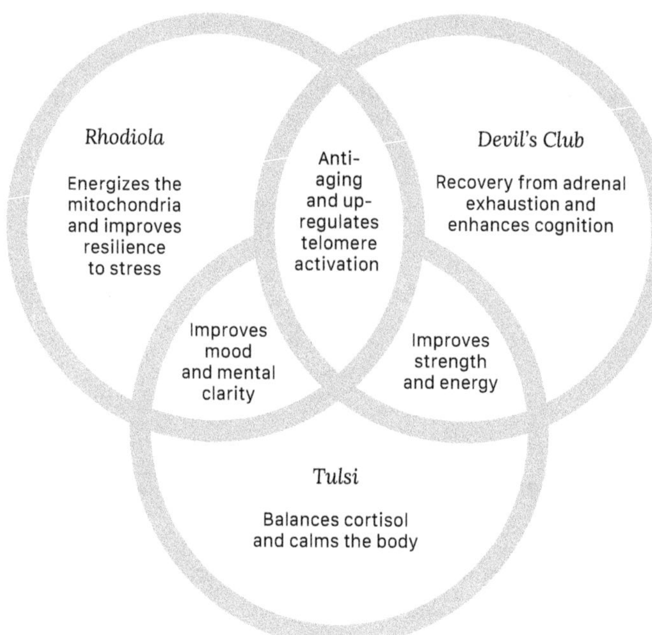

NOURISH THE ADRENALS – LIGHT WHEELS

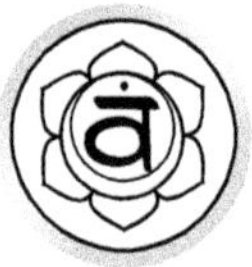

LIGHT WHEELS

MAJOR ARCHETYPE

THE 2nd LIGHT WHEEL, SVADHISTHANA

Svadhisthana is the sacral light wheel and connects the seat of sexuality with the heart. This light wheel aligns with the water element creating a flow of sexual energy up from the base to the heart. Svadhisthana releases walls of pain or hurt you may have put up around you as a defense mechanism from sexual trauma or violence. When this light wheel is activated you will feel the power of true self-expression and intimacy. It is time to release any thoughts or patterns you may have of embarrassment and shame related to your sexuality.

The second light wheel nourishes your creativity and aligns you with inner euphoria. We suggest making a list of things in your life that are creative – past, present, and future – and what you can do to take action. It brings in the life force of the sixth light wheel of inspiration to fuel your creative endeavors. Some ideas of creative expression: dance, music, writing, painting, drawing, cooking, gardening, and sex – anything your heart desires.

MINOR ARCHETYPES

∞ The 8th light wheel, Pancaka

Pancaka is the Soul Star light wheel joining your creative outlet with the community of the planet. It opens a doorway of compassion for all living creatures and the knowledge that we are one, we all come from the same source, one of love. It extinguishes all planetary hate, racism, sexism, bigotry, and violence. You are now able to see the light in everyone you meet.

COLORS

MAJOR ARCHETYPE

TERRACOTTA

Terracotta is the color of nature and embodies a deeper connection to it. If you are attracted to this color, it is time to put on those hiking boots and hit the trails. This is a color to wear or have in your surroundings if you are looking for new love or nurturing a new relationship. The warmth of this color will help you express your true feelings.

SOUND

∞ LAM

Lam is the deep note of C sounding like "larm." Use this sound frequency and vibration by either playing a recording – or by saying it aloud in repetition for five or ten minutes. You can also use it in conjunction with nourishing the adrenals mudra and meditation for extra attunement. Lam helps ground deep into the center of the Earth and feel its embrace.

NOURISH THE ADRENALS – CRYSTALS AND STONES

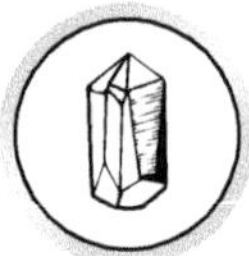

MAJOR ARCHETYPE

FLUORITE

Fluorite assists in creating fundamental change in the way the physical body accepts the life force. Fluorite is excellent for reducing anxiety, facilitating peace, and breaking free from the third dimensional matrix of fear and control. Fluorite soothes the nerves and helps to activate the parasympathetic nervous system for the body to be able to relax and realign with the Earth, bringing balance to the lower chakras. The calming nature of this crystal is also helpful to dissipate anxiety, frenetic behavior, and sexual angst. This crystal offers potent medicine at the cellular level, particularly where there is a high level of toxins and systemic inflammation. With its varied colors, fluorite lends itself to the unification of the higher and lower aspects of being, helping to balance the auric field.

MINOR ARCHETYPE

∞ Jasper

Jasper assists in releasing fears, both conscious and those hidden within the subconscious. This crystal brings healing to the masculine aspects with and through the father bloodline, particularly those connected to fear of not having enough money to support self and family. This crystal also brings strength to your will to live and thrive through the challenges that life offers, bringing vital energy up through the dantian to the adrenals. Jasper stimulates the thymus gland and helps to bolster immunity.

∞ Copper

Copper is a highly versatile element for healing. It helps to protect from radiation and advanced technological interference. Copper amplifies energy and strengthens the masculine aspect. It brings resilience and greater flexibility to the bones and tissue. It activates the electrical charge within the cells and brings alignment to the energy bodies and the hara line. Copper enhances all glandular functions. It also aligns the astral and physical body and balances emotions, lifting depressive energy and weakness to persevere in life.

NOURISH THE ADRENALS CRYSTAL GRID

Do this crystal attunement grid for 30 minutes as soon as you wake up in the morning. You may listen to music - drumming connecting to the native rhythm of the earth. Immediately after the treatment cleanse the crystals and stones. Drink a glass of Fluorite charged water throughout the day after this attunement. (See Appendix C)

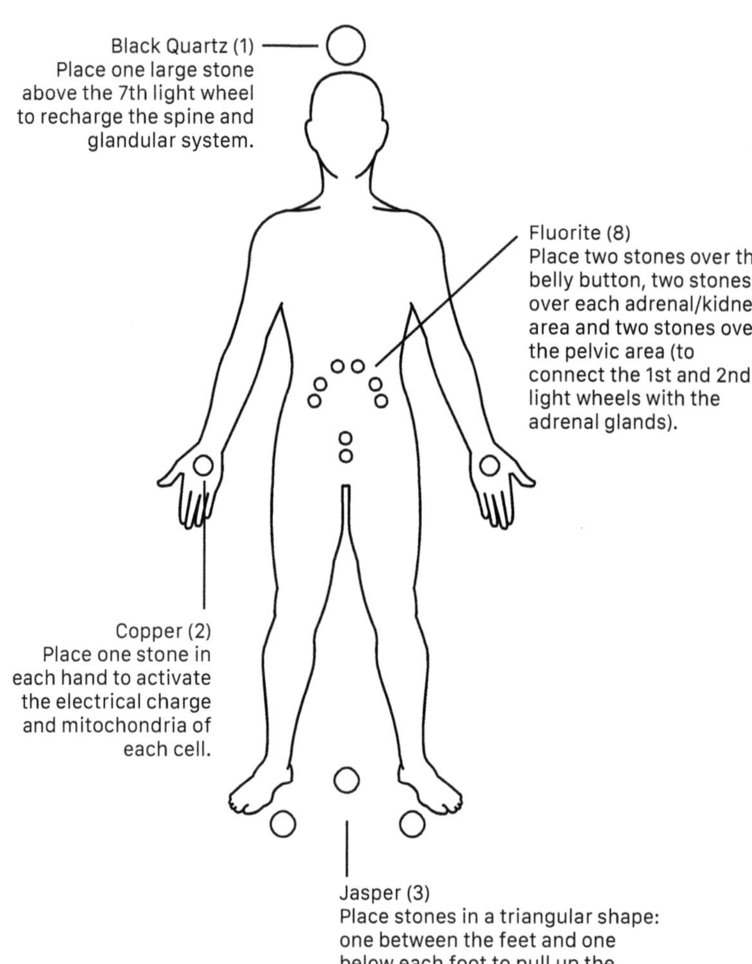

NOURISH THE ADRENALS – ENERGETIC AND VIBRATIONAL TECHNIQUES

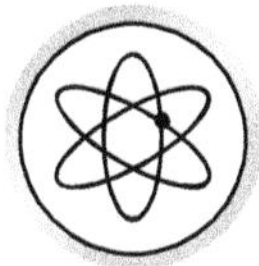

MAJOR ARCHETYPE

ADRENAL NOURISHING HYDROTHERAPY

- ∞ 4 drops of Carrot Seed essential oil (*Daucus carota*)
- ∞ 3 drops Bergamot essential oil (*Citrus bergamia*)
- ∞ 2 drops Sandalwood essential oil (*Santalum austrocaledonicum*)
- ∞ 2 drops Frankincense essential oil (*Boswellia carterii*)
- ∞ 10 drops Self Heal Flower Essence
- ∞ Fluorite Crystal (you can hold this while in a bath, or place it in the tub)

Add to a bath of warm water and soak for 20 minutes.

Nourish the Adrenals – Golden Light Visualization

Envision your adrenal glands as two glorious temples. The one on your right side represents your masculine aspect and connects into the DNA of your father bloodline. The one on your left represents your feminine aspect and holds all accesses to the DNA of your mother bloodline. Now invite in the golden light of divine consciousness to permeate each temple until it completely pulsates golden light. The liquid light continues to run through all your generations on each bloodline. You may feel a tingling sensation or even a lightness in your body: this is natural. Allow this golden light to charge all the levels of your auric field and cells until you sense your entire being is filled with the golden light of divine consciousness.

Nourish the Adrenals EOBT

Place one drop of carrot seed essential oil between the first two fingertips of the right hand, inhale deeply and tap the Kidney-3, Great Mountain Stream, Source point of the Kidney Meridian for 30 seconds with the intention of regenerating your entire being with vibrant energy.

Location: On the inside (medial aspect) of the ankle in the valley formed between the Achilles tendon and the prominence of bone that is the medial malleolus. Use your right hand to locate the point on the left ankle, and the left hand to locate the point on the right ankle. Place the flat of your fingers across the ankle with the fourth digit over the malleolus. The point will be under the second digit.

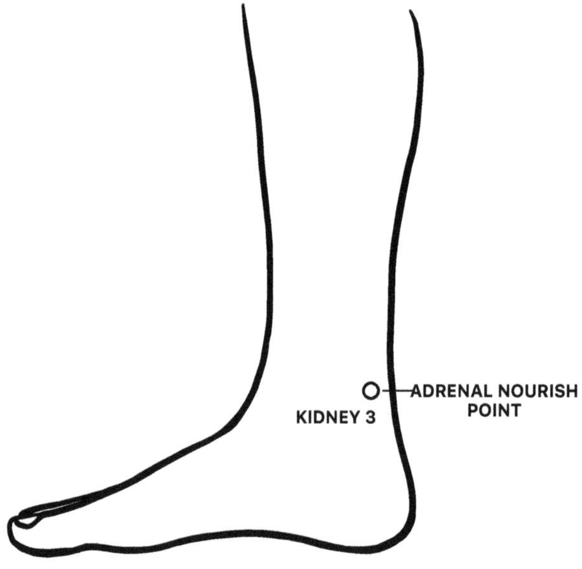

NOURISH THE ADRENALS – FLOWER AND GEM ESSENCES

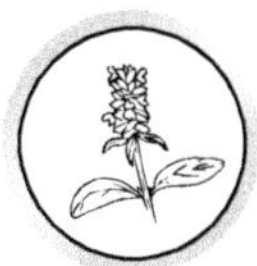

FLOWER ESSENCES

MAJOR ARCHETYPE

SELF HEAL

Self heal is a master healer in the realm of essences. It offers potent medicine to address deep trauma at the cellular level, nourishing the blood and bone marrow after deep release, particularly past life karmic aspects. Self heal brings healing through our genetic lineage, specifically current family dynamics with power struggles and sibling rivalry.

MINOR ARCHETYPES

Bergamot

Bergamot brings the energy of lightness, joy, and simplicity back into your life. It encourages authenticity and intimacy in friendships and love relationships. Invite bergamot essence medicine into your life when you feel depleted physically, disconnected from others, and drained by the responsibilities and expectations of your day-to-day life.

Bloodroot

Bloodroot offers the energy of strength and endurance. It is beneficial for clearing ancestral trauma where there has been an impurity of intention regarding control over others. This essence also helps to clear karmic ties to lower energies that have been allowed to influence decision making in relation to power and money.

GEM ESSENCE

MAJOR ARCHETYPE

TIGER'S EYE

Tiger's eye is helpful for sexual healing, sexual dysfunction, and connecting and opening the kundalini channel. It allows us to remember that juicy feeling of being in our physicality. It realigns the merkaba. Tiger's eye purifies the blood. Use externally on the third toe which activates and stabilizes the Earth connection. This essence elicits a sense of safety and strength in the body.

NOURISH THE ADRENALS – INTENTIONS AND AFFIRMATIONS

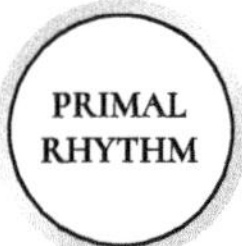

MAJOR ARCHETYPE

PRIMAL RHYTHM

MINOR ARCHETYPES

∞ My adrenal glands are nourished fully by each cell of my body
∞ I am grounded into the flow of life
∞ My connection to the Earth is circular and flowing

ADDITIONAL INTENTIONS

∞ In am in sync
∞ Every cell in my body is at ease and connected
∞ I am connected to the life force within
∞ I am nourished and full of life
∞ I am nourished by my deep connection to the Earth
∞ I am fluid

NOURISH THE ADRENALS – MEDITATION MUDRA

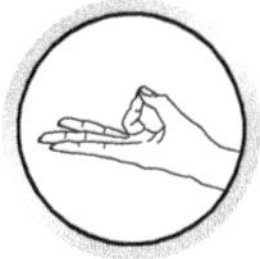

Jala Mudra

My heartbeat is one with the rhythm of the Earth.
I am fluid and flexible, floating in the river of life.

The Jala mudra is the gesture of water and connects you to the circulatory waters of the Earth, hydrating and nourishing the cells of the body. This mudra creates a nourishing wave moving through the adrenal glands, urinary system, reproductive system, and the bowel system, filling this lower chakra or physical bowel with light and nutrients for the DNA. This mudra aligns with the second chakra, Svadhisthana, and ignites hidden energy, inspiring sexual creativity. As you begin to use this mudra more frequently, you will notice how you are able to adapt more easily to life's situations with ease and grace.

Jala Mudra Alignment

1. Touch the tips of the little fingers of each hand with the thumb off the same hand.
2. Extend the other three fingers of each hand straight out.
3. In a relaxed seated position, rest the hands on top of the knees or thighs.
4. Take a deep breath, let your body relax.
5. You may now either do the meditation below or 10 minutes of *Water Breathing* (to access the water breathing technique please go to www.zenergymedicinals.com).
6. You may also use this mudra when you are seeking more fluid and flexible solutions to complex situations and nourish your body when it feels depleted physically and emotionally.

∞ To access the mudra meditation please go to www.zenergymedicinals.com

∞ Take a deep breath, inhaling your essential oil, relaxing the body, opening the heart, settling the mind.
∞ Hold the Jala mudra and take several breaths to align to the center of the Earth and the element of water. With each breath, feel the fluidity and flexibility of your body. Feel the water coursing through your system nourishing each cell and organ.
∞ Connect with the amber light of the core of Mother Earth, nourishing every cell and particle, restructuring within your cellular matrix.
∞ The light begins to change into gold and circling each adrenal gland with golden light revitalizing, recalibrating, and regenerating the adrenal system.
∞ Envision a golden elongated vertical infinity symbol coming down through the higher realms and all the levels of your auric field, down through the crown, the heart.
∞ The concentric point settles in the dantian while the bottom sphere moves down through the root, connecting in the core crystal.
∞ Envision the very top of the infinity symbol connected in from the cosmic realms of divine light, the concentric point and the dantian below your navel and the bottom ring connected into the core crystal of the Earth.
∞ Breathe in and allow the recalibration and vibration to lift within your energy field. We call forth the DNA infinity teams of light to ignite the cellular consciousness with this remembrance of freedom.
∞ Envision a horizontal, much smaller infinity symbol that comes in horizontally to the concentric point again, meeting at the dantian, but now each adrenal organ will be surrounded by the left and right sphere of the infinity sign.
∞ With each breath the lower body is bathed in soothing energy, nourishing the adrenal glands, the kidneys, and the bladder. Your lymphatic system is hydrated and opens to releasing toxins and assimilating all nourishments. Repeat the intention three times either silently or aloud: "My heartbeat is one with the rhythm of the Earth. I am fluid and flexible, floating in the river of life."
∞ And we call forth a purification into the DNA, into the mother and father bloodlines through each adrenal organ.
∞ Held in infinite protection in light within this symbol, the sacred geometric form, we call for a full disconnection and unwinding of all constriction around life force, freedom, prosperity, energy, self-mastery.
∞ Envision your adrenal organs pulsating with life force, with strength, with vigor, with renewed vibrancy.

- ∞ Continue to breathe in this light until you envision both the vertical and horizontal infinity symbols pulsating at the same frequency, same resonance of vitality and freedom.
- ∞ May all beings upon this great and vast planet free themselves from the past.
- ∞ Walk in the light within you from this moment forward with the full frequency of your freedom and vibrancy.

NOURISH THE ADRENALS – SACRED GEOMETRY

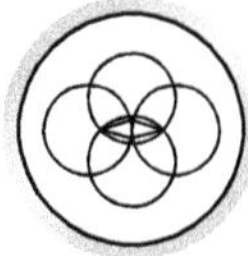

MAJOR ARCHETYPE

NOURISH THE ADRENALS SACRED GEOMETRY

In this intentional and original depiction of sacred geometry, the diamond light of the cosmic consciousness connects both adrenal glands, filling them with regenerative frequency of divine light and the energy of the fire element. The circular formations unite the energy of Heaven and Earth along with the elements of water to create a continuous circuit of nurturing connection.

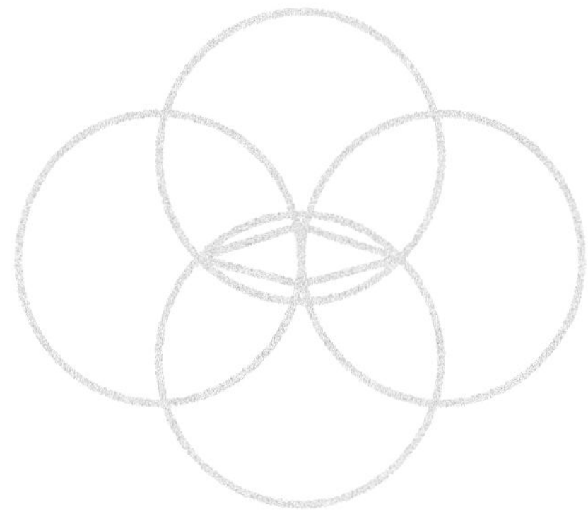

NOURISH THE ADRENALS – NUTRITION

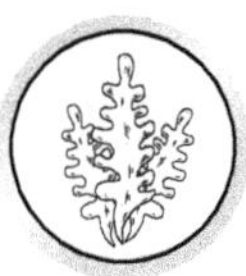

MAJOR ARCHETYPE

SEA LETTUCE

This bright green sea ally is a type of algae that looks like lettuce leaves. It can be consumed raw as a condiment, added to salads or cooked in healthy soups. Sea lettuce is the longevity vegetable of the ocean providing rich minerals for the minor mineralocorticoids of the adrenal cortex regulating the absorption of water and other electrolytes. It also contains a high amount of chlorophyll protecting against DNA damage and aiding the mitochondria in storing energy.

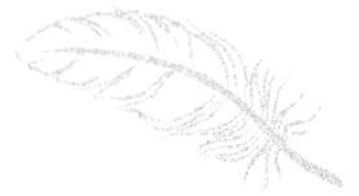

Sea Lettuce Salad and Cucumber Salad

Ingredients
½ cup of sea lettuce
1 cucumber
1 small fennel bulb
2 tablespoon finely diced shallots
1–2 tablespoons rice vinegar
2 tablespoons avocado or other light oil
1 teaspoon sweetener of choice (optional)
Garnish with smoked sea salt and pepper

Directions
Cut thin slices of the cucumber and fennel bulb.
Whisk the vinegar, oil, and sweetener together in a bowl.
Add the sea lettuce, cucumber, fennel, and shallots to the bowl.
Mix all ingredients together and top with smoked sea salt and pepper.
Eat immediately and enjoy!

MINOR ARCHETYPE

Carrots

Carrots are an excellent source of vitamins and minerals including: B6, biotin, vitamins A and K1, and potassium. The B6 component of carrots is especially connected to the adrenal glands because it assists the body into converting food into energy. Carrots, when eaten raw or blanched, provide a constant supply of energy as they are low on the glycemic index and balance blood sugar regulation. When the adrenal glands are taxed or fatigued during constant states of stress, it is common to experience bouts of low blood sugar and challenges in blood sugar control. Eating a healthy mid-afternoon snack, like carrots, will help nourish the adrenal glands for the rest of the day.

Borage Seed Oil

Borage Seed Oil comes from the seeds of the borage plant with its brilliant blue flowers. It is high in GLA, Gamma Linoleic Acid. This fatty acid helps to nourish the adrenal glands hormonally, providing relief from exhausting adrenal fatigue and many other health conditions. Borage oil, via prostaglandin, helps the adrenal glands to relax and to stop overworking in terms of long-term stress.

NOURISH THE ADRENALS – DISCOVERY DIVE – RECHARGING THE INTERNAL BATTERY

Take a deep breath in and tune in to your adrenal glands. Place your hands on your low back over the kidneys to increase your connection. Feel the energy moving up through the Earth, through both of your feet, through the sacrum, and up into the adrenal glands. Feel the pulse of the life force of the Earth charging your life force and spinal energy. Now imagine the yellow light of the sun shining upon your body. These solar rays begin to swirl and combine with the energy of that flowing back and forth through the adrenal glands in the shape of the infinity symbol. For the audio version of this meditation and visualization please click the link below.

∞ To access the meditation please go to www.zenergymedicinals.com

Now with the feel of this life force beginning to pulse through your system, from this place, answer the following questions.

How much energy do I have to do the things in my life that bring me joy and passion? Do I feel so burned out that I feel disconnected from my life and relationships?

How do I recharge, rejuvenate, and replenish my energy?

How much do I prioritize spending time on myself and on my dreams? How much of my day is spent with "have tos" versus "want tos"?

How do I deal with stressful situations? Do I tend to worry a lot? How does stress manifest in my body?

How much energy do I have every day?

Am I stuck in the same pattern or loop of running on empty or over-working myself?

Am I physically fit? What story do I tell myself and others about my physical health and vitality? Is my will to live strong? – If the answer is no, what are the reasons why not?

DIVE DEEPER – explore what emotions and feelings came to the surface as you answered these questions.

FREEDOM PHOTON WHEEL™

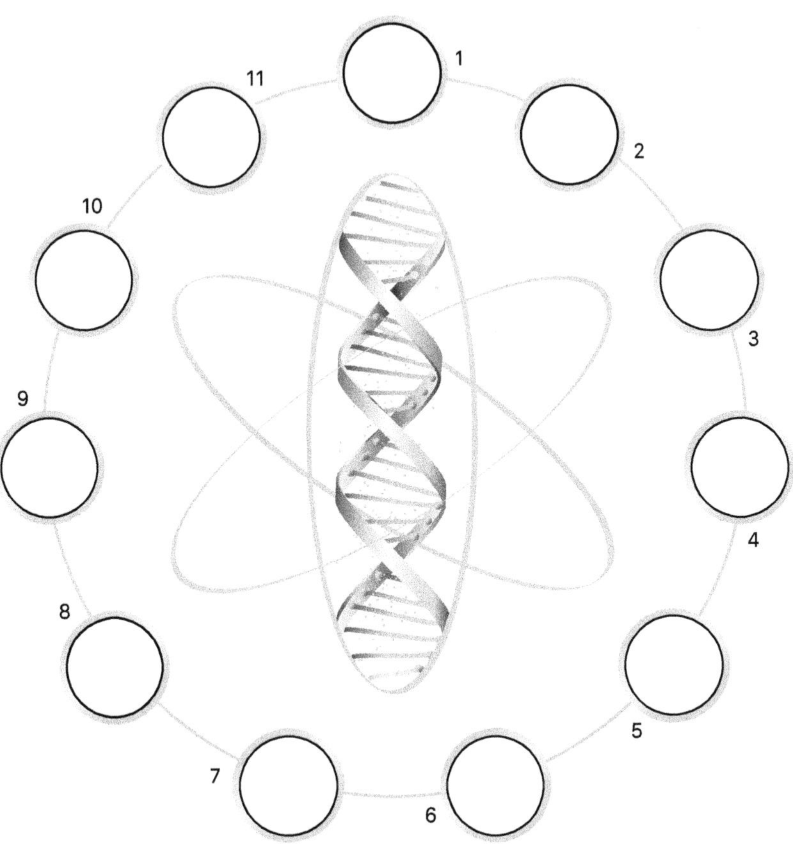

NOURISH THE ADRENALS
YOUR PERSONAL FREEDOM PHOTON RITUAL

Moon Phase

Perform your ritual during any moon phase.

Intention

"My connection to the deep reservoir of vital life force fills and nourishes every part of my being down to the DNA level and through my genetic lineage."

Select, Align, and Activate

Select your interventions according to the instructions in Chapter Five. Inhale and apply your chosen essential oil for 30–45 seconds. Use your botanical tincture or tea as directed. You may also listen to the meditation and use the mudra from this chapter while attuning your FPW.

Affirm

"Divine Consciousness, assist me in allowing the vibration of regeneration love to permeate my cells, particles, and all structures of my body, physical and nonphysical, of all that I have carried through my lineage. Allow the flow of the connection to the life pulse of humanity, and the sacred drumbeat, the heartbeat of Mother Earth, to fluidly and consistently nourish me."

ACTIVATE THE ADRENALS

Activating the adrenal glands will light up your superhero power pack and allow your entire system to flow with regenerative life force. In the preceding chapters, you have explored and experienced the transformative process of deeper introspection. Able now to understand how your current state of health and well-being is directly related to your habitual patterns and your genetic lineage, you have let go of the old and found healthier new ways to fill these parts of yourself with love and self-care.

Now you are ready for your entire column of light to open anew. You may be thinking right now, "What? These two tiny glands I have barely even heard of before have that much power?" It is true, activating the adrenal glands is a critical step to moving from a life of "surviving" to a life of "thriving." This activation completely resets your main energy channel, or vertical power current to connect in with the Earth and receive a consistent flow of vital life force to fuel your soul purpose thriving in all facets of life: energy, vibrancy and vitality, abundance, and the freedom to fully self-actualize, mastering the Earth game of soul evolution.

Activating the adrenal glands opens your being to the freedom of living as a fully sovereign divine being of light in human form. This process activates the DNA stranding and original blueprint held deep within your cells, freeing your spirit and physicality to expand beyond the limitations of the third dimensional construct of reality.

ADRENAL ACTIVATE FREEDOM PHOTON WHEEL

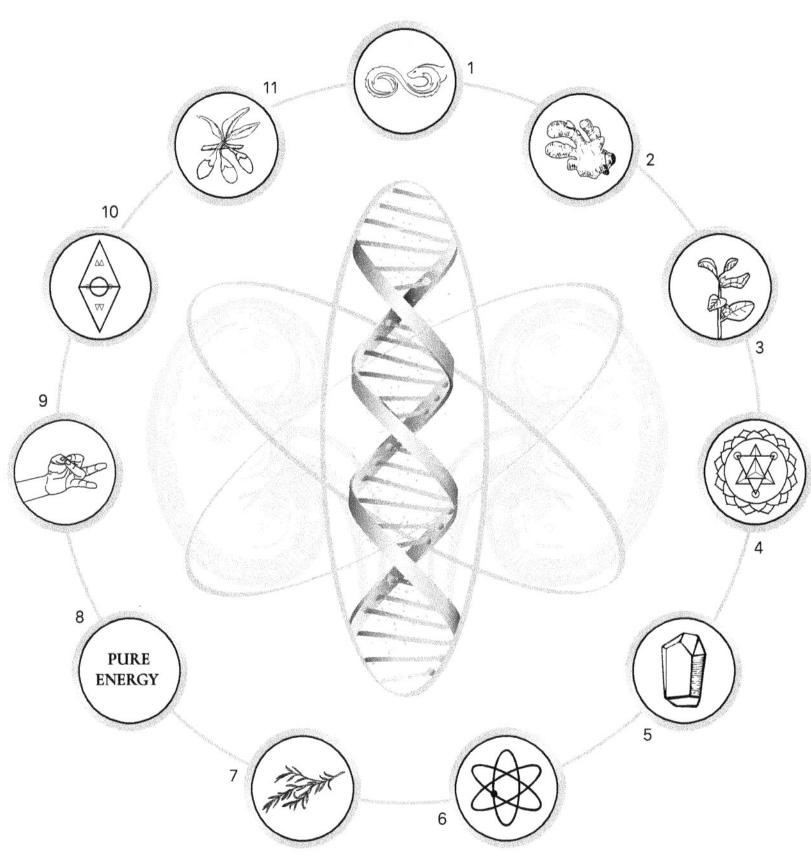

1 Alchemy Animal: White Dragon
2 Aromatherapy: Ginger
3 Botanical: Ashwagandha
4 Light Wheel: Aajaadee
5 Crystal: Aquamarine
6 Photon Vibration
7 Flower or Gem Essence: Rosemary
8 Intention: Pure Energy
9 Meditation Mudra: Rudra
10 Sacred Geometry
11 Nutrition: Goji Berry

ADRENAL ACTIVATE
INFINITY INFLUENCERS

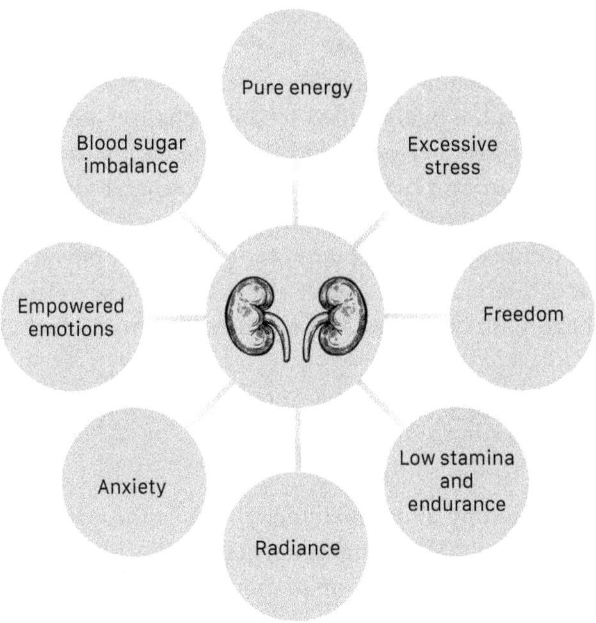

ACTIVATE THE ADRENALS – ALCHEMY ANIMALS

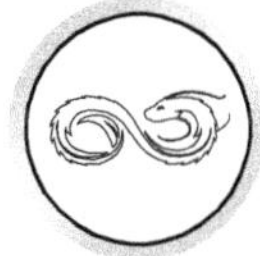

The activate alchemy animals of the adrenals embody the element of ether. Ether is the element of expansiveness and of unlimited boundaries, the space of freedom. These alchemy animals are bright with energy and boundless power, able to transform or shape-shift into new forms with ease.

MAJOR ARCHETYPE

WHITE DRAGON

The white dragon is one of the most powerful totems for strength and courage. The energy of the dragon is of purification and protection burning with a bright flame of endless magic. She heals negative emotions: sorrow, regret, grief, hate, and any emotions holding your cells back from true freedom. The white dragon asks you to question your life for exploration and adventure and to seek out new journeys of mystery and power through her eyes.

This mythical creature is deeply rooted in the stories and folklore of our elders. If you are being called to this alchemy animal, we suggest reading a great folk story or legend from the region of your ancestors, connecting to your family bloodline of healing and wisdom. This will ignite the power of the dragon within you.

Creature Connection: "I call upon the primordial power of the white dragon. I feel the boundless power rise within me. I welcome the new journey ahead with fierce passion, mystery, and magnetism."

MINOR ARCHETYPES

Tiger

The tiger is known by all for its ferocity. This is the energy to call forth now to activate the DNA of the adrenal glands. The tiger ignites the adrenal dynamism at the cellular core of determination yet patience. Imagine you as the tiger in the meadow. Crouching in the grass, seeing but not seen. Feel the momentum of the life force. Now take that vitality and absorb it through every adrenal cell. Feeling the rush of adrenaline. The power that you have to manifest and become all your desires.

The tiger is also the alchemy connection to the night realm. If you are feeling the call of the tiger, we suggest taking some night walks in your neighborhood or a camping trip where you lay under the stars. Listen with your night senses. Notice the transition the world takes as it moves from light to dark. How does it make your soul feel to lay under the stars or moon?

Creature Connection: "I roar with determination. I am strong. I am fierce. I am the person I have been longing for."

Scarlet Tanager

Have you seen this colorful and brilliant bird in the wild? It is really one of the most breathtaking moments. You gasp and scream with inner delight at this glorious vision.

When this impressive bird is calling out your name, it is a time to add color to every aspect of your precious life. Let go of the hardship and the struggle, knowing that you don't have to go through struggle in life but can be free to fly like a bird in the wind of happiness. He calls you to remember that everything you do here in this life is of importance and all the intentions you are setting forth are coming into reality.

Creature Connection: "I am free. I am free to live. I activate my DNA with the coding of freedom."

ACTIVATE THE ADRENALS – AROMATHERAPY

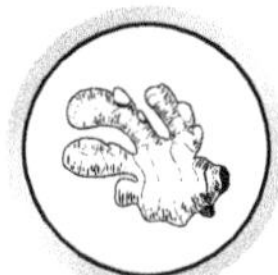

MAJOR ARCHETYPE

GINGER – *Zingiber officinale*

Part extracted: Rhizome

Core Properties: anti-inflammatory, anticoagulant, digestive aid (carminative), anesthetic, antimicrobial, and expectorant
Safety: nontoxic, nonirritant

Ginger, the root of life with its spicy earthy aroma, is a messenger of warmth bringing the nourishment of the Earth to places of frigidity and sluggishness from our emotional nature to the sexual arena. This oil invites energy flow in places where we become stuck and closed and disconnected from the Earth, ourselves, and each other.

Ginger alchemy encourages us to communicate from a place of warmth and connection and extend that care to those around us.

Ginger with its root medicine reminds us that we are connected to the core and that the separation we see in the world comes from places within. Ginger medicine helps us unite those disjointed places. Where we have crossed intentions of negative and positive desire. It unites the emotions of rejection and hate, bringing them to understanding and love. It unifies parts of ourselves that we have lost along the way, and as a key oil to bring healing along the male bloodline where rejection and betrayal have created a split and injured relationships along the genetic line.

Ginger invites us to break the belief systems held in our lineage related to life having to be hard, working ourselves to the bone, and that there's not enough to go around. This is an ally for those with mental and emotional disconnections, creating cohesion and unification. It improves circulation and digestion, strengthens the adrenal glands, and is aphrodisiac in nature.

Activate the Adrenals – Ginger Warming Body Oil

- ∞ 5 drops Ginger essential oil (*Zingiber Officinale*)
- ∞ 2 drops Vetiver essential oil (*Vetiveria zizanioides*)
- ∞ 3 drops Patchouli essential oil (*Pogostemon cablin*)
- ∞ 1 drop Oakmoss absolute (*Evernia prunastri*)
- ∞ 3 drops Myrrh essential oil (*Commiphora myrrha*)

Blend into 30 ml of jojoba or your favorite carrier oil and infuse it with your intention to bring warmth everywhere within you to each cell, deep into the bones, deep into your mind, your heart, and your emotions. Massage a 5 ml amount onto the body as desired.

MINOR ARCHETYPES

Geranium – *Pelargonium graveolens*

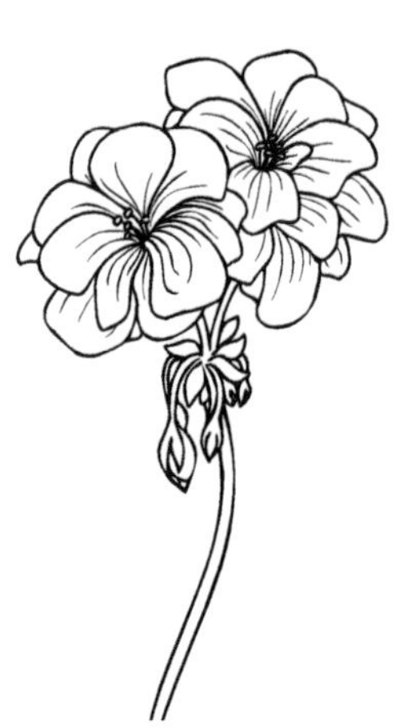

Part extracted: Leaves

Core Properties: astringent, hemostatic, cicatrisant, cytophylactic, diuretic, deodoranttonic, vermifuge, and vulnerary
Safety: nontoxic, nonirritant

Geranium is one of the greatest allies for healing the feminine aspects. It's rich and full aroma invites you to swim in the sea of the divine feminine. It assists to open an endless reservoir of creativity, sensuality, and intuition. This oil brings us to the threshold of our own inner wise one, the ancient voice of knowing that resides within our DNA.

Geranium is a potent alchemy for healing female-based trauma of a sexual nature, particularly when there is a family pattern of incest or other perceived impropriety. This oil funnels its healing vibration through the DNA and female bloodline, with the reverence of the feminine in all her beauty, glory, and power. Geranium opens us with a gentle reminder to love oneself, to be compassionate, to be kind, and to release the guilt and shame held within the cells and to fill them with a strong sense of empowerment.

Geranium balances hormonal levels and thus is a key oil for PMS (premenstrual syndrome), endometriosis, menopause, and other female based imbalances. Geranium is also an oil of beautification reminding us that with our heart and mind open, we can access our inner goddess.

Geranium invokes fullness of life. Breathing in this oil dissipates anxiety and the uncertainty of the future, replacing it with a fullness of presence rooted in the moment. Geranium invites us to embrace the beauty of our ability to feel the joy, the wonder, and all the intimate opportunities life has for us to explore.

This oil speaks to us with a reminder of the richness of life, love, and loving oneself first.

Activate the Adrenals – Geranium Body Oil for Healing the Feminine

- ∞ 7 drops of Geranium essential oil (*Pelargonium graveolens*)
- ∞ 3 drops of Patchouli essential oil (*Pogostemon cablin*)
- ∞ 1 drop Rose Otto essential oil (*Rosa damascena*)
- ∞ 2 drops Ylang Ylang essential oil (*Cananga odorata superior extra*)

Blend into 30 ml Gardenia monoi and infuse with your longing to heal the divine feminine within. Massage a silver dollar size amount onto the body daily.

Black Pepper – *Piper nigrum*

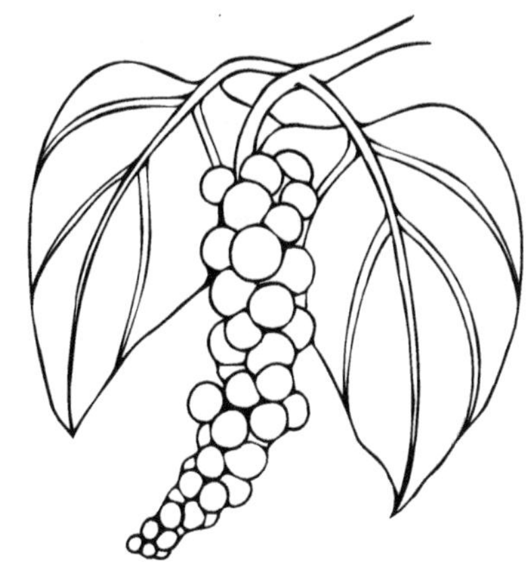

Part extracted: Fruit

Core properties: analgesic, antiseptic, antispasmodic, antitoxic, aphrodisiac, diaphoretic, digestive, diuretic, febrifuge, laxative, rubefacient, and tonic
Safety: nontoxic, nonirritant, and nonsensitizing

Warm, spicy, and invigorating, black pepper medicine is circular in nature. It activates the electrical charge in the cells and clears the density, or "stuck" energy to increase energy flow and facilitate circular completion. Consider the infinity symbol representing physical and psycho-spiritual aspects from the cells to the energy bodies. Also note that each ellipse in the infinity symbol represents the mother and father bloodlines, meeting in the middle, representing the zero-point field, the place of limitless creation.

Black pepper is a most potent alchemy to clear energy "blocks" in the auric level and toxins at the cellular level to allow for greater flow and completion of the energy circuit. This also applies to aspects of our physicality where we have two glands, like the adrenal or two appendages, like the legs. It opens and expands energy flow between the two aspects to generate greater life force, strength, and endurance.

This also applies to the emotional nature of black pepper: it breaks up patterns of fatigue related to depression. This oil is beneficial for the type of exhaustion that feels as though it originates from deep within the bones. Black pepper clears places of procrastination and vacillation, releasing the inability to decide and act towards your intentions and soul's longings.

Activate the Adrenals – Black Pepper Foot Oil to Get "Unstuck"

∞ 4 drops of Black Pepper essential oil (*Piper nigrum*)
∞ 3 drops of Lemon essential oil (*Citrus limonum*)
∞ 1 drop Cinnamon essential oil (*Cinnamomum cassia*)
∞ 2 drops Frankincense essential oil (*Boswellia carterii*)
∞ 4 drops Tulsi essential oil (*Ocimum tenuiflorum*)

Blend into 30 ml of jojoba oil and apply to the soles of your feet in the morning while envisioning your day filled with clarity, vitality, and drive. Massage a half dollar sized amount to the soles of feet.

ADRENAL ACTIVATE AROMATHERAPY
DNA BLUEPRINT BENEFITS

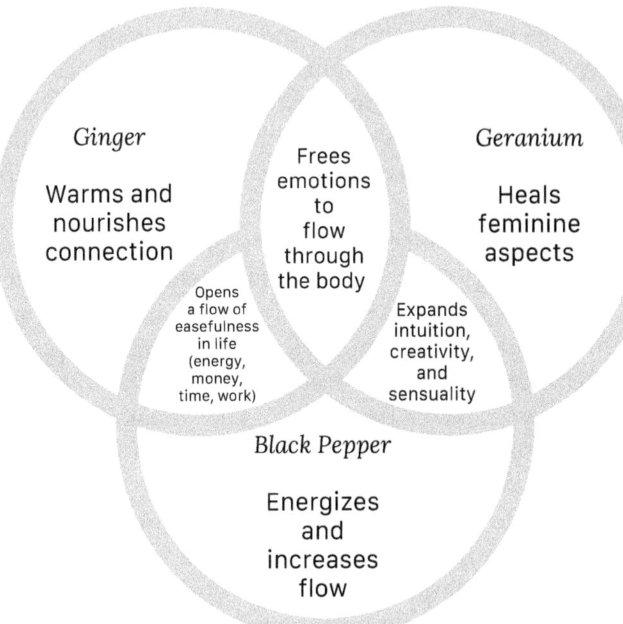

ACTIVATE THE ADRENALS – BOTANICAL MEDICINE

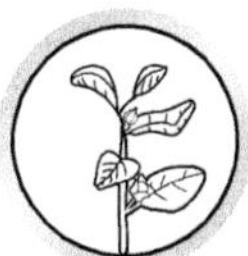

MAJOR ARCHETYPE

ASHWAGANDA – *Withania somnifera*

Parts used: Root and Leaf

Ashwagandha is an ayurvedic botanical with a well-known reputation as an herb for longevity and elixir for increasing vitality. In Sanskrit ashwagandha means "the smell of a horse," indicating that the herb has the potential to impart the vigor and strength of a stallion, and it also has a smell reminiscent of horse sweat.

This powerhouse adaptogen is for exhaustion and debilitated states of stress. It works in alignment with the nervous system, coping with excessive stress: easing mental strain, enhancing memory, and increasing endurance. It decreases anxiety and stress by lowering cortisol levels and mimicking the inhibitory neurotransmitter GABA in the brain. Ashwagandha also strengthens the immune system after illness, surgery, or cancer treatment.

Turn to this magnificent herb when you are so exhausted you can't even muster the energy to feel better or take action to feel better. Have you ever felt like that? Or are you even feeling like that now? It's becoming more and more common as we find ourselves pushing and pushing to get more things done faster and faster throughout the day. Ashwagandha says, "Take a breath, rest. Let me take over and be the surge of power you need to sustain and strengthen you. Go live your life with energy and vitality!"

Energetically Ashwagandha balances the kundalini life force energy between the first and fifth light wheels. This is a very important connection. As you begin to trust and listen to your inner voice or intuition and download information from your spirit guides you will need to be connected to the Earth. This way you don't feel unstable and flighty but instead you feel safe and secure.

Activate the Adrenals – Ashwagandha Physical Uses

Activate: Increases mitochondrial energy and replication. Strengthens the DNA of the neurotransmitter GABA

Adrenal System: Restores health to the adrenal system – for exhausted and debilitated states of stress as a rejuvenating tonic

Cardiovascular System: Increases circulation and anemia

Nervous System: Mental clarity, improves memory, adaptogen (eases stress), persistent anxiety, early dementia and Alzheimer's prevention

Musculoskeletal System: Bone building, anti-inflammatory, rheumatism, joint pain, and neuralgia

Immune System: Promotes recovery during convalescence and in inflammatory chronic diseases, anti-tumor and strengthens the immune system after chemo increasing white blood cell count.
Endocrine: Thyroid based eating disorders
Reproductive: Aphrodisiac, antispasmodic, and impotence with aging or due to stress
Integumentary: Topically for wound healing

Activate the Adrenals – Ashwagandha Emotional Uses

Feeling disconnected from yourself and others
Decreases worry of basic needs (food, money, and shelter)
Feeling at home and safe anywhere you are or go

Activate the Adrenals – Ashwagandha Energetic Uses

Grounding for the first light wheel
Activates the fifth light wheel for awakening intuition
Alignment for direct downloads from the astral plane

Activate the Adrenals – Ashwagandha Dosage

Powder: 1–2 g per day
Decoction: 1 tablespoon of Ashwagandha root per cup water. Drink 3–5 cups/day
Tincture: 60 drops 3x/day
Topically: Make a paste made from the powdered root and apply topically to boils, ulcers, and skin irritations.
See Appendix B for instructions on how to make a decoction

Activate the Adrenals – Ashwagandha Cautions and Contraindications

Pregnancy
May cause digestive discomfort in high doses

Activate the Adrenals – Ashwagandha Freedom to Infinite Energy

Combine equal parts of the following tinctures or liquid extracts: Ashwagandha, Eleuthero, Rehmannia, Schisandra
If you like to spice things up add a little splash of ginger tincture or a few drops of cayenne tincture.
Dosage: 60 drops 4x/day in a small amount of water.

MINOR ARCHETYPES

Rehmannia – *Rehmannia glutinosa*

Parts Used: Root

This adrenal activating botanical, rehmannia, has been used traditionally in Chinese herbal medicine as an herbal tonic for longevity with specific benefits for the adrenals, kidney, and liver. It works in harmony with the adrenal system by increasing and nourishing blood circulation, balancing blood sugar, and, most importantly, replenishing exhausted reserves. Rehmannia also assists the liver in hepatoregeneration and supports the adrenal glands with hormonal production. The herbal constituents of rehmannia, phytosterols, influence the liver and intestinal genes' transcription factors. These phytosterols are key players or regulators in the transport and expression cholesterol genes forming the backbone of adrenal hormone production.

As a blood nourisher, it acts similarly to the kidney hormone erythropoietin, stimulating the maturation of erythrocytes. Erythrocytes are red blood cells containing hemoglobin transporting oxygen and carbon dioxide to and from the cells and tissues of the body. Now you might be asking, why is this important for the adrenal system? Well, when the cells are more oxygenated, they produce more ATP (Adenosine 5′-triphosphate) the dynamic molecule for transferring and storing energy for the cells. You want more ATP when in a state of adrenal exhaustion and fatigue.

Emotionally rehmannia connects the adrenal system in two ways. One, it connects to the metals of the molten core of the Earth, engaging this deep strength of Gaia to strengthen and empower the energy of the adrenal glands. Especially the metals: gold, copper, platinum, and meteorites or other universal fire. Cosmically or spiritually, rehmannia connects the bright shining lights of these earthly metals to your inner being or spiritual being. Lighting your spirit and lightening the dark or drained spiritual cocoon or aura which takes place during adrenal exhaustion. It's time for you to let go of the disappointment of not feeling well, for rehmannia is here to guide you and be your ally on the road to vitality and freedom from stagnation.

Activate the Adrenals – Rehmannia Physical Uses

Activate: The ATP base of energy for the RNA and DNA
Adrenal System: Trophorestorative – adrenal burnout
Cardiovascular System: Cardioprotective, antioxidant, and anemic states
Nervous System: Adaptogen (for long term stress)
Urinary System: Kidney tonic
Musculoskeletal System: Prevents bone loss (Osteoporosis)
Immune System: Aids in recovery from chronic illness and allergies
Endocrine: Hyperthyroidism, diabetes, and boosts metabolism
Reproductive: Menopause, hormonal balancing, night sweats, vaginal dryness, and prostate support

Activate the Adrenals – Rehmannia Emotional Uses

Releases blocked and suppressed anger
Support when you have lost the will to fight for your life
Frees the heart from resentment

Activate the Adrenals – Rehmannia Energetic Uses

Grounding to the molten core of the metallic Earth and manifesting abundance – place dried herb and metals on your sacred altar
Channeling the longevity and hormonal potency of the forests and trees
Opens the higher light wheels connecting to the universal pool of unlimited cosmic energy

Activate the Adrenals – Rehmannia Dosage

Decoction: 1 tablespoon of Rehmannia root per cup water.
Drink 3 cups/day
Tincture: 60 drops 3x/day
See Appendix B for instructions on how to make a decoction

Activate the Adrenals – Rehmannia Cautions and Contraindications

Pregnancy and Lactation

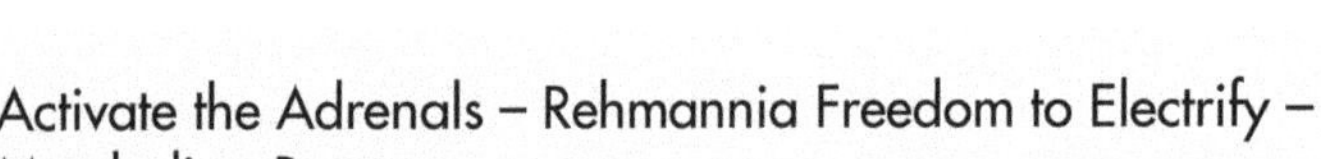

Activate the Adrenals – Rehmannia Freedom to Electrify – Metabolism Booster

This energizing decoction will boost your internal power and vitality.
Make a decoction in 473 ml of water.
1 tablespoon Rehmannia root – *Rehmannia glutinosa*
1 tablespoon Ashwagandha root – *Withania somnifera*
1 teaspoon Fenugreek seed – *Trigonella foenum-graecum*
Drink 1 cup 3x/day
See Appendix B for instructions on how to make a decoction.

Schisandra – *Schisandra chinensis*

Parts Used: Fruit

This activates the adrenals and as an ally is an antioxidant, hepatoprotector, and adaptogen. It has a great affinity with the adrenals and the mind, increasing resilience to stress in anxiety related health conditions. Schisandra tones the vessels and muscles of the heart increasing function and circulation. It also promotes vitality and increases memory and cognitive functions. Schisandra is known for tremendous sexual strength and stamina and is used for loss of sex drive, reigniting passion, and for enhancing fertility.

Schisandra's antioxidant features support the DNA by not only preventing further damage during times of high stress but it also reduces the damage experienced from environmental and emotional toxins, especially heavy metals. We always recommend taking it while traveling to reduce stress and cellular toxic load from organophosphates.

Emotionally schisandra is the herbal mediator. It softens the heart after arguments and creates the entryway to let the love in. Think of using this herb when you are in a "drama mama" state. What this means is you are stuck in the loop making something out of nothing and then the nothing becomes bigger and bigger and bigger. Schisandra brings the nervous system back down or turns the volume down on the situation by providing you with an open perspective.

Activate the Adrenals – Schisandra Physical Uses

Activate: DNA protection against pollutants
Adrenal System: Promotes vitality and adaptogen
Cardiovascular: Antioxidant, palpitations, cleanses blood
Nervous System: Increases memory and cognitive function, depression, irritability, and insomnia
Immune System: Increase resilience to illnesses
Liver: Facilitates detoxification, hepatoprotection, and hepatitis
Digestive System: Stimulates digestive juices
Urinary System: Increases urine flow and kidney tonic
Reproductive: Strengthens the uterus
Integumentary: Skin conditions and rashes
Vitality: Endurance, stamina, strength, and sexual tonic

Activate the Adrenals – Schisandra Emotional Uses

Quiets the spirit and softens the heart
Soothes an emotional melt down or "drama mama"
Soothes you to sleep after a late night argument

Activate the Adrenals – Schisandra Energetic Uses

Enhances the dream world
Increase memory of past life experiences in meditation
Connection of the second and fourth light wheels

Activate the Adrenals – Schisandra Dosage

Infusion: 1 cup 3x/day
Tincture: 2–3 ml 2–3x/day

Activate the Adrenals – Schisandra Cautions and Contraindications

Pregnancy

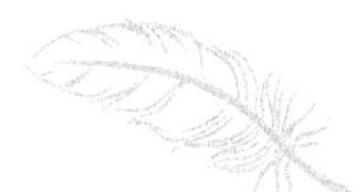

Activate the Adrenals – Schisandra Freedom to Feel

To revitalize your love life and sexual stamina soak ¼ cup Schisandra berries with 236 ml of water each night before bed. Make a decoction with the berries each morning and drink. Continue this ritual for 30 days.

Also place a few of the berries on the Freedom Photon Wheel for your sacred intentions.

See Appendix B for instructions on how to make a decoction.

ADRENAL ACTIVATE BOTANICAL MEDICINE
DNA BLUEPRINT BENEFITS

Ashwagandha
Increases mitochondrial replication and taps into limitless energy

Rehmannia
Upgrades ATP production and DNA synthesis

Adrenal burnout and deep-rooted stress

Rehabilitation of exhausted and poor functioning DNA

Adapts to habitual stress

Schisandra
Protects the DNA and improves liver DNA detoxification

ACTIVATE THE ADRENALS – LIGHT WHEELS

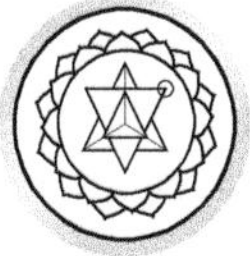

LIGHT WHEELS

MAJOR ARCHETYPE

THE 38th LIGHT WHEEL, AAJAADEE

This ascending light wheel Aajaadee, meaning freedom, relates to the seventy-seventh light wheel of past life karma and your soul journey. We each have come to this planet incarnated in this life for a purpose.

This light wheel recognizes the many lifetimes of the past and brings forward all the necessary creative tools for healing. For example, in many times we have had lives of healers, magicians, warriors, and more, and by working with this light wheel we are able to access all this information, like a book in the akashic records. This light wheel releases the past life negativity of persecution and allows you to be free.

MINOR ARCHETYPES

∞ The 33rd light wheel, Suraksha

Suraksha, meaning protection, is the thirty-third light wheel. As one of the ascending light wheels it connects us back to a time when we were victimized or violated for our beliefs and sexuality. We all have had many past life experiences where, unfortunately, our power was taken away from us. This light wheel returns this power to you, unconditionally: it is rightfully yours.

LIGHT WHEEL COLORS

MAJOR ARCHETYPE

TURQUOISE

Turquoise is the color of intuition and of a forward thinker. With this color activation it's time to let your brilliance and weirdness shine. The world needs your creative input. You are different and there is a reason; you are a magnificent being of light, a star seed. You might be afraid to express your thoughts and visions but now is not the time to hold back, you are needed. Be clear in your expressions for they are valid and powerful.

SOUND

∞ VAM

Vam is the deep note of D sounding like "Varm." Use this sound frequency and vibration by either playing a recording or by saying it aloud in repetition for 5–10 minutes. You can also use it in conjunction with activating the adrenals mudra for extra attunement. Vam helps activate the circular energy from the first light wheel to the second light wheel kindling the power of the Earth with the adrenals.

ACTIVATE THE ADRENALS – CRYSTALS AND STONES

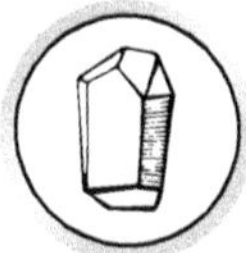

MAJOR ARCHETYPE

AQUAMARINE

Aquamarine ignites your internal fountain of youth with a renewed excitement and innocence of life. It heightens awareness to all levels of the auric field and expands our connection to the divine consciousness. It helps to release stuck emotions and fears, healing the deep grief that is held within and in the collective for the pain and suffering experienced generationally. Aquamarine allows your cells to remain in an energy state, regenerating your entire body and activating the original intent of the cell as the representation of the perfected blueprint for humanity. Aquamarine is deeply connected to the sea and the water element, and therefore offers this quintessential element for purification, nourishment, and activation at the energetic and cellular level.

MINOR ARCHETYPES

∞ Red Coral

Red Coral is great for connecting to the water element, crucial for optimum cellular vitality of the adrenals. It supports healing at the blood and bone marrow level, production of red blood cells, and increasing oxygen in the blood in the system; it's helpful for anemia, asthma, the optic nerves, joints, bones. This stone is beneficial for a spinal clearing and easing nervous tension held in the back.

∞ Blood Stone

Blood stone enhances grounding and helps to integrate the ever-changing Earth vibrations. This stone is beneficial for those who are intrinsically rigid and have difficulty adapting to change. Blood stone activates your inner courage and strengthens the will to live life from your own internal GPS versus the expectations of your family of origin, helping to dissolve projected opinions on the way you "should" be in the world. Blood stone is a power stone that invigorates the cells with pure energy and purifies and strengthens the blood. It supports the release of toxins and bolsters the physical and etheric bodies.

CRYSTAL ADDITIONS

- ∞ Agate
- ∞ Gaia Stone

ACTIVATE THE ADRENALS CRYSTAL GRID

Drink a glass of clean water with 3 drops each of Aquamarine & Calendula essences. Tribal music including drumming can be enjoyed during this session. This crystal attunement is best done in the morning or early afternoon for 20-30 minutes.
Cleanse crystals immediate after use. (See Appendix C).

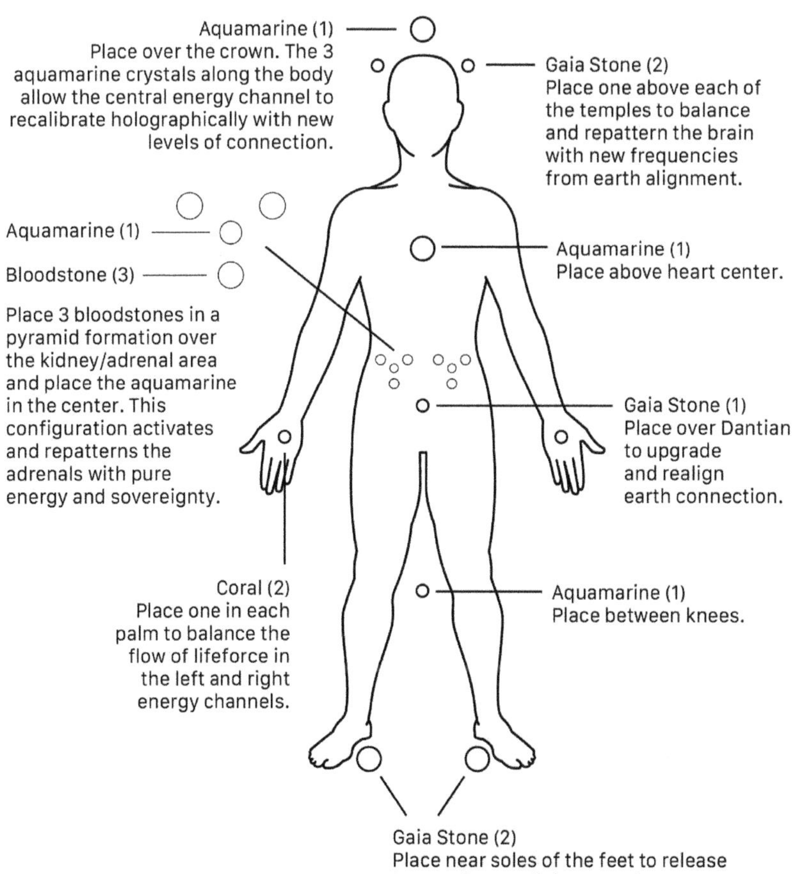

ACTIVATE THE ADRENALS – ENERGETIC AND VIBRATIONAL TECHNIQUES

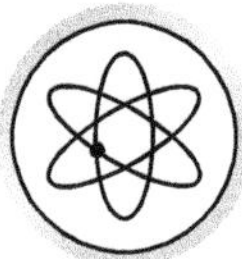

MAJOR ARCHETYPE

ACTIVATE THE ADRENAL HYDROTHERAPY

- ∞ 5 drops of Geranium essential oil (*Pelargonium graveolens*)
- ∞ 2 drops of Black Pepper essential oil (*Piper nigrum*)
- ∞ 3 drops Ginger essential oil (*Zingiber officinale*)
- ∞ 10 drops of Rosemary flower essence
- ∞ 10 drops of Gold gem essence

Add all ingredients to a warm bath and soak for 20 minutes.

MINOR ARCHETYPES

Activate the Adrenals Visualization

See, feel, allow, or imagine yourself seated deep in the forest in front of a fire. In this fire sacred herbs and spices like cinnamon, sandalwood, and ginger are infusing the air with their aromatic molecules. As you breathe in the aroma, you begin to feel entranced by the flames, journeying with your spirit to intertwine with the spirit of the flame. You begin to see the flame within each cell igniting and illumined. This light pulsates between turquoise and then gold and now penetrates each adrenal gland. As the light moves into the center of each gland, the shape of a diamond forms and ignites each gland to its full vibration.

Activate the Adrenals EOBT

Place one drop of ginger essential oil between the first two fingertips of the right hand, inhale deeply and tap the Kidney -1, Bubbling Spring, entry point of the Kidney Meridian for 30 seconds to ignite the sacred fire within.

Location: On the centerline of the sole of the foot, between the second and third toes, in the depression formed by curling the toes (plantar flexion). This will be just off the pad of flesh over the metatarsals.

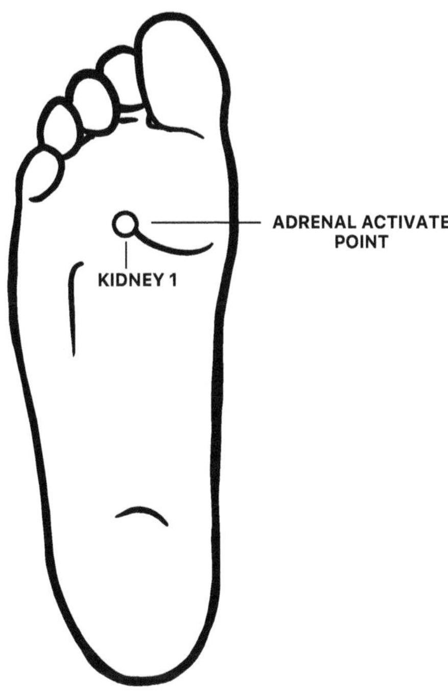

ACTIVATE THE ADRENALS – FLOWER AND GEM ESSENCES

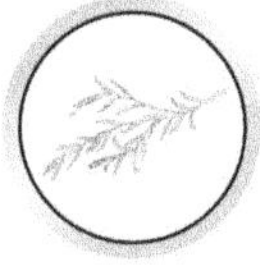

FLOWER ESSENCES

MAJOR ARCHETYPE

ROSEMARY

Rosemary is a powerful actuator and activator of balance, positive energy, and clarity from the cellular to the emotional, mental, and spiritual bodies. It helps us to clear karmic entanglements and brings deeper understanding to the challenges held in the child consciousness and past life experience for the evolutionary integration at your soul level. Rosemary is a potent dream medicine and can stimulate creative ideas through the night. It helps to dissolve worry and overthinking, energizing the auric field for those who tend to feel nervous exhaustion, frailty, or lack determination. This essence fuels the adrenal glands with the energy of vitality and resilience.

MINOR ARCHETYPES

Calendula

Calendula activates the passion and desire to fully enjoy life. It activates immunity and generates a balanced flow of life force along both energy channels, the ida and the pingala. This is a great essence to open desire at multiple levels: sensual, sexual desire, vibrancy, beauty, and greater abundance. This essence encourages laughter and lifts emotional heaviness from the energy field. It is also helpful for weight loss and activating physical vitality. Calendula also heals patterns of betrayal from the mother and through the female bloodline in the DNA.

Sunflower

Sunflower is filled with the bright, potent energy of the sun. Sunflower also holds the energetic connection to the Great Central Sun, activating higher levels of consciousness and universal understanding. Sunflower is one of the best essences to lift us from the doldrums, especially mood imbalances that run through the genetic bloodlines. This essence clears and balances the emotional body, quells anxiety, and reminds you of the simple joys of life.

FLOWER ESSENCE ADDITIONS

∞ Almond

ACTIVATE THE ADRENALS – INTENTIONS

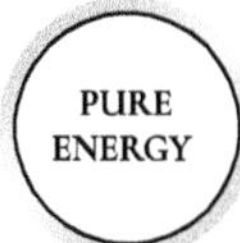

MAJOR ARCHETYPE

PURE ENERGY

MINOR ARCHETYPES

∞ I receive the element of fire to charge my adrenal glands with energy
∞ I am a free sovereign being of light
∞ I thrive in all my endeavors

ADDITIONAL INTENTIONS

∞ I am deeply connected to the Earth and my personal power

ACTIVATE THE ADRENALS – MEDITATION AND MUDRA

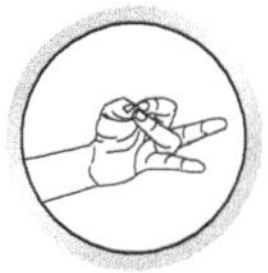

Rudra Mudra

I ignite the powerful fire within me, manifesting my life's vision and purpose.
I am pure energy.

The Rudra mudra is named after Lord Shiva, the destroyer and creator, cleansing the path so we may reach our highest potential. This is an extremely powerful mudra manifesting true cellular transformation and shifts in the DNA. This mudra is connected to the third chakra, Manipura, and is the power center or lustrous gem. When activated, this mudra illuminates the brilliant gem or diamond within and breaks through all obstacles in the way of healing. This mudra energizes the entire body. When using this mudra daily you will feel empowered.

Rudra Mudra Alignment

1. Touch the tip of your thumb of each hand to the tip of the forefinger and ring finger of the same hand.
2. Keep your pinkie and middle finger straight.
3. Take a deep breath, let your body relax.
4. You may now either do the meditation below or 10 minutes of *Fire Breathing* (To access the Fire Breathing technique please visit www.zenergymedicinals.com).
5. You may also use the mudra any time you want to recharge the body when feeling fatigued, overworked, or depleted.

∞ To access the mudra meditation please go to www.zenergymedicinals.com

∞ Inhale your essential oil, breathing deeply for 30–45 seconds.
∞ Hold the Rudra mudra and take several breaths to attune and activate your adrenal glands. With each breath, feel the energy and power of the adrenals like the warm rays of the sun and moon.
∞ Connect with the core of the Earth, allowing the light to come back up through the layers of the Earth, filled with golden geometric forms and golden symbols, light language and sacred codes that have been held deep within the Earth.
∞ Engage the moment of receptivity as we shift collectively to a new Earth, a unified Earth.
∞ Fully grounded and aligned with Mother Earth, receive the full spectrum of her life force to thrive. Thrive in vibrancy, energy, abundance.
∞ Adopt joy of life, of living fully on this planet currently. This very precious moment of time and space, here and now.
∞ Invite in both elements of fire and water and their highest form to energize the adrenals. Now we call forth the infinity teams of pure light and the activation sequence through the DNA, through the mother and father bloodlines.

- ∞ On your next breath see, feel, allow, imagine a triangular shaped symbol with the point facing down, coming down from the higher realms, pulsating and golden light, infinite light.
- ∞ The pyramid shaped symbol comes down to the crown of the head and splits into two. Sacred symbols of golden light, the shape of a pyramid with the point facing down, come down now through the energy bodies to encapsulate each of the adrenal organs.
- ∞ In each of these two pyramids, you can see the double helix of golden amber light at the very center of each adrenal organ, recalibrating, revitalizing, and reconfiguring each of the organs.
- ∞ Activation throughout the DNA and mother and father bloodlines and allowing now all energy centers: reconfigure, revitalize, and realign.
- ∞ With each wave of empowerment and light, your body feels rejuvenated and realigned with its true purpose. Repeat the intention three times either silently or aloud: "I ignite the powerful fire within me. Manifesting my life's vision and purpose. I am pure energy."
- ∞ Your energy is sacred. Your life on this Earth is sacred.
- ∞ Invite in the intention and affirmation: I am a free, sovereign, divine being of light.

ACTIVATE THE ADRENALS – SACRED GEOMETRY

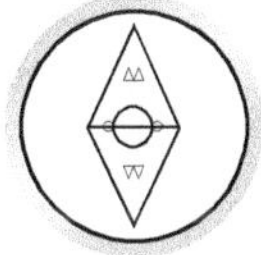

MAJOR ARCHETYPE

ACTIVATE THE ADRENALS SACRED GEOMETRY

This intentional and original depiction of activate the adrenals sacred geometry continues with the diamond light frequency, activating the adrenals to a new frequency of Heaven and Earth connection, allowing the sacred temple of Gaia to illuminate in between the two glands, honoring the Earth as a living, breathing force and ally to cocreate with.

This sacred geometric form connects the auric field and hara line to higher dimensional energy beyond the third, recalibrating the body and activating the genetic blueprint of freedom for the individual.

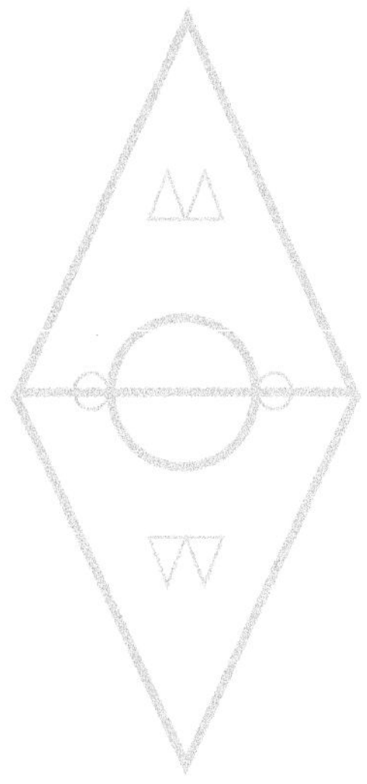

ACTIVATE THE ADRENALS – NUTRITION

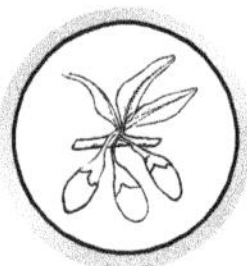

MAJOR ARCHETYPE

GOJI BERRY

The goji berry, as you learned about in the Activate the Heart section, is a golden nugget of power and energy. These small but energetically charged fruits contain amino acids, vitamins A, B1, B2, B6, C, and E and are rich in iron, zeaxanthin, and lutein. The B vitamins of the goji berry provide cellular protection for the adrenal and immune cells, especially important during times of adrenal stress and exhaustion. The impressive goji is such a powerful stimulant we recommend not eating them too late in the afternoon or evening or you might find yourself wired before bed.

Goji berries are also plentiful in tryptophan, the precursor to the neurotransmitter serotonin. It's common during times of adrenal fatigue and exhaustion to experience periods of depression and dissatisfaction with life. The goji berry provides and stimulates the release of more tryptophan from the brain and you quickly feel lighter and happier.

MINOR ARCHETYPES

Hijiki

Hijiki is a dark brown or black seaweed high in many minerals including magnesium. Magnesium acts like a lightning rod to each cell, activating the hypothalamic-pituitary-adrenal axis exemplifying the body's ability to deal with stress. When the adrenal system is stressed, the emotional body is more easily stressed, tending to frustration and anger. Magnesium helps soften this blow and stress response.

Horseradish

Horseradish is a powerful and pungent cruciferous vegetable containing the key constituent, glucosinolate. Glucosinolate has been studied for its profound ability to protect the cells against cancer as well as promoting apoptosis or cell death. This spicy root really packs a punch and increases blood circulation and reduces cellular inflammation. We recommend using it pickled, in small amounts, as an addition to your meal 1–2 times per day to activate the heart (Herz et al., 2017).

NUTRITIONAL ADDITIONS

- ∞ Avocado
- ∞ Beet
- ∞ Kidney bean
- ∞ Liver
- ∞ Sea salt

ACTIVATE THE ADRENALS – DISCOVERY DIVE – IGNITING YOUR INTERNAL FIRE

This Discovery Dive is about igniting your internal fire within. Many of us continue to burn and function without that spark and fire. You are now called to move from a state of surviving to a state of thriving. This internal spark gives you your charisma, your dance in life, your physical and spiritual flow. Do you ever notice how, when you are in rhythm with yourself, everything flows and falls into place? This is the spark or flame we want you to connect with in this Discovery Dive. The clearing of your tribal and genetic tangled energy is no longer a drain on your life force, you are liberated to live life to the fullest.
Let's Ignite!

What would it be to live from the perspective of unlimited energy? Energy to act, make connections, and freely live life on your own terms.

Start by making a list of ten (or more) things you would do if you had all the energy you desire?

Would you have a baby, start a new job, write a book, quit your job, travel the world?

Would you go back to school, change your career, learn to dance the tango, speak Italian? Reevaluate and invigorate your relationship or consider starting over?

Remember, this process is ongoing, and your desires will change with every layer you bring to the surface to transform. You are a diamond that continues to shine brighter with every stroke of polishing, further illuminating your great light within.

FREEDOM PHOTON WHEEL™

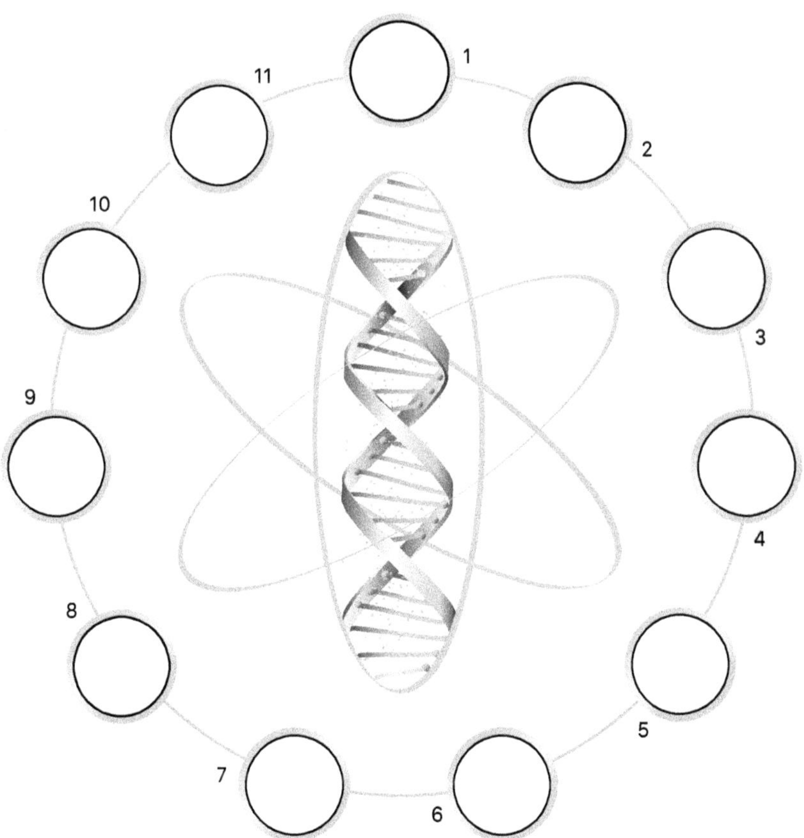

ACTIVATE THE ADRENALS
YOUR PERSONAL FREEDOM PHOTON RITUAL

Moon Phase

Moon Phase: Perform your ritual when the moon is waxing – from the new moon to the full moon.

Intention

"I call forth, activate, and allow the full DNA sequence for INFINITE energy, connection, and flow, igniting my vital life force to fuel the passion of my purpose on this planet."

Select, Align, and Activate

Select your interventions according to the instructions in Chapter Five. Inhale and apply your chosen essential oil for 30–45 seconds. Use your botanical tincture or tea as directed. You may also listen to the meditation and use the mudra from this chapter while attuning your FPW.

Affirm

"Divine Consciousness, please assist me in healing that I have carried through my lineage, my mother and father bloodlines so that I allow the highest experience of freedom and sovereignty, thriving in all areas of my existence."

CHAPTER 8

Mood Boosting Bliss – The Brain

As a civilization, we are at a pinnacle of mood-based discontent. We are experiencing increases in stress, anxiety, addiction, suicide, depression and distress, pandemics, injustice, and riots, contributing to confusion, uncertainty, and overload. We are being invited and, in some ways, forced to confront ourselves as a global community from the individual perspective. Every aspect of our humanity, held in shadow through the collective consciousness, is rising and demanding a voice. There is a deep calling for freedom rising from within, and, through turbulence, deep shifts of awareness are unfolding all around us. We stand at a critical juncture of unfoldment where the future is currently in flux and ever evolving from our beliefs, thoughts, actions, and emotional responses.

How can we sift through the cloudiness, the confusion, the extremity of emotion, and the propensity to feel bad, less than, not good enough, and ultimately separate and alone? Somewhere within we know that feeling good is empowering and that when we feel good, we experience greater clarity, competency, strength, and purpose. When we view life and create experience from this paradigm, that good feeling spills over into every other area of our lives, our relationships, our careers, and the greater world around us. Why can't we simply stay in a place of feeling good?

Furthermore, what is the difference between the brain and the mind? Consider the brain to be like a supercomputer; all data from your life experience is stored in your cells. Certain thoughts, emotions, and memories trigger chemical responses that flood the body. Like when you click on a file in your computer a wealth of information and often other programs and files surface with one click. When we experience a benevolent belief, thought, and then a feeling, a chemical release of serotonin floods the body, and our mood begins to elevate.

Now let's look at the mind. There was a point in time historically where the mind was thought to be entirely separate from the body and from this Cartesian philosophy, the systems, functions, and diseases thereof were considered finite and isolated from other parts of the physicality.

It was not until new and expanded scientific exploration of physics and then quantum physics that the nature of the mind–body connection and holographic healing were discovered and understood. All physical disease is rooted and connected to the mind and the emotions.

The mind has two main aspects, conscious and subconscious. The conscious mind represents our thinking and logical nature. And as we have discussed previously, our subconscious mind holds all unresolved emotional experiences resulting from trauma. Strain trauma occurs prior to language development and affects our entire physiological system including our perception of the world and human nature as well as our emotional responses and in some cases mood disorders. Shock trauma represents a traumatic experience after one has formed a sense of self. Consider the nature of PTSD (post-traumatic stress disorder), where the mind recalls previous trauma in a repetitive nature and reacts in specific patterns. This trauma is imprinted in the cells and can be reexperienced in the form of dreams, flashbacks, behavioral patterns of withdrawal and numbing, as well as physiological responses of extreme emotional outburst, insomnia, anxiety, and depression.

AW I have experienced chronic anxiety from an early age. Both strain and shock trauma exist in my trauma timeline. Chronic anxiety also runs through my mother's bloodline. So does depression on both bloodlines. From the perspective of a healer, I understand that I have incarnated to bring about healing within my being, my DNA, and my mother and father bloodlines, so that it is not passed through to further generations. There is understanding.

When I have those over the shoulder moments of looking back along my life path, I can see how far I have come. And then there are moments from my personality aspects when the anxiety and depression feel debilitating, and I sink. The knowing of the healer within reminds me of the power of the alchemical interventions woven throughout this book, that I have the herbs, oils, energy medicine, meditation, nutrition, and exercise at my disposal to lift myself up again. The healer reminds me that this is not something to be ashamed of, feel guilty about and that I am not alone, and for those of you out there that are experiencing similar challenges, you are not alone either.

The supercomputer of our brain needs the support of these interventions, especially nutrition, exercise, herbs, and essential oils so that it can create the optimum chemical balance and ultimate conditions for our consistent nature of feeling good and better than good: blissful, loving, connected, and illuminated.

THE INNER WORKINGS OF THE BRAIN

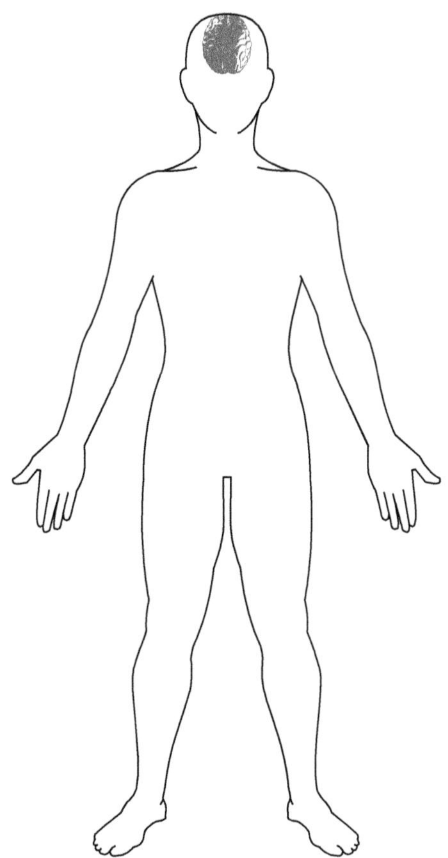

∞ To access the brain meditation please go to www.zenergymedicinals.com

THE BRAIN

The brain is our station for all cognitive function and neurotransmission for mood, ranging from pleasure to peace. The physical function of the brain is important for letting go of memories that are causing a shift in your daily emotions and memory. As we age, we often see a decline in memory and cognitive function, but we can achieve longevity with the right interventions. While you read through these next sections of the book you will enhance your brain function and improve long term retention with the archetypes and Discovery Dives. Specific energy healing techniques and meditation will facilitate opening to new levels of awareness, spiritual connection, and the elevation of consciousness.

The brain is one of the most complex and magnificent organs in the human body. Our mind gives us awareness of ourselves and of our

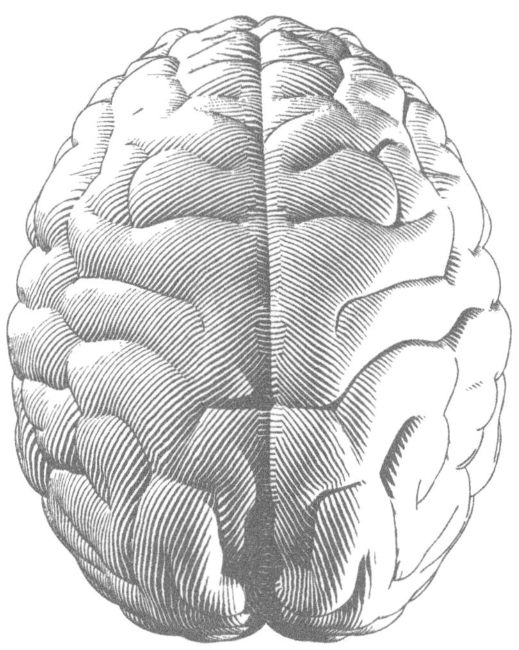

environment, processing a constant stream of sensory data. It controls our muscle movements, the secretions of our glands, and even our breathing and internal temperature. Every creative thought, feeling, and plan is developed by our brain. The brain's neurons record the memory of every event in our lives.

ANATOMY OF THE BRAIN

BRAIN CELLS

Brain cells can be broken into two groups: neurons and neuroglia. Neurons, or nerve cells, are the cells that perform all the communication and processing within the brain. Sensory neurons entering the brain from the peripheral nervous system deliver information about the condition of the body and its surroundings. Most of the neurons in the brain's gray matter are interneurons, which are responsible for integrating and processing information delivered to the brain by sensory neurons. Interneurons send signals to motor neurons, which carry signals to muscles and glands. Neuroglia, or glial cells, act as the helper cells of the brain; they support and protect the neurons. In the brain there are four types of glial cells: astrocytes, oligodendrocytes, microglia, and ependymal cells.

DIVISIONS OF THE BRAIN

There are different ways of dividing the brain anatomically into regions. Let's use a common method and divide the brain into three main regions based on embryonic development: the forebrain, midbrain, and hindbrain. Under these divisions:

- The forebrain is made up of our incredible cerebrum, thalamus, hypothalamus, and pineal gland among other features.
- The midbrain, located near the very center of the brain between the interbrain and the hindbrain, is composed of a portion of the brainstem.
- The hindbrain consists of the remaining brainstem as well as our cerebellum and pons.

PHYSIOLOGY OF THE BRAIN

METABOLISM

Despite weighing only about three pounds, the brain consumes as much as 20 percent of the oxygen and glucose taken in by the body. Nervous tissue in the brain has a very high metabolic rate due to the sheer number of decisions and processes taking place within the brain at any given time. Large volumes of blood must be constantly delivered to the brain in order to maintain proper brain function. Any interruption in the delivery of blood to the brain leads very quickly to dizziness, disorientation, and eventually unconsciousness.

SENSORY

The brain receives information about the body's condition and surroundings from all of the sensory receptors in the body. All of this information is fed into sensory areas of the brain, which put this information together to create a perception of the body's internal and external conditions. Some of this sensory information is autonomic sensory information that tells the brain subconsciously about the condition of the body. Body temperature, heart rate, and blood pressure are all autonomic senses that the body receives. Other information is somatic sensory information that the brain is consciously aware of. Touch, sight, sound, and hearing are all examples of somatic senses.

MOTOR CONTROL

Our brain directly controls almost all movement in the body. A region of the cerebral cortex known as the motor area sends signals to the skeletal muscles to produce all voluntary movements. The basal nuclei of the cerebrum and gray matter in the brainstem help to control these movements subconsciously and prevent extraneous motions that are undesired. The cerebellum helps with the timing and coordination of these movements during complex motions. Finally, smooth muscle tissue, cardiac muscle tissue, and glands are stimulated by motor outputs of the autonomic regions of the brain.

PROCESSING

Once sensory information has entered the brain, the association areas of the brain go to work processing and analyzing this information. Sensory information is combined, evaluated, and compared to prior experiences, providing the brain with an accurate picture of its conditions. The association areas also work to develop plans of action that are sent to the brain's motor regions in order to produce a change in the body through muscles or glands. Association areas also work to create our thoughts, plans, and personality.

LEARNING AND MEMORY

The brain needs to store many different types of information that it receives from the senses and that it develops through thinking in the association areas. Information in the brain is stored in a few different ways depending on its source and how long it is needed. Our brain maintains short-term memory to keep track of the tasks in which the brain is currently engaged. Short-term memory is believed to consist of a group of neurons that stimulate each other in a loop to keep data in the brain's memory. New information replaces the old information in short-term memory within a few seconds or minutes, unless the information gets moved to long-term memory.

Long-term memory is stored in the brain by the hippocampus. The hippocampus transfers information from short-term memory to memory-storage regions of the brain, particularly in the cerebral cortex of the temporal lobes. Memory related to motor skills (known as procedural memory) is stored by the cerebellum and basal nuclei.

HOMEOSTASIS

The brain acts as the body's control center by maintaining the homeostasis of many diverse functions such as breathing, heart rate, body temperature, and hunger. The brainstem and the hypothalamus are the brain structures most concerned with homeostasis.

In the brainstem, the medulla oblongata contains the cardiovascular center that monitors the levels of dissolved carbon dioxide and oxygen in the blood, along with blood pressure. The cardiovascular center adjusts the heart rate and blood vessel dilation to maintain healthy levels of dissolved gases in the blood and to maintain a healthy blood pressure. The medullary rhythmicity center of the medulla monitors oxygen and carbon dioxide levels in the blood and adjusts the rate of breathing to keep these levels in balance.

The hypothalamus controls the homeostasis of body temperature, blood pressure, sleep, thirst, and hunger. Many autonomic sensory receptors for temperature, pressure, and chemicals feed into the hypothalamus. The hypothalamus processes the sensory information that it receives and sends the output to autonomic effectors in the body such as sweat glands, the heart, and the kidneys.

SLEEP

While sleep may seem to be a time of rest for the brain, this organ is extremely active during sleep. The hypothalamus maintains the body's 24-hour biological clock, known as the circadian clock. When the circadian clock indicates that the time for sleep has arrived, it sends signals to the reticular activating system of the brainstem to reduce its stimulation of the cerebral cortex. Reduction in the stimulation of the cerebral cortex leads to a sense of sleepiness and eventually leads to sleep.

In a state of sleep, the brain stops maintaining consciousness, reduces some of its sensitivity to sensory input, relaxes skeletal muscles, and completes many administrative functions. These administrative functions include the consolidation and storage of memory, dreaming, and development of nervous tissue.

PSYCHO-SPIRITUAL ASPECTS OF THE BRAIN

BRAIN NERVOUS SYSTEM
PSYCHO-SPIRITUAL PATHWAY

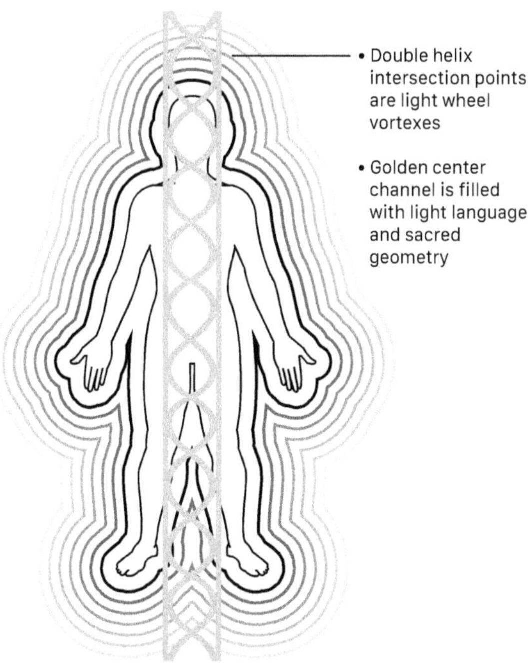

This design depicts a golden column of light descending through the higher light wheels, through the central energy channel, to the root light wheel and connecting to the core of the Earth. The double helix within the channel represents both the male and female pathways of energy flow. The points of intersection represent the center of each light wheel.

The central energy channel is flooded with the golden light of Divine Consciousness, light language and sacred geometric codes, directly correlated to the level of consciousness and the degree of healing embodied by the individual.

From an energetic and emotional perspective, the brain and nervous system drive more than just our thought process. In addition to being a key transmitter and receiver of consciousness, the brain also houses a power center for healing. The limbic system, which is a lock and key mechanism, regulates much of our physiology including mood, memory, and emotion. It is here we have one of the greatest opportunities to shift our mood and feeling experience in the moment, shifting the trajectory of our emotional responses. The more we can control our emotions in the moment, the more we can continue to elevate our feeling response. This creates a domino effect to empower and harness the clarity of our thoughts and ultimately create our life experience from a higher paradigm. Imagine this process as a bridge, the better you feel in the moment the more the bridge extends to actualize your greatest self.

AW I have been enamored by scent, since I was a young child. The wafting scent of lilacs in the spring has always moved me. In the same way the certain smell of burning wood can take me back to the countryside of India and all of the wondrous discoveries about myself and the world that I unearthed in that distant land.

The smell of neroli orange blossoms and the night air brings me immediately back to the magic of Giza and my experience in Egypt. These are powerfully evocative moments transcribed in my memory banks that transcend space and time and offer immediate psycho-spiritual and physiological responses.

This is the significant and far-reaching power of the limbic system at work. And a reminder that the memory and feeling of these experiences is tangible. A simple example of the limbic connection would be how scent can trigger memory and therefore emotion. In my youth, I spent a great deal of time at my grandparents home. It was a warm and loving, nurturing and safe environment where I experienced the excitement of learning how to read and play pinochle. It is where I grew in appreciation for America's favorite pastime, baseball. My grandmother had a soap or lotion in the scent of roses mixed with lavender. Today, whenever I smell something similar, I'm immediately transported back to their home. A sense of feeling safe and loved is evoked and my entire being reacts to this positive experience, physically, emotionally, and spiritually.

The limbic system allows us to make decisions that are in our best interest. It is through the system we learn how to engage and integrate with the world around us. The limbic system is intimately involved with memory, behavior, sexual function and attraction, learning, and the full gamut of emotions from anger and sadness to joy and so forth.

Through the limbic system, the brain creates an internal subjective experience of the senses and from the feelings that arise. Interestingly, it takes only a single change or damage to an individual nucleus or neurotransmitter in the brain to disrupt homeostasis and, therefore, emotionally how we relate to the world around us.

DETOX THE BRAIN

What if we were to ask you to take the leap of faith, that everything you may believe to be true about yourself, your life, your health, and your actual ability to create and experience life is not even half the truth.

Although our belief system can be held in various parts of the body, including the auric field and therefore the cells and our DNA, their chemical reactions take place in the brain, affecting our neurochemistry and directly formatting our neural pathways. What we feel, we think. What we think, we believe. What we believe, whether conscious or subconscious, forms our experience of reality and indirectly our perception of humanity. Science now understands that our beliefs and thoughts create chemical reactions in the body. The emotions that are created from this process contribute to our overall frequency, vibration, and greater understanding of life as well as how we feel on a day-to-day basis.

We have an enormous opportunity by detoxing the brain and being able to release the belief systems that are affecting our neurochemistry. We can then reformat our neural pathways for a new story of health, of vibrancy, of love, of abundance, of joy, and of creating beyond a limited perception of reality or our third dimensional existence. All the patterns of distortion, habits, images, and limiting thought processes create the energy of disharmony and resistance. The kicker is that when we have unrealistic expectations about ourselves or another, we create further resistance. The good news is that we have the power to change for the better.

When we think about the brain and the mind–body connection and detoxification, let's again come back to the holographic perspective. We have talked about belief systems from the energetic perspective, now let's come back to the physical and talk about clutter. Yes, we said clutter. Take a moment to look around your house, your office, and even we dare say, your car.

Clutter in our external environment represents the clutter of thoughts, emotions, and energetic dissonance that exists within. You may know where we are going with this. It brings us full circle, back to the holographic, infinity perspective of healing. Sustainable healing invites us to complete all the circuits within us and outside of us. When we address healing from the physiological perspective, we shift. In parallel, when we heal through the energy field, and all that exists as energy around us, we shift. When we view both pathways as necessary and balance our approach, we complete the circuit and quantum leaps along our healing spiral are tangible.

Completing the circuit is crucial for our cells and consciousness to anchor the new information and intelligence and then assimilate it to soul level. When our cells and our soul resonate at the same frequency, we arrive at the threshold of self-mastery and the physical actualization of our soul purpose. This is an important element in the understanding of holographic healing.

In direct relationship to quantum physics, when we allow an observer into our experience, and process, we complete the circuit. The observer is your ally, another human to share the depth of your perspective, your healing, and understanding of yourself. This circuit completion allows the anchoring of the life lesson or experience, shifts you holographically, and imprints this new information down to the DNA level and then onto the web of the collective consciousness.

This is part of the design of the human experience. In turn, your ally receives the transmission of this new information, shift in consciousness, and healing energy to plant the seed and accelerate your awakening process. This is relative, of course, to where you are on your journey. You get the idea; this is how we evolve, and it all starts with you. So, go ahead, clean out that closet, desk, or cluttered surface, invite in the principles of feng shui and take this first step of many. Let's get clear!

BRAIN DETOX FREEDOM PHOTON WHEEL

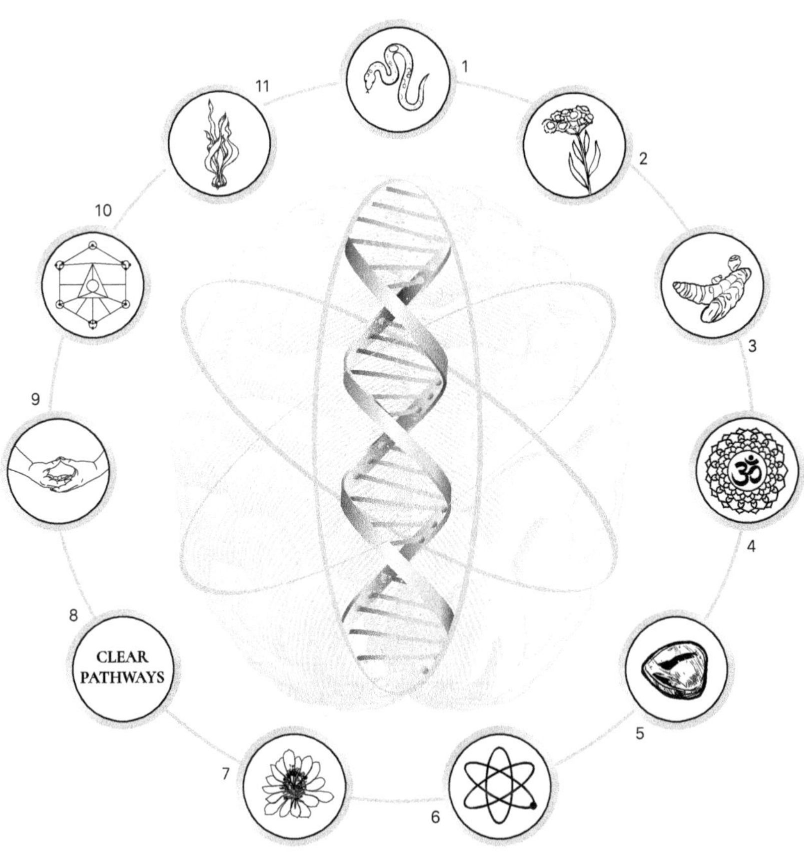

1 Alchemy Animal: Boa
2 Aromatherapy: Immortelle
3 Botanical: Turmeric
4 Light Wheel: Sahasrara
5 Crystal: Shungite
6 Photon Vibration
7 Flower or Gem Essence: Night-Blooming Cereus
8 Intention: Clear Pathways
9 Meditation Mudra: Dharmadhatu
10 Sacred Geometry
11 Nutrition: Spirulina

BRAIN DETOX
INFINITY INFLUENCERS

Inner critic
Pain and inflammation
Denial of divine connection
Pharmaceutical toxicity
Disconnected from body
Dementia and Alzheimer's
Anxiety and depression
Addictions

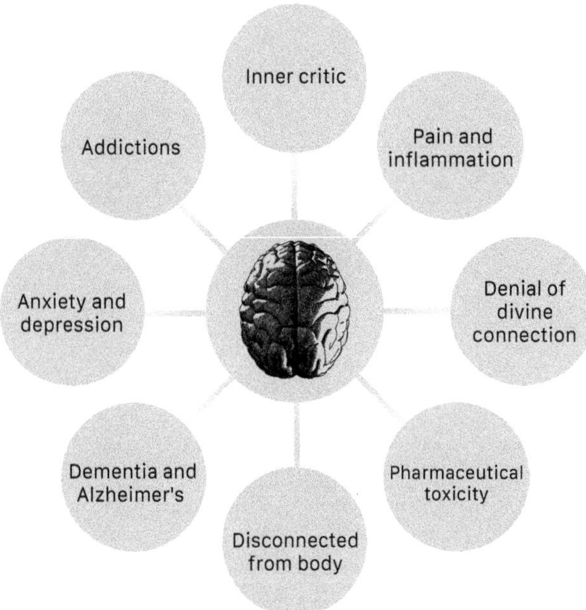

DETOX THE BRAIN – ALCHEMY ANIMALS

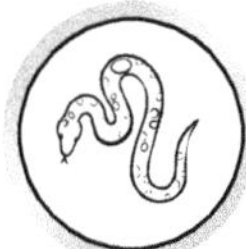

The detox alchemy animals of the brain symbolize a path of metamorphosis is ahead. They will be the guardians of your sacred emotional treasures. The road between the old and the new might be filled with rocks and take you down branches and over creek crossings and sinkholes. For each of you this path will be unique. These alchemy animals will guide you along the bridge during this transition.

MAJOR ARCHETYPE

BOA CONSTRICTOR

The boa constrictor is an alchemy ally of stupendous emotional and genetic rebirth. The boa challenges and supports you to shift and let go of all aspects that are no longer in alignment with the new you and your thought patterns. The snake sheds its skin four to twelve times per year. This is a symbol for shedding old nervous system patterns: depression, sadness, anxiety, worry, or any repetitive depleting emotional loops.

As this transformation begins, you will feel the core energy of the Earth, kundalini, activating all the light wheels in the etheric body. You will feel lighter and able to glide more easily through the understory or terrain of your life.

Creature Connection: "I call upon my eternal guardians to light the way for my rebirth and metamorphosis. I am safe and thrive with the new me!"

MINOR ARCHETYPES

Peacock

This colorful and magnificent bird is well known for its brilliant plumage. Have you heard the call of the peacock? It's quite different and lighthearted. Some almost say it's an outcry or shriek to the world. This cry symbolizes taking your new transition and changing with a little laughter. When was the last time you had a laugh? A really good laugh where you cried? It's time! So, lighten up!

The other important message the peacock imparts is the vision of wisdom. On the end of each of the tail feathers is an "eye." The peacock will be your guardian watching out for obstacles blocking your path ahead, surrounding you with a glow of radiant blue and green. Let your guard down and know all is well.

Creature Connection: "I call upon the brilliance and wisdom of the peacock. I trust my intuition and inner voice. I believe in my instinctive wisdom. I show my true self to the world."

Spider

The spider is a great weaver of imagination, linking to the past and future and allowing a new road or path to be chosen. The spider is deeply connected to the number eight or the infinity symbol, opening the path towards infinite possibilities and creations. Since the spider weaves its own web, it is also a symbol to remember you are the creator of your own destiny and reality. Have you forgotten your truest desire and vision? Now is the time to refocus and choose a new direction – create your own destiny. The spider also asks you to connect with symbols or writings that are meaningful to you – keep a journal, write, draw, or whatever else gets those magic desires flowing. How are you using your creative brain? Are you using your words in a creative and powerful way?

Creature Connection: "Dear spider, come into my consciousness and help me to weave a new story of creative vision expressing my truest desires and love."

ANIMAL ADDITIONS

- ∞ Giraffe
- ∞ Centipede
- ∞ Howler monkey
- ∞ Sloth
- ∞ Dolphin
- ∞ Koi

DETOX THE BRAIN – AROMATHERAPY

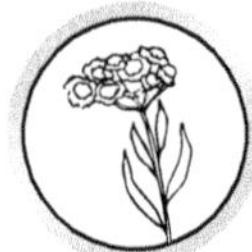

MAJOR ARCHETYPE

IMMORTELLE – *Helichrysum italicum*

Part Extracted: Flower

Core Properties: Antiallergenic, anti-inflammatory, antispasmodic, astringent, diuretic, analgesic, expectorant, cytophylactic, cholagogue, and nervine

Safety: Nontoxic, nonirritant

Immortelle has one of the most curious, multifaceted, and resounding deep aromas. It speaks volumes about its versatility. Also known as Everlasting, this oil has the strength and "everlasting" perseverance to permeate the deepest of traumas. Its nature as a potent anti-inflammatory and antispasmodic lends a unique ability to move through frenetic energy and inflamed emotions of outrage towards individuals or establishments as well as rage turned inward. Immortelle encourages us to source strength from within. Inhaling its aromatic molecules connect us with ancient wisdom within our DNA. With a nature of courage and fortitude supports our ability to pull that forward to the present moment, the place of power where we can bring light, love, and healing holographically to shift our past and our future. Invite the medicine of immortelle to all the places of doubt and pain and forge ahead with courage.

Immortelle is a key oil for accessing and healing deep pain associated with soul level disappointment of not finding a true match or partner in a primary relationship. This degree of disappointment can also relate to the incomplete search for soul purpose and expression of the high self, in which immortelle can assist in opening the connections within our cells and consciousness for the deep clearing and illumination of the core, authentic self to surface.

This oil is also a great ally in addressing the pain related to fibromyalgia and neuralgia that comes from a sense of constriction and separation of living life with purpose, heart, and expression feeling misaligned.

Immortelle medicine is potent alchemy for healing and clearing the masculine aspects through the DNA and father bloodline of past failures of providing and protecting. It also clears the energy of being dishonored, whether actual or perceived.

Detox the Brain – Helichrysum Alchemy for Releasing Disappointment

∞ 2 drops Immortelle essential oil (Helichrysum italicum)
∞ 3 drops Ylang Ylang essential oil (Cananga odorata superior extra)
∞ 1 drop Cistus essential oil (Cistus ladaniferus)

Blend into 15 ml jojoba oil or coconut oil and apply sparingly to palms and breathe in for 30–45 seconds with your intention and apply to the heart and as a perfume as desired.

MINOR ARCHETYPES

Frankincense – *Boswellia carterii*

Part Extracted: Resin

Core Properties: Anti-inflammatory, antiviral, antiseptic, antifungal, anticatarrhal, expectorant, and antidepressant
Safety: Nontoxic, nonirritant

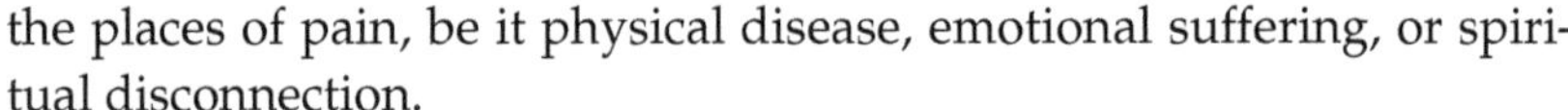

Frankincense medicine is deeply spiritual. It offers a balm of tranquility, inviting spirit to soothe the places of pain, be it physical disease, emotional suffering, or spiritual disconnection.

Frankincense bathes all the places of starvation within us with its healing light. It feeds those places where what we truly crave is connection, and instead attempt to fill it with food, sex, alcohol, drugs, and other addictions. Frankincense brings the energy of unification, unifying mind with body. For those that tend to overthink or worry with anxiety loops that become mentally exhausting, this is good medicine.

The earthy resonance of its aroma connotes spiritual awakening. Frankincense is an oil of ceremony and is beneficial for anointing to awaken the sleeping soul and engage it through the rapture of mystical inspiration. Frankincense is soul medicine, deepening connection and understanding of the lessons we have chosen in the current incarnation and the ability to assimilate the wisdom from them at the cellular level through unifying emotion and experience. This oil of unification, unifies breath with spirit, unifies our male and female aspects, and unifies Heaven and Earth within and around us.

Frankincense helps to bridge the loneliness from not being fully seen for the totality of who you are, particularly by your family of origin. Through the process of deepening the breath, frankincense reminds us that spirit is all around us: in the trees, the plants, the animals. Spirit is even in those around us that trigger our defenses as great mirrors and teachers of the emotional edges and shadow aspects we have brought into this life to be healed and transformed.

The tranquil nature of frankincense encourages us to release the patterns and habitual self-talk that limits our experience of life. It invites a deeper communion with the universe and divine mind and reminds us that we are never alone. It assists us to break down family bloodline belief systems and patterns of addiction, resistance, and misunderstanding of the divine and the places where we have experienced a weakness of will to live fully, wholly, and healthfully.

Detox the Brain – Frankincense Meditation Oil

- ∞ 3 drops Frankincense essential oil (*Boswellia carterii*)
- ∞ 1 drop Cistus essential oil (*Cistus ladaniferus*)
- ∞ 1 drop Sandalwood essential oil (*Santalum austrocaledonicum*)
- ∞ 1 drop Jasmine absolute (*Jasminum grandiflorum*)
- ∞ 2 drops Myrrh essential oil (*Commiphora myrrha*)

With its invitation to deeply connect with the divine consciousness, frankincense medicine helps to enhance and deepen meditation. Blend all ingredients into 15 ml of coconut oil. Apply sparingly to palms and inhale for 30 to 45 seconds. Apply to temples and third eye area prior to meditation.

Lavender – *Lavandula angustifolia*

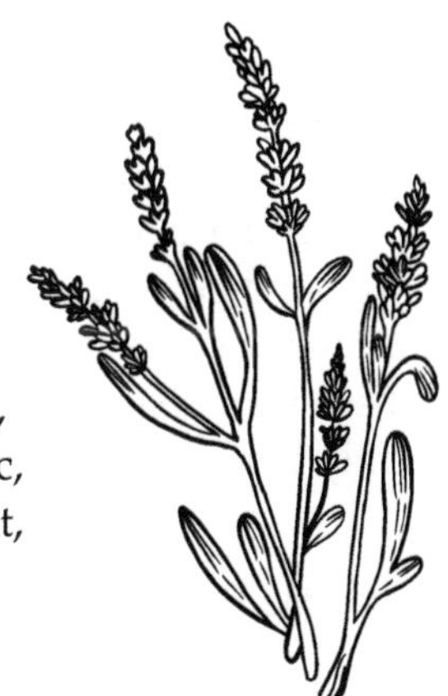

Part Extracted: Flower and Leaf

Core Properties: Antiseptic, analgesic, anticonvulsant, antidepressant, antirheumatic, antispasmodic, anti-inflammatory, antiviral, bactericide, carminative, cholagogue, cicatrisant, cordial, cytophylactic, decongestant, deodorant, diuretic, emmenagogue, hypotensive, nervine, rubefacient, sedative, sudorific, and vulnerary
Safety: Nontoxic, nonirritant

Lavender is the great shape-shifter of plant medicine. Its versatility is perhaps unparalleled. There are over forty species and hundreds of varieties.

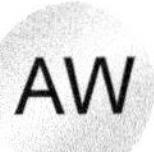

I recall training at a Rutgers University program many years ago. We were blindfolded and asked to identify more than ten different lavender species. It was a beautiful opportunity to continue to build my scent differentiation "muscle." We highly recommend this process for all oils: it is how you will come to a deeper understanding and relationship regarding species and chemotype nuances and more importantly quality and rampant adulteration. Your nose and other organoleptic senses will become your best guide.

Lavender is an excellent nervine and is a quintessential calming and balancing plant medicine for all aspects of the self that are out of alignment. It quells an overactive mind, gently settles emotions, and is an excellent oil for conflict resolution in relationships and business, even the boardroom. Lavender can ease the need of the ego to be right or in control and thus is an oil for peaceful communication.

Lavender brings an ease and grace to one's perspective on life, dissolving tension, anxiety, and an unsettled nature. This oil can gently ease its way into the trauma "energy blocks" in the auric field as well as at the cellular level to bring the healing energy of peace to places of deep emotional holding, through the DNA and particularly to the male bloodline where feelings of pain, loss, and betrayal have been "depressed" along the timeline.

Its regenerative nature makes it excellent for wound healing and is a must have for your "aromatic arsenal" for burns, cuts, scrapes, emotional outbursts, and family conflict resolution. We recommend choosing three lavenders from different countries to begin to explore the vast alchemy of this plant medicine. Our favorites are French Highland, Kashmiri, and Bulgarian.

Lavender's ability to amplify the holistic healing effect of any synergy is potent. It lends the medicine of "relief" and freedom to every formula it is blended into. Relief from any overactive, underactive, or otherwise imbalanced nature of thinking or feeling, and freedom to gently ease into a greater expression of self.

Detox the Brain – Soothing Lavender Sleep Spray

- ∞ 11 drops Lavender essential oil (*Lavandula angustifolia*)
- ∞ 2 drops Mandarin essential oil (*Citrus reticulata*)
- ∞ 1 drop German Chamomile essential oil (*Matricaria recutita*)
- ∞ 2 drops Geranium essential oil (*Pelargonium graveolens*)

Blend into 30 ml of distilled water and shake well before use. Mist bedroom and pillows before retiring for a restful night's sleep.

ESSENTIAL OIL ADDITIONS

German chamomile – *Matricaria chamomilla*

BRAIN DETOX AROMATHERAPY
DNA BLUEPRINT BENEFITS

Immortelle
Heals masculine aspects
Awakens courage, fortitude, and conflict resolution
Lavender
Peace and balance
Connects spirit with the soul to heal loneliness, divine disconnection, and addictions
Understanding and assimilation of soul level lessons
Frankincense
Spiritual connection and unification

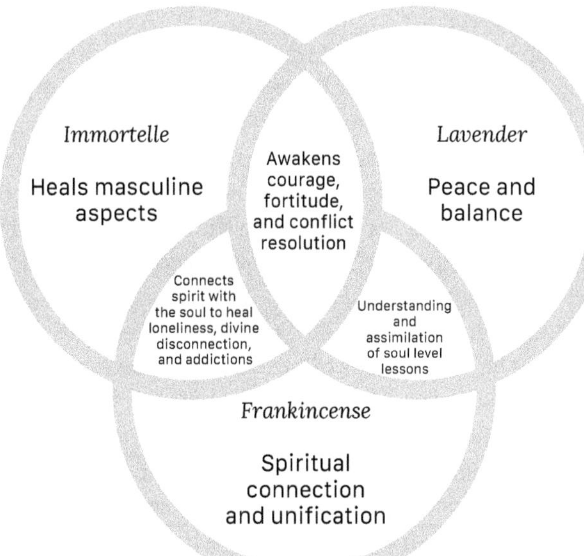

DETOX THE BRAIN – BOTANICAL MEDICINE

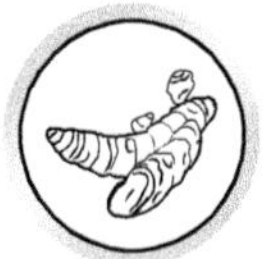

MAJOR ARCHETYPE

TUMERIC – *Curcuma longa*

Parts used: Rhizome

Turmeric, the vibrant yellow root, has so many benefits for detoxifying the entire body and specifically the nervous system. Each day in your environment you are exposed to environmental and emotional toxins, and these substances are not generally present in the human body. These substances and emotions are often associated with increased inflammation when specific inflammatory neurons or pathways of communication to immune cells are released from the brain. Turmeric assists the body with detoxification from xenobiotics by aiding the liver in Phase I and Phase II detoxification.

Turmeric also has been studied for its benefit in reducing symptoms of depression. Of course, as you have learned throughout this book so far, most of our chronic emotional disorders are connected to genetic and emotional trauma. Treating just the symptom suppresses the emotional or physical problem deeper and deeper into the body. Turmeric has the profound ability to lift this "symptom" to the surface by impacting neurotransmitter function through the brain-derived neurotrophic factor.

Call upon this majestic herbal ally for its ability to aid in all aspects of inflammation. Especially the anti-inflammatory effects on the brain and nervous system. The constituents of turmeric have been studied for many cognitive conditions and as a possible treatment for Alzheimer's disease.

Turmeric has long been considered to hold the energy of the divine and was used in ancient India and other cultures for sacred ceremonies, cleansing the light wheels and purifying the emotional and energetic channels of the body. It can be applied to the forehead (ajna light wheel) during sacred ceremonies or when wanting to connect to the divine source of the universe.

Detox the Brain – Turmeric Physical Uses

Detox: Remove cellular debris of the nervous system and brain
Nervous System: Mental dullness and clarity, depression, Alzheimer's, removes toxins from the pineal gland and brain
Cardiovascular: Antioxidant and circulatory stimulant
Adrenals: Alterative and trophorestorative
Musculoskeletal System: Anti-inflammatory and antiarthritic
Digestive: Anthelmintic, carminative, IBS (Irritable Bowel Syndrome), flatulence, and protection of the digestive mucosa
Liver: Choleretic, hypolipidemic, and hepatoprotector
Immune System: Anticancer, antimicrobial, and antibiotic
Integumentary System: Inflammation and rashes

Detox the Brain – Turmeric Emotional Uses

Purify emotional toxicity and reclaim your power
Release limiting thought patterns of chronic pain
For birthing a new you in times of great emotional shift

Detox the Brain – Turmeric Energetic Uses

Third Light Wheel: Healing and empowerment of self
Sixth Light Wheel: Awakening third eye vibrational energy
Connects to the divine energy and power of the sun

Detox the Brain – Turmeric Dosage

Powdered Herb: 4g 2x/day
Decoction: ½–1 cup 3x/day
Tincture: 2 ml 3–4x/day
Topical Poultice: Apply as needed for inflammation
Note: Best absorbed with fat and black pepper

Detox the Brain – Turmeric Cautions and Contraindications

Caution with biliary obstruction, gallstones, or stomach hyperacidity/stomach ulcer
Contraindicated during pregnancy

Detox the Brain – Turmeric Freedom from Inflammation

Ingredients:
1 part Turmeric powder – *Curcuma longa*
1 part Lemongrass – *Cymbopogon citratus*
1 part Ginger root powder – *Zingiber officinale*

Directions:
Combine all ingredients in a small bowl
Make a paste by adding water a small amount at a time until the right consistency forms.
Apply over the area of pain or rash.
Avoid open wounds
Note – may turn skin yellow temporarily

MINOR ARCHETYPES

Milk Thistle – *Silybum marianum*

Part used: Fruit/Seed

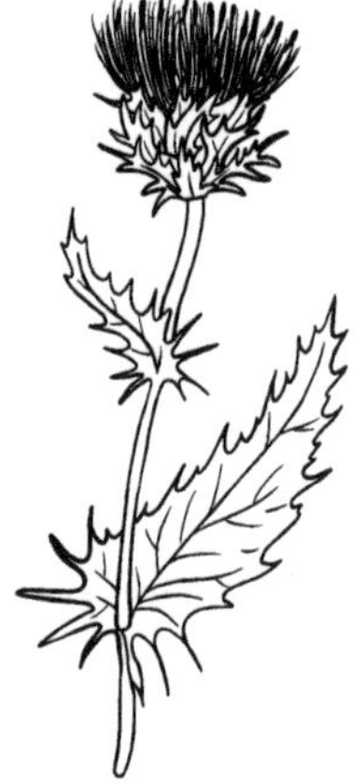

Milk thistle is a palatial nervous system cellular detoxifier and restorative. Have you met this plant in person? If not, we suggest you find some in your area and introduce yourself. It is regal, spiky, and loves to spread around the garden. Plants have a vibration they resonate with from seed to blossom and milk thistle is boisterous in expressing her medicine. The spiky seed blossoms resemble the protective nature of this plant. She realigns the DNA of the cell, strengthening the cellular membrane and assisting in the regeneration and creation of a more robust cell.

One of the most important aspects of milk thistle is its ability in detoxifying the body from cellular imprinting. You might be asking yourself, "What's cellular imprinting?" Cellular imprinting is a memory or "ghost" genetic aspect that is left behind in the DNA and membrane of the cell. For example, milk thistle is especially useful when recovering from a drug addiction. Drugs, including mental health pharmaceuticals, leave behind this imprint in the cell causing cellular damage. Once this damaged cell has been created, the system continues to duplicate this damaged cell causing disruption in cellular and physiological functioning. Milk thistle not only facilitates the detoxification of the damaged cells but rebuilds the cellular membrane for optimal functioning.

Detox the Brain – Milk Thistle Physical Uses

Detox: Releasing the genetic imprint of drugs, toxins, and anesthesia
Nervous System: Regeneration and protection of the neurons, increases cognitive function, and improves mood
Cardiovascular: Antioxidant and improves blood circulation
Adrenals: Protects the adrenals from heavy metal toxicity
Digestive: Aids the liver and gallbladder to break down fat
Urinary: Demulcent and kidney restorative
Liver: Jaundice, hepatitis, gallstones, hepatoprotective, hepatorestorative, and cholagogue
Immune System: Congestion of the spleen, recovery from a debilitating illness
Reproductive: Pelvic congestion and stagnation

Detox the Brain – Milk Thistle Emotional Uses

Releases emotional attachments to addictions
Uplifts mood during chronic illnesses and "feelings of defeat"
Unbind and detach from feelings of anger

Detox the Brain – Milk Thistle Energetic Uses

Emotional support and protection from toxic energy
Nurtures the loving feminine energy within
Absolves karmic anger within the DNA and bloodline

Detox the Brain – Milk Thistle Dosage

Powdered Herb: 80–200 mg 3x/day
Infusion: 1 teaspoon per cup of hot water, infuse 15–30 minutes. Drink 1 cup 3x/day
Tincture: 2 ml 3–4x/day

Detox the Brain – Milk Thistle Cautions and Contraindications

Pregnancy

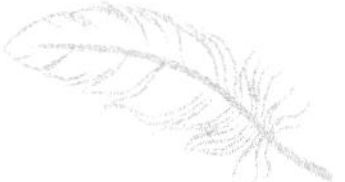

Detox the Brain – Milk Thistle Freedom from Addiction Elixir

Ingredients:
56 g Elderberries – *Sambucus nigra*
14 g Milk Thistle seed – *Silybum marianum*
14 g Anise seed – *Pimpinella anisum*
14 g Dandelion root – *Taraxacum officinale*
10 g Sarsaparilla root – *Smilax ornata*
118 ml honey
473 ml cold water
See Appendix B on how to make this elixir.

Ginkgo – *Gingko biloba*

Part used: Leaf

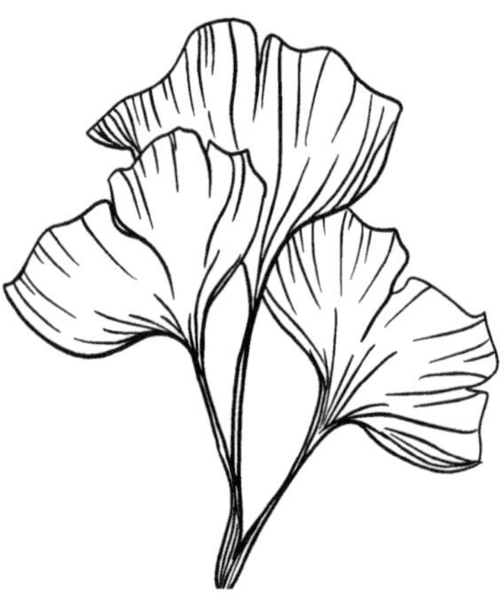

Gingko is one of our dearest and most revered ancient plant allies. It has been on this gorgeous planet for over 190 million years. The DNA and genetic wisdom run deep through its leaves and core and tapping into this ancient knowledge works miracles on the body.

Ginkgo promotes blood flow to the brain and heart improving memory, brain function, and circulation. It's useful in peripheral vascular disease and disorders of restricted blood flow. Its strong antioxidant and anti-inflammatory effects can increase energy and are useful for allergies. Use ginkgo when you are looking for clarity and improved cognitive function – great for a day of creative learning and studying.

We all come to Earth with a higher purpose and along our journey through life our goal is to remember this purpose and live it. Through the ancient genetic wisdom of ginkgo, we can tap into this truth of who we really are. If you are lost on your life's path, we recommend using the ginkgo tea in your sacred ceremonies prior to the meditations throughout the book and it will help to activate your inner wisdom and truth. If you can use the fresh leaf, it will make your ceremony magical.

Detox the Brain – Ginkgo Physical Uses

Detox: DNA nerve healing
Nervous System: Cerebral circulation, dementia, Alzheimer's, depression, nerve tissue damage, and neuroprotective
Cardiovascular: Circulatory stimulant, tonic, antioxidant, thins the blood reducing clots and prevents strokes
Respiratory: Asthma and allergies
Musculoskeletal: Headaches and migraines

Detox the Brain – Ginkgo Emotional Uses

Self-acceptance of the multitude of love
Softness – loving with an open and warm heart
Abundance of universal love

Detox the Brain – Ginkgo Energetic Uses

Remember the truth of who you are
Opens the connection bridge of the fourth and seventh light wheels
Reclaim your ancient wisdom and intuition

Detox the Brain – Ginkgo Dosage

Infusion: 1 tablespoon per cup of water.
Drink 3x/day
Tincture: 3–5 ml 2x/day

Detox the Brain – Ginkgo Cautions and Contraindications

Hypotension and hemorrhagic stroke
Pregnancy

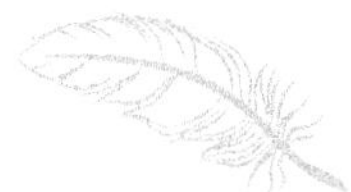

Activate the Heart – Ginkgo Freedom to Recall Memories – Chocolates

Melt 128 g dark chocolate in a double boiler
Add 32 g dried Gingko powder – *Gingko biloba*
Add 2.5 g crystalized Ginger – *Zingiber officinale*

Mix all ingredients.
Drop by spoonful onto a cookie sheet lined with parchment paper or silicone chocolate molds.
Refrigerate, cool, and place in a glass storage container.
Dosage: 1–2 chocolates per day for memory boost

BOTANICAL ADDITIONS

- ∞ Blue vervain – *Verbena hastata*
- ∞ Valerian – *Valeriana officinalis*
- ∞ Lousewort – *Pedicularis*
- ∞ St. John's wort – *Hypericum perforatum*
- ∞ Lavender – *Lavandula angustifolia*
- ∞ Passionflower – *Passiflora incarnata*

BRAIN DETOX BOTANICAL MEDICINE
DNA BLUEPRINT BENEFITS

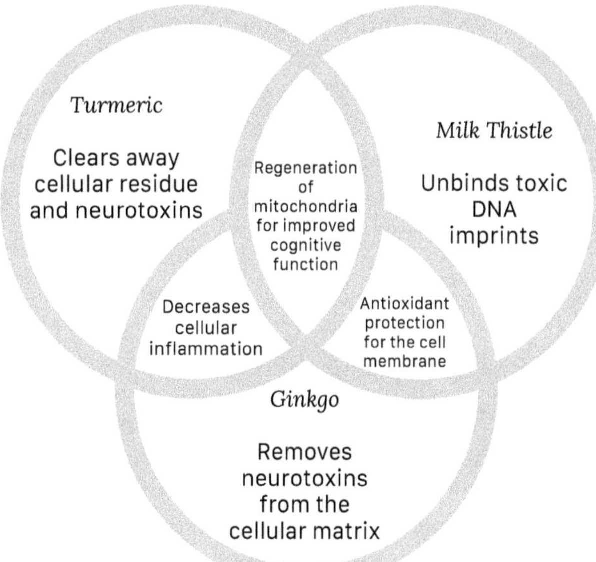

DETOX THE BRAIN – LIGHT WHEELS

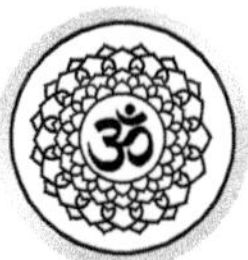

The light wheels or chakras of the brain are to open up your body, mind, and spirit for healing. You might find you experience tingling, light-headedness, euphoria, or greater intuition. These observations are all normal. If you are feeling "spacy" go back to the adrenal light wheel interventions and connect to the grounding of the Earth for balance. Invite in these light wheels to connect, open, expand, and balance for your highest good.

MAJOR ARCHETYPE

THE 7th LIGHT WHEEL, SAHASRARA

The seventh light wheel, Sahasrara, thousand-petaled lotus, is the connection to the Divine and your inner being or soul. Sahasrara is the control center or command station of two very important glands of the body: the pineal, maintaining regular sleep patterns, and the pituitary gland, influencing and regulating every hormone in the body. It also connects the brain with the spine and central nervous system, balancing communication between the physical and emotional body.

MINOR ARCHETYPES

∞ The 88th light wheel, Ashtaasheetihi

Ashtaasheetihi is the gateway light wheel, and it connects the cells of the body holographically with the cells of the universe. This light wheel fully activates the call of humanity to your soul purpose and the purpose of the planet. When aligned and opened, this chakra connects you to unlimited joy and connects the alignment of the fourth, eighth, and eight-eighth light wheels. It attunes your nervous system with all the living creatures of the planet and all the beings of the universe.

LIGHT WHEEL COLORS

MAJOR ARCHETYPE

GOLD

Gold is well known as a symbol of luxury and divinity. It is the color of true knowledge and learning tapping into the wisdom within your DNA and the wisdom of your soul. When using this color in your life and on your sacred altar, it is a time to share your wisdom with others around you and to share your brilliance. You will experience a clear focus of what you want and desire in your life. Gold is also a symbol of abundance and we suggest you get a gold coin (gold chocolate coin) and place it in your sacred space to increase and manifest abundance. Refer to Chapter Four for allowing more abundance into your life.

SOUND

∞ Mauna or Silence

Mauna is the Sanskrit word for silence. When was the last time you took a day of silence? We don't' mean a day where you are not hearing sound but where you are not speaking. We suggest you try this as an experiment and see how this affects you. Pick a day when you can be in an environment of ease and peace, not at a busy workplace where you are having to communicate with many people. Take the time to listen to your inner being, to YOU. In the silence your brain is given the space to decompress and heal and for the "realness" of life to surface.

DETOX THE BRAIN – CRYSTALS AND STONES

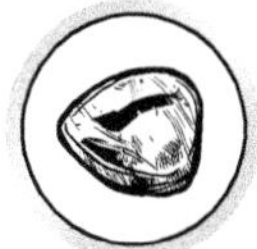

MAJOR ARCHETYPE

SHUNGITE

Shungite is a powerhouse of protection and purification. It encases and strengthens the auric field with a force field of high frequency light by flowing this frequency from the cosmic perspective to the ketheric template and then floods the auric field permeating down to the cellular and DNA level. It is helpful to block EMF (Electromagentic Field) including 5G networks. Shungite also shields from emotional negativity and projection from others. It cleanses and purifies energy in your personal space. It helps to calm the overactive mind and break apart ancient energies of separation from the Divine in the auric field.

MINOR ARCHETYPES

∞ Serpentine

Serpentine medicine supports rousing kundalini energy like the serpent. Place this stone at root chakras and crown for activation of the nervous system. When applying to the points on the body, it will clear the blocked energy of the brain and nervous system. It works on the reptilian part of the brain. Serpentine medicine carries the blueprint of evolution for the Earth. Working with stone will open the higher aspects of your consciousness to connect you holographically at the DNA level to the highest ultimate reality for Earth and humankind. This stone carries the history of all the elemental realms. It connects the brain and heart of the body with that of the Earth. It helps us to see the broader vision of the planet in the span of the history of Gaia. Serpentine supports cellular regeneration and a rebalancing of the nervous system.

∞ Mother of Pearl

Mother of pearl offers a deep healing to the female aspects and the mother bloodline in the DNA, assisting to resolve a sense of abandonment and unfulfilled emotional or physical needs from childhood. Offering the love and nurturance of the cosmic mother aspect, this crystal calms and soothes the emotional body releasing the anger and sadness from the early childhood dynamics with the mother. Pearl brings healing energy to imbalances in the reproductive system and restores purity to the feminine principle within.

CRYSTAL ADDITIONS

∞ Amethyst

DETOX THE BRAIN CRYSTAL GRID

Drink a glass of clean water with 3 drops each of Sapphire and Buttercup essences. Indian flute music can be enjoyed during this session. This crystal attunement is best done before bed or a good long nap for 20-30 minutes. Cleanse crystals immediately after use. (See Appendix C).

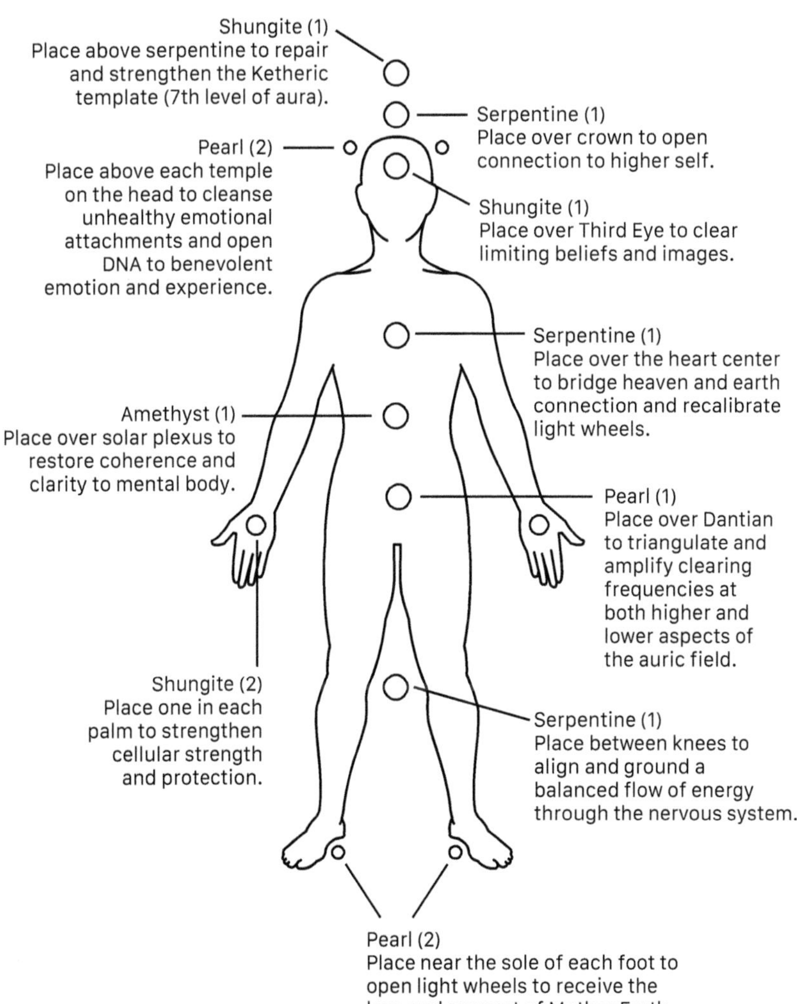

DETOX THE BRAIN – ENERGETIC AND VIBRATIONAL TECHNIQUES

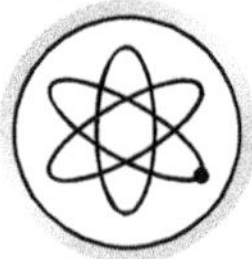

MAJOR ARCHETYPE

DETOX THE BRAIN HYDROTHERAPY

- ∞ 1 drop Immortelle essential oil (*Helichrysum italicum*)
- ∞ 6 drops of Lavender essential oil (*Lavendula angustifolia*)
- ∞ 3 drops German Chamomile essential oil (*Matriciaria recutita*)
- ∞ 480 ml fresh Turmeric tea
- ∞ 453 g Epsom salt
- ∞ 226 g Dead Sea salt

Soak in this lovely and lightly tinted bluish-yellow water for at least 20 minutes.

MINOR ARCHETYPES

Detox the Brain Visualization

See, feel, allow, or imagine yourself seated deep inside a shungite crystal pyramid as you deepen your breath, envision all limited patterns, the repetition of your old story, the places of trauma and genetic imbalance being dissolved into the shungite pyramid then releasing out to the universe. With each breath in you begin to feel lighter, calmer, and more centered. The healing vibration of shungite fills every structure within your brain, all cells, and neural pathways, clearing away the old energy to renew and revitalize your entire being.

Detox the Brain EOBT

Place one drop of immortelle essential oil between the first two fingers of the right hand, inhale deeply and tap the Bladder-63, Golden Gate point of the Bladder Meridian for thirty seconds with the intention of letting go of all patterns, thoughts, emotions and energy that no longer serves you.

Location: On the lateral side of the foot, in the depression posterior to the tuberosity of the fifth metatarsal bone. Run the flat of your finger down the front shin bone of the leg until it hits onto the foot, then slide the finger down to the lateral edge of the foot and feel for the depression.

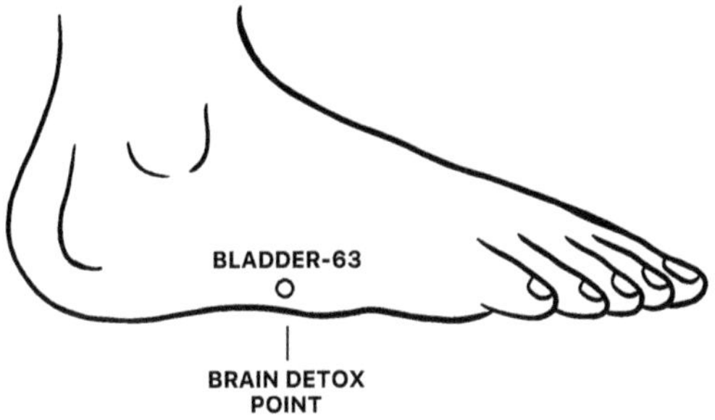

DETOX THE BRAIN – FLOWER AND GEM ESSENCES

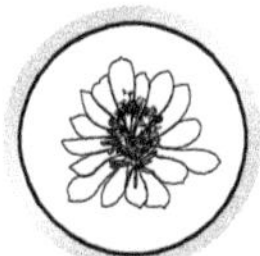

FLOWER ESSENCES

MAJOR ARCHETYPE

NIGHT-BLOOMING CEREUS

Night-blooming cereus opens the crown chakra or light wheel and anchors the I AM presence. It rejuvenates at the cellular level, opening the heart to joy of life and authentic self. This essence engages our playful nature and frees creativity. It activates the soul seat or high heart where all the longings of your soul for this incarnation are held.

MINOR ARCHETYPES

Comfrey

Comfrey energizes the auric field and opens the third eye. This is an essence of strength. It increases physical resilience and enhances all glandular function, including the adrenals. Comfrey strengthens the nervous system, mental memory and balances both hemispheres of the brain. It brings clarity and healing to past life karmic issues, allowing the current life connection to the past to be illuminated and assimilated.

Buttercup

Buttercup reminds us of the innocence of our youth. This essence is helpful when innocence was lost too young from dysfunction in the family environment or when there have been patterns of abuse, physically, emotionally, or sexually that robbed the vital life force early in life. This essence helps to free the playful and pure aspects of the child consciousness held deep within.

GEM ESSENCE

MAJOR ARCHETYPE

SAPPHIRE

Sapphire opens your inner and innate wisdom of knowing what is truly right for your healing. If you are drawn to this stone, it also is a time to learn new tools and modalities to awaken and access your inner healer. This essence is great for opening the crown light wheel to a broader understanding of universal connection. It encourages the channeling chakra to open and expand (located at the back of the neck), accessing the higher self and the esoteric teachings of the Akashic records and sacred language. It also opens the third eye connection with high frequency sacred geometry.

DETOX THE BRAIN – INTENTIONS

MAJOR ARCHETYPE

CLEAR PATHWAYS

MINOR ARCHETYPES

∞ I release all trauma of brain injury, inflammation, and neuronal dysfunction.

- ∞ My body is as light as a feather and moves effortlessly.
- ∞ I let go of all the old patterns that no longer serve the truth of who I AM.

ADDITIONAL INTENTIONS

- ∞ The cells of my nervous system are filled with light and travel with ease through my body for elimination and release.
- ∞ I OPEN to divine mind.
- ∞ I clear and cleanse all pathways that do not serve my highest good.

DETOX THE BRAIN – MEDITATION MUDRA

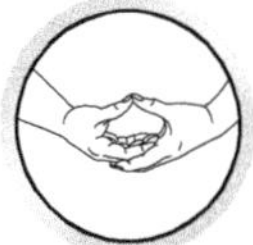

Dharmadhatu Mudra

I connect to the cosmic light of the universe,
enlightening and harmonizing all pathways of my brain and being.

Dharmadhatu mudra opens the brain and invokes a sense of calm and serenity. It allows us to clear all pathways of communication in the brain that have become distorted or damaged and are in need of repair. This mudra is often used as a meditation mudra, called the cosmic mudra, because it not only connects our seventh chakra to the planetary and universal chakras, but it also connects the brain and body to the soul. This is the mudra of bliss connecting the front of the body with the back of the body creating an endless circuit of energy throughout the spine and nervous system. A level of complete serenity can be achieved when using this mudra on a daily basis – especially while in meditation.

Dharmadhatu Mudra Alignment

1. Place the left hand onto the lap with the palm facing upward.
2. Rest the back of the right hand on top of the left hand.
3. Take the tips of the thumbs and lightly touch them together forming the shape of an oval.

4. Take a deep breath, let your body relax.
5. You may now either do the meditation below or ten minutes of *Brain Breathing* (to access the Brain Breathing technique please visit www.zenergymedicinals.com).
6. You may also use the mudra any time you want to align your brain and body or your seventh chakra with the other chakras and harmonize the nervous system.

∞ To access the mudra meditation please go to www.zenergymedicinals.com

∞ Take a deep breath in, inhaling your essential oil for 30–45 seconds.
∞ Hold the Dharmadhatu mudra and take several breaths to align and attune to your nervous system and brain. With each breath, feel the circular connection of energy flow down the front of the body to the root chakra or pelvis and up the back side of the body back to the brain.
∞ With each breath, feel yourself melting into a state of bliss. Repeat the intention three times either silently or aloud: "I connect to the cosmic light of the universe. Enlightening and harmonizing all pathways of my brain and being."
∞ See, feel, allow, or imagine an opalescent light coming down from the higher realms.
∞ Envision this light raining down upon the higher levels of your energy field, as it begins to pour down into your brain and nervous system, filling all the neurons and the neural pathways with opalescent light.
∞ Cleansing, clearing, balancing. This light moves all the way down the spine.
∞ Feeding all the nerves, all the meridian points, all the energy centers with this light.
∞ See, feel, allow, or imagine a horizontal infinity symbol pulsating this opalescent light, illuminating in the very center of your brain. A golden light moves through each of the circular pathways of the symbol in its figure of eight formation. This golden light is balancing both hemispheres of the brain and bringing more light into the brain, into the neurons, into the structures and cells and receptor points.

- ∞ We invite this opalescent light to come into all the structures of the brain, the amygdala, the hypothalamus, the singular gyrus, the prefrontal cortex, all the structures within the brain.
- ∞ Inviting all that no longer serves you, all the old stories, beliefs, images, emotions, and memories to dissolve into this opalescent light and be returned to the Source. Cleansing, purifying all neural pathways and any areas of our deep grooves of dysfunctional patterning.
- ∞ This light rebalances the areas just as the frequency of the infinity symbol is balancing and communicating deeply and directly into the cells, into the DNA, the mother and father bloodlines.
- ∞ Let go of the stories of pain and struggle that have been passed through generation to generation.
- ∞ Release cellular cultural imprints throughout the DNA of abuse of power, of struggle, of domination, lack of determination, allowing the old emotions and feelings that have been suppressed through the ages to be embraced and accepted and transmuted by the light.
- ∞ Release patterns of expectation, of disappointment, disease, discomfort, and lack.
- ∞ Invite in permission to feel good, to feel light.
- ∞ Release confusion and invite in a greater understanding of self, of the universe, of the past, the places of holding, letting go of the illusion of control, the pressure of having to know.
- ∞ Invite in the permission to be. Be here now in the soothing quiet. In all the magnificence of who you are. In the silence the monkey mind is quiet.
- ∞ Breathe into the opalescent light and feel it lift the essence of your spirit.
- ∞ Offer a breath of gratitude to yourself for the great courage to incarnate here and now. To bring the light of healing throughout your DNA, your lineage, and to fully change and lift the experience for all those that come after you, vibrating higher with the light of divine consciousness.
- ∞ Breathe in this light into the new spaces created within your brain, your nervous system, and every cell within your body, every place within your physicality and your non physicality. Lighter. Calmer.

DETOX THE BRAIN – SACRED GEOMETRY

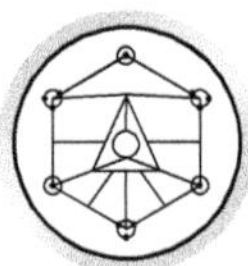

MAJOR ARCHETYPE

DETOX THE BRAIN SACRED GEOMETRY

This intentional and original detox of the brain sacred geometry depicts a hexagon with six small spherical points and a diamond in the center. The energetic configuration of the diamond represents clearing at the core level of the brain, nervous system, and at the cellular and DNA level. The hexagon represents the connection to divine mind, with the points along the hexagon representing neural spheres of connectivity to this divine consciousness. As we allow the frequency of the diamond to expand and absorb all the old patterns, energy, and trauma, the six spheres can expand to receive more light from the Divine.

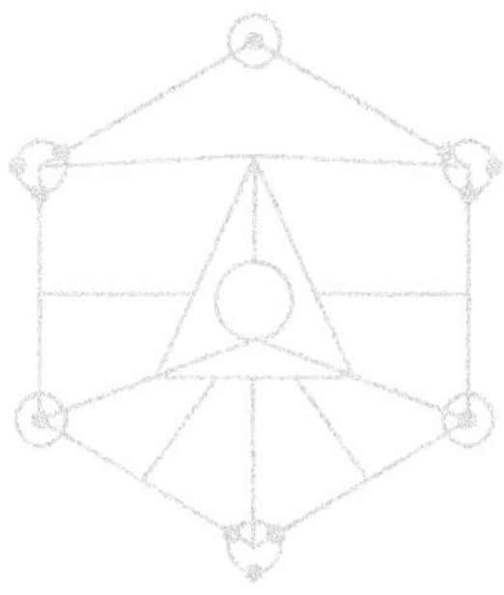

DETOX THE BRAIN – NUTRITION

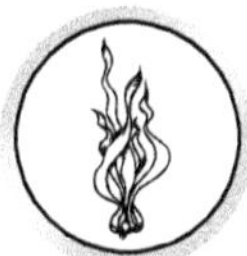

MAJOR ARCHETYPE

SPIRULINA

Spirulina is a vibrant blue green algae first consumed by the ancient Aztecs. Since this ancient food has a tie to a civilization rooted in healers and spiritual medicine, spirulina still carries this alchemy that we may tap into for detoxing the brain. Gram per gram, this superfood is one of the most nutrient dense foods on our planet.

This powerful archetype assists the brain in releasing neurons that are no longer functioning because they have been damaged. It goes even a step further and helps to repair this oxidative damage with its active constituent, phycocyanin, a powerful antioxidant (Farooq et al. 2014).

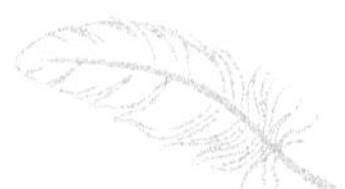

Detox the Brain Spirulina Infused Water

Ingredients:
680 ml filtered water at room temperature
½ juiced grapefruit or lemon
15 ml apple cider vinegar
2 g organic spirulina powder

Directions:
Add the water to a mason jar or glass shaker jar.
Whisk all the ingredients, until well combined.
If desired, add sweetener, pour over a glass of ice or drink at room temperature.

Enjoy!

MINOR ARCHETYPES

Mango

Just thinking of this tropical fruit makes us want to make mango smoothies – you? This oval shaped fruit is rich in vitamin E and hydrates the nervous system. Mango increases nervous system circulation, preserves brain tissue and DNA, and slows down the aging process. The brilliant yellow color connects the pathways in the brain and enhances brain power by shedding old thoughts no longer needed. AKA brain dump!

Cantaloupe

When was the last time you held a cantaloupe? The rough outside and smooth fleshy fruit of the inside reminds us of the brain – law of similars. This sweet fruit is high in the powerful antioxidant, Vitamin C. It's very helpful for detoxing the brain from addictions, that is, pharmaceutical detox, as well as shifting the brain from a state of mental imbalance to a healthy one.

NUTRITIONAL ADDITIONS

∞ Cod liver oil
∞ Omega-6 fatty acids
∞ Mussels
∞ Oyster mushrooms
∞ Pecans

DETOX THE BRAIN – DISCOVERY DIVE – THE BRAIN BODY CONNECTION

Systemic inflammation is the precursor to disease forming in the physical body. The catch-22 here is that inflammation causes pain and pain causes fluctuations in mood responses such as withdrawal, depression, and unbalanced emotional reactions. As you explore each question, consider the brain–body connection and in particular your sense of mood and well-being. Furthermore, how do your mood and emotions affect your relationships? Your choices? Or the way you honor and take care of yourself?

What are your thoughts like daily? Moment by moment? Write down the repeating pattern of thoughts you have – for example, do your thoughts run endlessly like a running hamster wheel or is it hard to find a thought?

What larger belief system do you sense this is connected to?

How can you break this repeating thought pattern and break down the connected belief system? It's OK if you don't have an answer for this yet, just brainstorm and let any thoughts that surface flow to the page.

Are you having pain and inflammation in your body? Where? Does it radiate or travel to other areas of the body?

Is this acute pain or chronic? Did it arise from an accident? If so, explore the emotions that rise and are connected to the memory of this trauma?

How long has it been there? Why do you sense it has been going on this long?

Did anyone in your genetic lineage experience something similar? What core belief do you feel this is connected to?

What are the emotional and physical connections attached to this pain and or inflammation? Do you feel angry, sad, or numb?

Are you depressed, anxious, or feeling helpless? How long has this been going on? Is it new? Is it connected to an experience or circumstance?

How and who can you ask for support in your healing journey?

Are you ready to release these areas? What is one step today that you can take to heal?

FREEDOM PHOTON WHEEL™

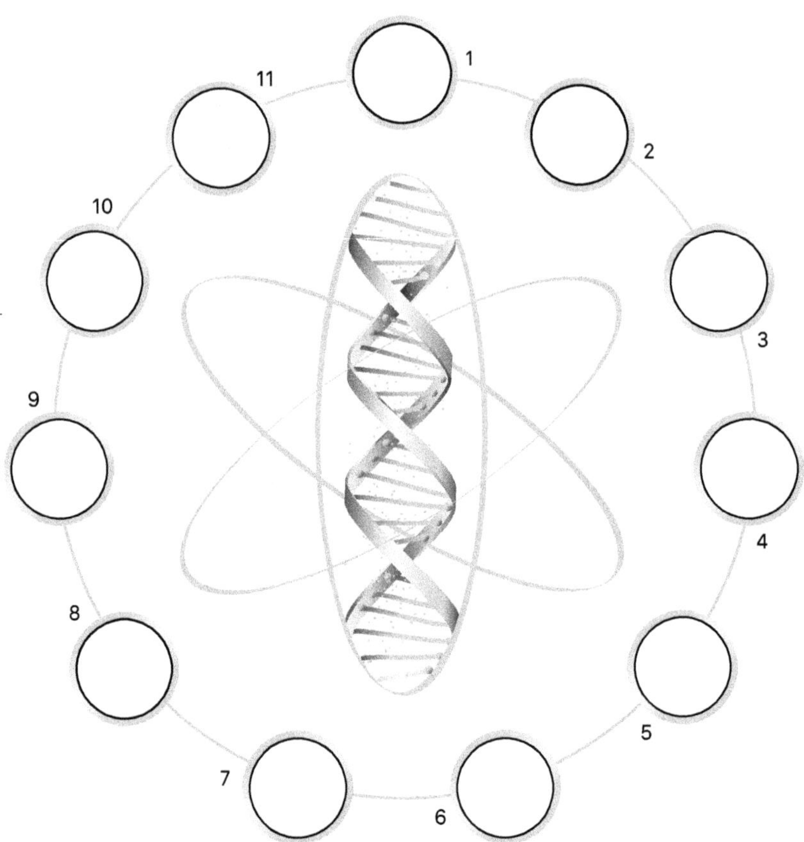

DETOX THE BRAIN
YOUR PERSONAL FREEDOM PHOTON WHEEL RITUAL

Moon Phase

It is best to perform your ritual when the moon is waning from the full moon to the new moon, to align with the phase. However, the power of your intention and momentum is key so if you are inspired at another time, go for it.

Intention

"I release all energy of confusion, of distortion, and dysfunctional patterns. I let go of the old stories of struggle, disconnection, and pain through my genetic lineage."

Select, Align, and Activate

Select your interventions according to the instructions in Chapter Five. Inhale and apply your chosen essential oil for 30–45 seconds. Use your botanical tincture or tea as directed. You may also listen to the meditation and use the mudra from this chapter while attuning your FPW.

Affirm

"Divine Consciousness, please assist me in healing all that I have carried through my lineage, my mother and father bloodlines so that I allow the highest degree of clarity, universal truth, and peace to permeate every level of my being."

NOURISH THE BRAIN

What nourishes the brain nourishes the entire body, the blood, the bone, every cell, every particle and subatomic structure down to your DNA. Just as our belief system, thought, and emotions cause chemical reactions to flood our system, when we nourish our brains we shift and evolve our core paradigm and perceptions.

Nourishing the brain requires us to return to our holographic infinity approach to sustainable healing. Finding what nutrition is right for your body is key. Exercise is as important. A healthy and safe, age-appropriate sex life in partnership or self-pleasure is also an important way to nourish the brain and body with healthful chemical release. Marinating the brain in meditation, prayer, and other sacred or energetic work is the other end of that spectrum and similarly just as needed. When grace fills your cellular consciousness, it feeds your system on all levels including purifying your nervous system and neural pathways and infuses your limbic connections with healing light.

BRAIN NOURISH FREEDOM PHOTON WHEEL

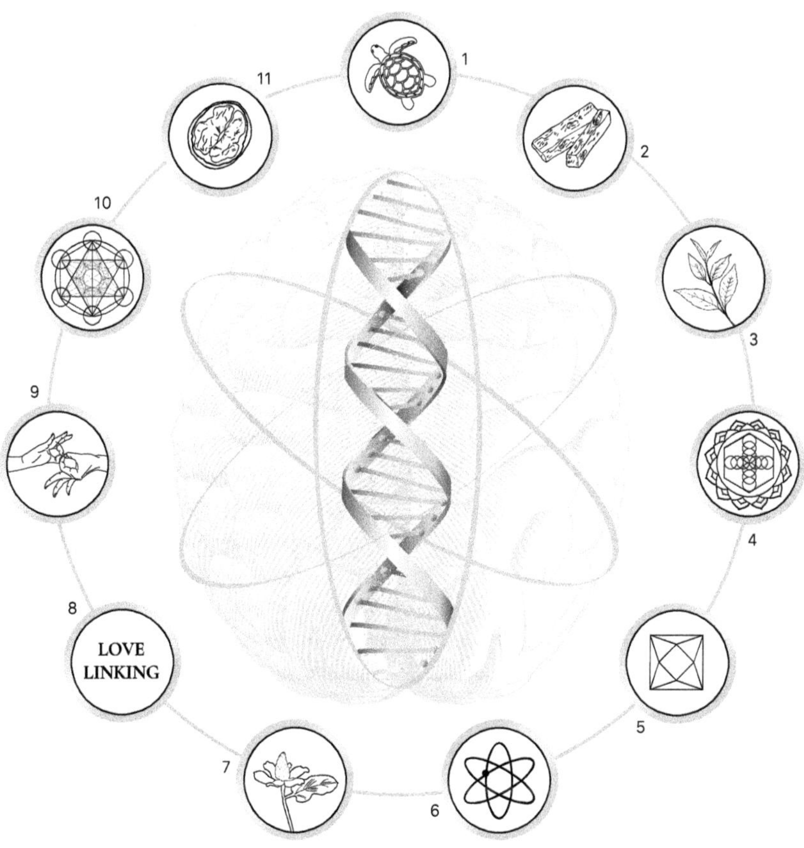

1 Alchemy Animal: Sea Turtle
2 Aromatherapy: Sandalwood
3 Botanical: Green Tea
4 Light Wheel: Mudita
5 Crystal: Herderite
6 Photon Vibration
7 Flower or Gem Essence: Yerba Mansa
8 Intention: Love Linking
9 Meditation Mudra: Dharma Chakra
10 Sacred Geometry
11 Nutrition: Walnut

BRAIN NOURISH
INFINITY INFLUENCERS

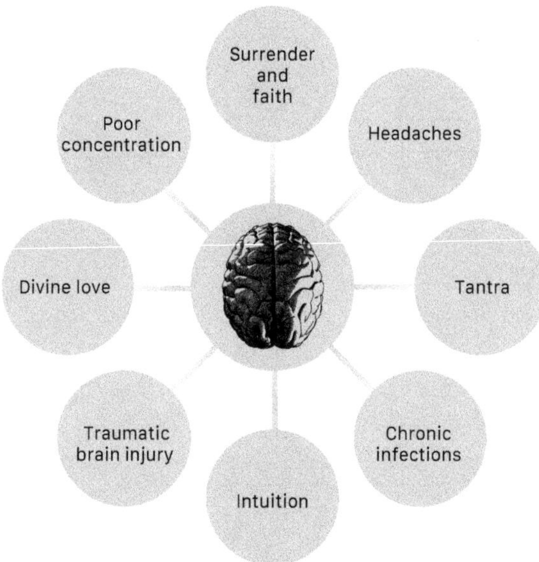

NOURISH THE BRAIN – ALCHEMY ANIMALS

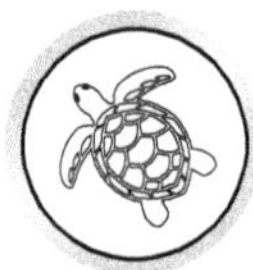

The nourish alchemy animals of the brain invite you to connect to the ocean and the heavens above. They open the doorway of unity between all realms, nourishing the deeper connection of your origination and your current manifestation. Feel the connection to the limitless ocean, the vastness of the desert, and the expansiveness of the air.

MAJOR ARCHETYPE

SEA TURTLE

Motherhood, longevity, awakening to opportunity, the sea turtle is an ancient ally connecting you to the immense spiritual connection of the ocean. The ocean and the creatures within carry a genetic code and history back to the beginning of time. The sea turtle accesses and shares the healing knowledge of the ocean to each cell of your being.

DL One time when I was camping on the beach as a young girl, I went for a family hike on the beach in the moonlight. We came across a group of baby turtles traveling along the beach to the ocean. I will never forget the freedom I felt as I watched them traverse the sand and first touch the waves. Do you remember the first time you met the ocean? This is the freedom the sea turtle invites you to embrace. The sense of joy you feel when you experience something for the first time. The sea turtle invites you to dive deep into your memories and bring to the surface of your brain a memory of such joy and freedom. Embrace this memory with every cell of your being – and live it again!

Creature Connection: "I call upon you, great creature of the sea. May I ride upon your back and feel the deep vibration of the ocean enriching each cell of my being."

MINOR ARCHETYPES

Camel

Have you ever ridden a camel? Well, it's quite the experience!

DL When I was visiting Jordan, I rode a camel up to the top of Mount Sinai in Egypt. The camel had a mind of its own and wanted to run the whole way down on its own. You can't control a camel! It was as if the camel had taken flight. The camel is a symbol you are on the right path and you will continue at the speed of light to your destination of success and prosperity.

We are sure you also know the other symbolism of the camel, the never-ending search for the oasis. During your journey don't forget to take time to nurture yourself – self care is key for without it your journey will not succeed. Of course, make sure you are hydrated!

Creature Connection: "I call upon the power and strength of the camel. As I speed closer to my destination, I take time to savor the journey each step of the way."

Honey Bee

The honey bee has long been known as a symbol of fertility and fulfillment. When this alchemy animal is called into your life, it's time to know that the dreams are ready to be fulfilled, no matter how far-fetched you might think they are. It's time to drink from the nectar of the gods, the elixir of life, and savor the sweetness.

The honey bee is also a symbol of busyness – the busy bee. Are you a workaholic? Are you busying yourself with distractions or are you pursuing your dreams? It's time to refocus your passion and dedicate your time to the messages of your heart.

Creature Connection: "I am the elixir of my dreams. I buzz with a restored fervor in pursuit of my unending and unimaginable happiness."

ANIMAL ADDITIONS

- ∞ Fox
- ∞ Otter
- ∞ Leopard
- ∞ Manatee
- ∞ Painted bunting
- ∞ Blue poison dart frog
- ∞ Fruit bat

NOURISH THE BRAIN – AROMATHERAPY

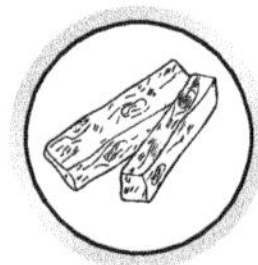

MAJOR ARCHETYPE

SANDALWOOD – *Santalum austrocaledonicum*

Part extracted: Heartwood

We recommend using the New Caledonian species of this endangered oil with reverence and gratitude for its potent medicine.

Core Properties: antiphlogistic, antiseptic, antispasmodic, astringent, carminative, diuretic, emollient, expectorant, sedative, and tonic
Safety: nontoxic, nonirritant

Sandalwood medicine is profound and expansive. It connects us to the higher realms of consciousness and then bridges them to the earthly. Once you inhale this central woodsy aroma, a place of reverence for the Divine is opened and remains open for you to cross that threshold for the rest of your life. Sandalwood is filled with the invitation from the Divine to open, to receive infinite light and through this, a reminder that you walk the Earth as a divine being. Every step is sacred and filled with the potential of the creator. Every moment in your life is a miracle of possibility, awaiting your gaze, your attention, and your intention to create an experience. Then to learn from that experience and assimilate the richness and wisdom from it. Sandalwood floods the brain with this richness and the ability to ease into our cellular consciousness and expand a sense of soothing connection and unification of the mind – body, to the cells, the organs, the blood, the bone, the thoughts, and the emotions, all uniting as one.

Sandalwood floods our neural pathways with tremendous healing energy and elicits a sense of greater universal understanding and presence. Sandalwood medicine assists us in opening our ajna light wheel, or third eye, expanding our inner vision, intuition, and ability to garner more abstract mental concepts and ideas and visions and ground them into the Earth, for it is only through this process that they can be actualized into physical reality.

Sandalwood quells anxiety and invites us to breathe deeply and fully. To trust the heavens above, the Earth below, and ourselves in the middle as conduits of sacred light. Sandalwood medicine deepens our experience of sacred work, ritual, and meditation. This oil brings pronounced healing through the male bloodline when there have been patterns of strife and rejection of the self as an expression of the Divine.

Nourish the Brain – Divine Masculine Healing Sandalwood Oil

∞ 2 drops of Sandalwood essential oil (*Santalum austrocaledonicum*)
∞ 2 drops of Ginger essential oil (*Zingiber officinale*)

- ∞ 1 drop of Immortelle essential oil (*Helichrysum italicum*)
- ∞ 1 drop Spikenard essential oil (*Nardostachys jatamansi*)
- ∞ 1 drop Cistus essential oil (*Cistus ladaniferus*)
- ∞ 2 drops of essential Vetiver oil (*Vetiveria zizanioides*)

Blend into one tablespoon coconut oil and infuse with the intention to bring sandalwood healing medicine through your masculine aspects and father bloodline. Use sparingly on the body as you would a cologne.

MINOR ARCHETYPES

Lemon – *Citrus limon*

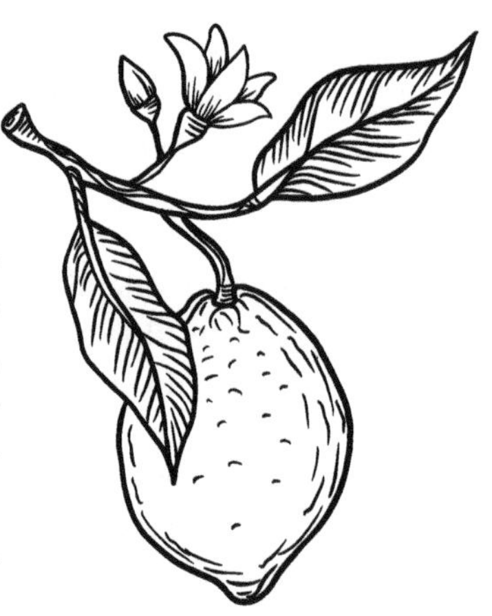

Part extracted: Peel

Core Properties: Antianemic, antimicrobial, antirheumatic, antisclerotic, antiseptic, bactericidal, carminative, cicatrisant, depurative, diaphoretic, diuretic, febrifuge, hemostatic, hypotensive, insecticidal, rubefacient, tonic, and vermifuge
Safety: Nontoxic, potential irritant and sensitizer, photo-toxic

Lemon is a medicine of freedom and liberation, clearing tangles of distorted energy from the mental and emotional bodies and illuminating the brain with clarity, focus, and concentration. Lemon's light and bright aromatic molecules help to energize at the cellular level, clearing away heavy or distorted energy and emotion.

This is particularly helpful to clear the solar plexus chakra or Manipura light wheel, where lower frequency energy and beliefs about the self are stored. This area also tends to have tangled relational chords from power struggles that were initiated by the early childhood and family dynamics and then repeated through current life patterns until cleared. Lemon is immensely helpful in this area with its laser focused clarity and cleansing vibration. The biochemical nature of lemon increases circulation and drainage for the lymphatic system and is also helpful to balance the digestive system, particularly when the pH of the terrain is unbalanced.

Lemon is an excellent oil for encouraging focus and concentration in the younger generation, many of whom experience ADD and ADHD symptoms. Children and adolescents respond well to aromatic medicine and it can become an ally of empowerment in their education process, supporting also the great range of emotional pressures they experience as great beings of light and change on the ever-evolving planet.

Nourish the Brain – Clear Ahead Lemon Study Ally

- ∞ 6 drops of Lemon essential oil (*Citrus limonum*)
- ∞ 4 drops of Rosemary essential oil (*Rosmarinus officinalis CT verbenone*)
- ∞ 6 drops of Wild Orange essential oil (*Citrus sinensis*)
- ∞ 5 drops of Lavender essential oil (*Lavendula angustifolia*)

Blend into a 10 ml roller ball (or another bottle) filled with jojoba. Encourage your student to inhale this blend for 40 seconds after applying it to the palms of their hands before study or homework. And then inhale at the end of study to complete the memory cell. Then because of the power of the limbic system, have them repeat the process for testing and other study preparation to access this memory and all the information encapsulated therein.

Patchouli – *Pogostemon cablin*

Part extracted: Leaves

Core Properties: Antidepressive, antiphlogistic, antiseptic, aphrodisiac, astringent, cicatrisant, cytophylactic, deodorant, diuretic, febrifuge, fungicide, insecticide, sedative, and tonic
Safety: nontoxic, nonirritant

Those that consider patchouli to be a hippie aroma of the 1960s have not experienced the true essential oil.

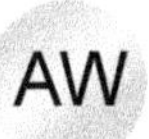

I happened upon patchouli for the first time in India and was thoroughly surprised by the level and longevity of euphoria created from inhaling the leaves between my fingers.

My friend and I laughed heartily for over an hour. About what? At this point, I have no idea. With its deeply intoxicating earthy aroma, patchouli medicine invites us to connect with the playful side of life. Immersing oneself in nature with the elemental intelligence of the Earth. This oil opens our sacral center to the sensual nature within, freeing sexual desire and dissolving the insecurity around the body.

It activates a primal nature of sexual connection, aligning the heart to open to greater levels of intimacy and tantra. The voice of patchouli invites us to open, and then to trust and open more deeply. It encourages us to expand our connection with the Earth to surrender and trust the ground beneath our feet, that all our needs are provided for and we can let go of the need to overcontrol people and situations around us.

Patchouli calms and grounds an overactivated brain and monkey mind and soothes the nervous system to open energy flow along the spine and at the cellular level. Patchouli alleviates anxiety from overthinking and the pressure of overwhelm felt commonly in the head and the heart.

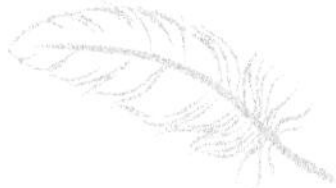

Every home aroma arsenal should have a bottle of patchouli as a versatile medicine for insect and snake bites, as a remedy for anxiousness and frigidity, as a bolster for immunity, and as a skin cell regenerator.

Nourish the Brain – Patchouli Synergy to Calm the Monkey Mind

- ∞ 5 drops of Patchouli oil (*Pogostemon cablin*)
- ∞ 1 drop of Carrot seed oil (*Daucus carota*)
- ∞ 1 drop of Vetiver oil (*Chrysopogon zizanioides*)
- ∞ 2 drops of Geranium oil (*Pelargonium graveolens*)

Blend into one tablespoon of coconut oil and apply sparingly to palms and temples and inhale deeply to generate a sense of calm and centeredness.

ESSENTIAL OIL ADDITIONS

Sea Pine – *Pinus pinaster*

BRAIN NOURISH AROMATHERAPY
DNA BLUEPRINT BENEFITS

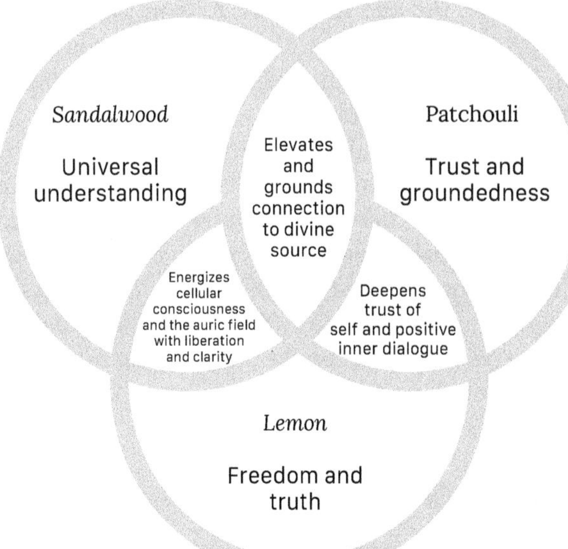

NOURISH THE BRAIN – BOTANICAL MEDICINE

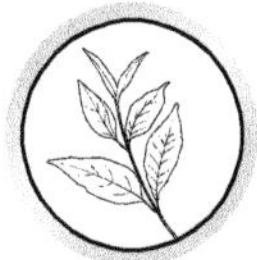

MAJOR ARCHETYPE

GREEN TEA – *Camellia sinensis*

Part used: Dried Leaf

Green tea is an antioxidant used for nourishing the nervous system with many therapeutic purposes: nervous system stimulant, and to combat fatigue and headaches. The main constituents of green tea, polyphenols, have widely been used for anticancer and cancer prevention especially related to imbalanced female hormonal conditions. Green tea supports the immune system by reducing inflammation and stimulates glutathione production as a protective cell barrier aiding the body in protection against fever, cough, flu, and infections. As you learned earlier in the heart section of this book, antioxidant botanical allies, such as green tea, are cardiotonics preventing cardiovascular disease and arteriosclerosis and decreasing high cholesterol.

From the genetic and cellular perspectives, green tea facilitates the release of two important cellular imprints. One, as an emotional function, green tea releases traumatic memories in the amygdala from abuse, specifically sexual abuse. Second, many of us have a genetic history on our bloodlines of STDs (sexually transmitted diseases), as they were much more common especially during the Industrial Revolution. These diseases leave an imprint on the cells that can cause other genetic malfunctions or mutations in the code.

Nourish the Brain – Green Tea Physical Uses

Nourish: Reduces and terminates DNA damage
Nervous System: Increases cognitive function, memory, cellular communication, and energy
Adrenal System: Improves energy in CFS
Cardiovascular System: Antioxidant and atherosclerosis
Respiratory System: Asthma
Reproductive System: Hormonal balancing and infertility
Endocrine: Weight loss and increasing metabolism
Liver: Liver disease prevention
Urinary System: Astringent
Immune System: Anticancer, antimicrobial, inflammation modulator, and allergies
Musculoskeletal System: Headaches
Integumentary System: Topically for HPV, atopic dermatitis

Nourish the Brain – Green Tea Emotional Uses

Clarity for tough decisions
Relief from withdrawal symptoms of drugs
Enriches gratitude and friendship

Nourish the Brain – Green Tea Energetic Uses

Releases the memory and trauma of abuse
Clears old energetic blocks and old belief patterns
Brings positive energy to a new project

Nourish the Brain – Green Tea Dosage

Infusion: 2 teaspoons per cup of water, infuse 3–5 min, drink 1 cup 3x/day
Tincture: 2–3 ml 3x/day
Capsules: 300–400 mg/day

Nourish the Brain – Green Tea Cautions and Contraindications

Caffeine intake in hypertension
Pregnancy

Nourish the Brain – Green Tea Freedom from Oxidation – Cellular Protection

Ingredients:
15 ml Green Tea – *Camellia sinensis* solid extract
10 ml Hawthorn – *Crataegus spp.* solid extract
10 ml Rose Hips – *Rosa canina* solid extract

Directions:
Combine the solid extract listed above.
Dosage: Take 1 teaspoon 3x/day

NOTE: a solid extract is different than a liquid extract or tincture

MINOR ARCHETYPES

Asian ginseng – *Panax ginseng*

Parts used: Root

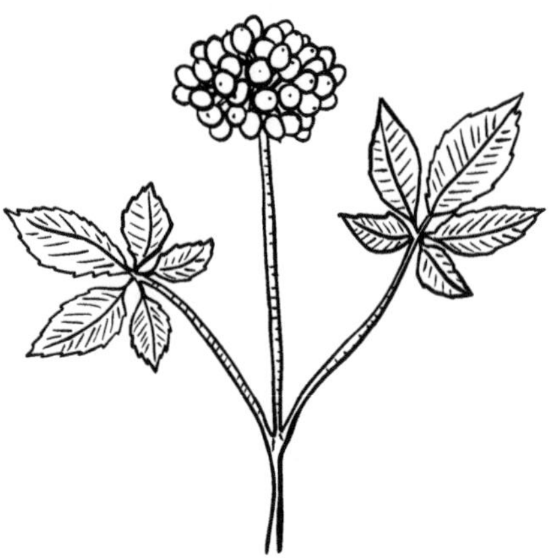

Ginseng is the ancient botanical ally of strength and longevity well known in alternative medicine for its phenomenal health benefits. It's used as a brain nourishing tonic to promote mental and physical stamina. It also works with the neurons of the brain by accelerating development, growth, and repair of the cells. Ginseng protects the cellular membrane by increasing the resistance of the cells to the environment and taxing emotional stress.

Emotionally ginseng gives you strength for states of emotional exhaustion or depletion. As the brain becomes imbalanced emotionally, ginseng harmonizes the etheric body by grounding the spinal chakras to the crystal core of the Earth. This creates a rod of light and strength in the system connecting all the chakras with the infinity energy we have discussed throughout the book.

Note about usage and protecting this sacred plant. Ginseng is an "at risk" plant. Populations have been overharvested and have not recovered and it takes six years before this plant is able to be harvested. Please be respectful and research the source before purchasing ginseng. You can still focus on the energetics of the plant by putting an image of ginseng on your altar or in your sacred space to honor this dear ally.

Nourish the Brain – Asian Ginseng Physical Uses

Nourish: Protects the cellular membrane from damage
Nervous System: Tonic, nervous system exhaustion, hysteria, and mental stamina
Adrenal System: Adaptogenic and improves life force

Cardiovascular System: Enhances circulation and heart function
Endocrine System: Balances blood sugar
Reproductive System: Stamina, infertility, libido, promotes estrogen, and menopause
Digestive System: Loss of appetite (nervous stomach)
Liver: Hepatoprotection
Immune System: Supports cancer therapy, increases white blood cell count, improves resistance to infection and chemical sensitivities

Nourish the Brain – Asian Ginseng Emotional Uses

Balances and harmonizes emotions
Grounding for nervous states of stress
Revitalizing for emotional depletion or apathy

Nourish the Brain – Asian Ginseng Cautions and Contraindications

Use with caution in acute asthma and hypertension

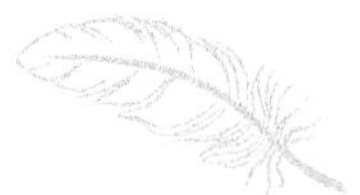

Nourish the Brain – Panax Ginseng Freedom for Vitality Tea

Ingredients:
15 g Asian Ginseng – *Panax ginseng*
10 g Burdock Root – *Arctium lappa*
5 g Rhodiola – *Rhodiola rosea*
5 g Dried Ginger *Root – Zingiber off*

Directions:
Combine all ingredients.
Decoct 1 tablespoon in 236 ml of hot water for 8 minutes.
Drink 1–3 cups/day

Rosemary – *Rosmarinus officinalis*

Part Used: Leaf

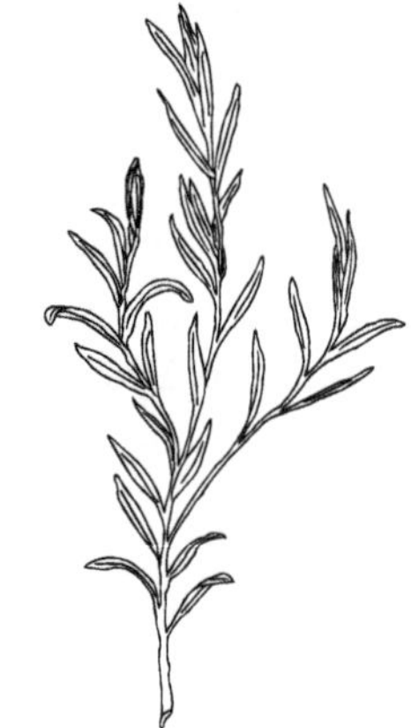

Rosemary opens all the senses of the nervous system. It increases circulation in the brain and throughout the body by enhancing blood flow. It's one of our favorite plants for all nervous system conditions of "density": improving memory, vision, and mental clarity. It's the go to botanical ally for nourishing and reviving the mind.

Rosemary is a cardio and nervous system tonic, making it therapeutically potent in chronic cardiac weakness including blood pressure conditions. Rosemary is exemplary as a botanical for antiaging, protecting the telomeres from shortening, and repairing nervous system DNA.

DL When I was in medical school, I placed stems of rosemary in my mask while working in the cadaver lab. This not only helped me to remember all the aspects of the human body, but it opened a direct line of refreshing smell and invigoration – much needed to block the smell of the formaldehyde. Rosemary is an energetic and environmental cleanser. Use it for ceremonies or burn it in your house to clear out old, dusty smells.

Nourish the Brain – Rosemary Physical Uses

Nourish: Uplifting – revives the DNA and brain
Nervous System: Tonic, improves memory and concentration, balances the nervous system, and chronic nervous states
Adrenal System: Energizing
Cardiovascular System: Antioxidant – increases circulation
Reproductive System: Dysmenorrhea and recovery form OCPs and implants
Mens' Health: Enlarged prostate
Digestive System: Regenerates the mucous membranes and intestinal gas
Liver: Hepatoprotective
Gallbladder: Antispasmodic

Immune System: Inflammation modulating, antiviral, anticarcinogenic and recovery from long term illness
Musculoskeletal System: Topically for pains, headaches, and rheumatoid arthritis
Integumentary System: Acne

Nourish the Brain – Rosemary Emotional Uses

Lifts the spirit and mood
Increases self confidence
Releases repressed anger

Nourish the Brain – Rosemary Energetic Uses

Cleansing and purifying your environment and aura
Connects to the power and energy of the sun
Removes worries and invigorates your inner spirit

Nourish the Brain – Rosemary Dosage

Tincture: 2–4 ml three times per day
Infusion: Drink 1 cup 2–3x/day
Topically: Apply essential oil in a carrier oil to the skin in a solution of 1 drop of essential oil to 5 drops of oil

Nourish the Brain – Rosemary Cautions and Contraindications

None

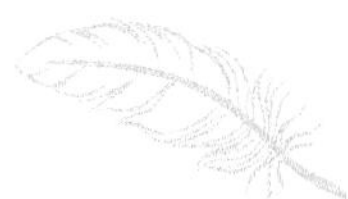

Nourish the Brain – Rosemary Freedom of Spirit

Drink one cup of rosemary infused tea 3–4x/day to lift the spirits. Add a bit of dried lavender for a stubborn headache.

BOTANICAL ADDITIONS

∞ Rhodiola – *Rhodiola rosea*
∞ Devil's club – *Oplopanax horridus*
∞ Hawthorn – *Crataegus oxycantha*
∞ Cottonwood – *Populus balsamifera*
∞ Thuja, White Cedar – *Thuja occidentalis*

BRAIN NOURISH BOTANICAL MEDICINE
DNA BLUEPRINT BENEFITS

NOURISH THE BRAIN – LIGHT WHEELS

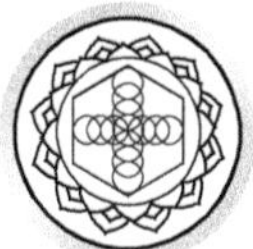

LIGHT WHEELS

MAJOR ARCHETYPE

THE 133rd LIGHT WHEEL, MUDITA

Mudita is the light wheel of spiritual enlightenment or illumination. Mudita in Sanskrit means joy. When this light wheel is "turned on" or activated you will feel a rush of energy through your brain and into your spine. You will have the heaviness of life lifted and delight in wonderment for this new vibration within your cells. At first this connection to the infinite might feel peculiar; this is normal, but as you continue your work with the other segments of the brain DNA in the book you will surrender easily to these new feelings and vibrations. Mudita is assisting the clearing and healing of your brain so it will feel a renewed.

MINOR ARCHETYPE

∞ The 17th light wheel, Chit

The seventeenth light wheel, Chit, is the Sanskrit word for "true awareness" or "consciousness." This light wheel connects your body to the atmospheric ring surrounding the planet called the exosphere. The exosphere is the upper limit of our atmosphere 6,200 miles above the Earth. Chit brings your awareness to the other energies of the universe swirling around you. It connects deeper into pathways or spaceways or universal highways to the other planets and other higher light wheels. This light wheel connects to the universal life source and connects this energy to you and to the core of the Earth, bringing a sense of peace like the feeling of floating in space without any gravity. Feel the lightness of Chit and tune your awareness inward.

LIGHT WHEEL COLORS

MAJOR ARCHETYPE

CHARTREUSE

Chartreuse green is the color of transformation, soothing and calming. Through this calming energy of love, you can give and receive love more fully with an open mind. If you are called to this color or are working with this section, Nourish the Brain, it is time to go outside and enjoy nature and the nourishing joy of wildlife around you. We suggest taking a walk in the park or taking a hike and picking a spot where you can sit with the trees and appreciate nature. If you can find a space by the water this is even better! Sit for at least fifteen minutes and tune into the trees around you. Listen to the subtle sound of the wind blowing through the trees. Soak in the magnificence of their large trunk and limbs. Feel the healing soak into every cell of your nervous system.

SOUNDS

∞ AUM

AUM is the sound that opens us to the higher realms and activates every cell with divine consciousness, and the perfected blueprint for humanity. This tones and harmonizes the energy field and aligns the light wheels, preparing you for meditation and deep healing. We suggest listening to a recording of the sound Aum in conjunction with Nourish the Brain mudra and meditation for extra attunement.

NOURISH THE BRAIN – CRYSTALS AND STONES

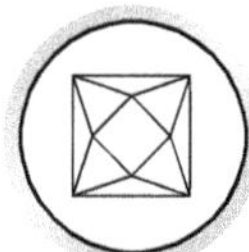

MAJOR ARCHETYPE

HERDERITE

Herderite is the crystal of inter-dimensional travel, communication with light beings, physical shift to the higher planes; it stimulates psychic abilities and activates the brain for opening ourselves to a higher vibration and communicating to higher dimensions. This stone assists you to gain a better outside perspective of emotional distress or blockages. It supports increased brain function. Supporting balance in aspects of the brain it is helpful to decrease or diffuse head pain, particularly in cases of brain injury. It supports the rewiring of the brain with higher levels of light and understanding.

MINOR ARCHETYPE

∞ Datolite

Datolite retrieves lost childhood memories and connects to the heart. It releases trauma and fears of being open to change and new choices. It soothes the nervous system and aids in the recovery of nervous system imbalance.

∞ Onyx

Onyx is a striking black stone connecting the heart and brain to the core of the Earth and the crystalline grid. It connects all the light wheels or chakras as brilliant rods of pure light activating each light wheel enabling them to open more fully. When your body is beginning to be activated, you may find it difficult to navigate through all the new information coming from your inner being and from source. Onyx stabilizes your energy, assisting you to shift easily from one thought or healing process to another with a grace of calmness.

Onyx physically connects the feet to the Earth, easing disorders of balance and instability. It also is a stone of science illuminating mysteries of illness. Are you troubled by an illness within and not sure of the root cause? Onyx is the stone to turn to.

CRYSTAL ADDITIONS

∞ Fluorite
∞ Black Tourmaline
∞ Malachite

NOURISH THE BRAIN CRYSTAL GRID

Drink a glass of clean water with 3 drops each of Gold and Yerba Mansa essences. Classical music can also be enjoyed during this session. This crystal attunement can be done at any time of the day for 20-30 minutes. Cleanse crystals immediately after use. (See Appendix C).

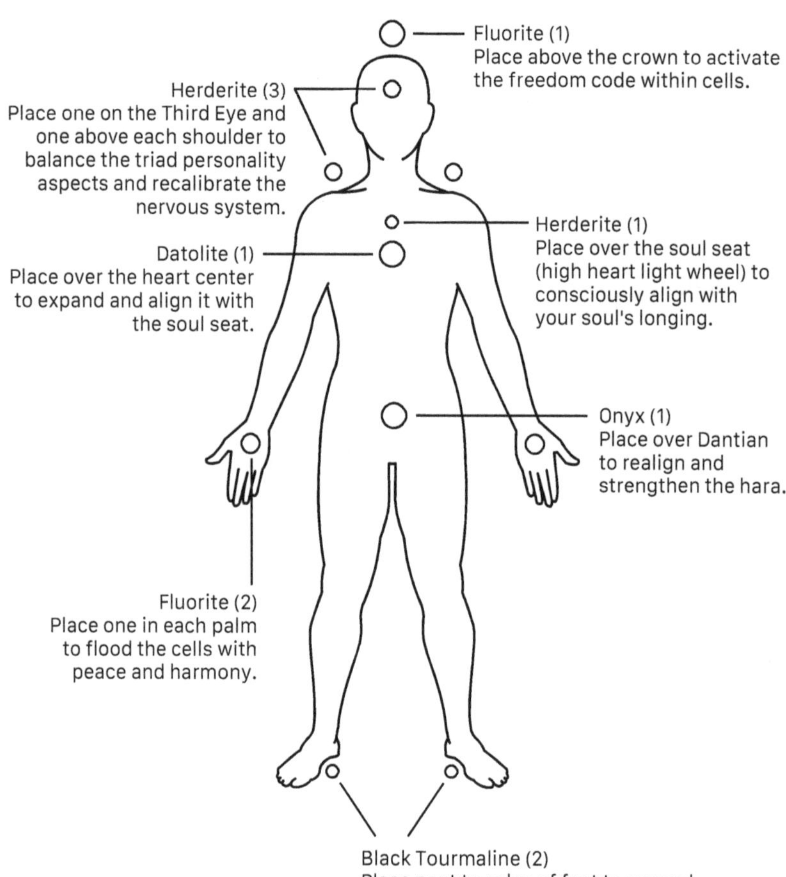

NOURISH THE BRAIN – ENERGETIC AND VIBRATIONAL TECHNIQUES

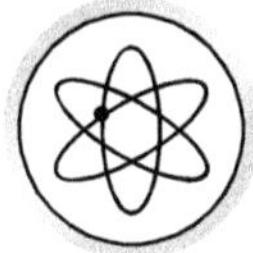

MAJOR ARCHETYPE

NOURISH THE BRAIN HYDROTHERAPY

∞ 4 drops of Patchouli essential oil (*Pogostemon cablin*)
∞ 3 drops of Vetiver essential oil (*Chrysopogon zizanioides*)
∞ 2 drops Lemon essential oil (*Citrus limonum*)
∞ 2 drops of Sandalwood essential oil (*Santalum austrocaledonicum*)
∞ 10 drops of Yerba Mansa Flower Essence

Directions:
Add the essential oils and flower essences to warm water. Choose a crystal from the Nourish the Brain section and place it in the bathtub or foot bath while focusing on your intention. Feel free to create your own intention or use one from this section.

MINOR ARCHETYPES

Brain Nourishing Visualization

Walking in the forest offers a tremendously nourishing and invigorating effect on all systems of the body, especially the brain. Taking the time to be in silence, connect with the Earth and allow nature to sing to you as it fills the mind with tranquility.

If you do not have access to a forest where you live, you can turn this into a visualization. You can add nature sounds, woodsy incense, and envision yourself on a forest walk too, connecting with the nurturing safety of the woods through your intention.

Wherever you choose to be for this meditation, seat yourself comfortably. As you take a relaxing breath, begin to envision pink rays of unconditional love beginning to flood your brain and fill your cells with the most delicious sensations of ease, comfort, and grace. Liquid love fills every structure and particle of your brain and then begins to rain down upon your spine like a glorious waterfall. Allow yourself to soak this in until you feel completely full and then notice how your body feels and shifts in your emotional disposition are experienced.

Nourish the Brain EOBT

Place one drop of sandalwood essential oil between the first two fingertips of the right hand, inhale deeply and tap the Bladder-66, Penetrating Valley point of the Bladder Meridian for thirty seconds with the intention of marinating the brain with unconditional love.

Location: Run your finger from the outside of the small toe along the lateral side of the foot until it falls into the depression over the prominence of the head of the metatarsal.

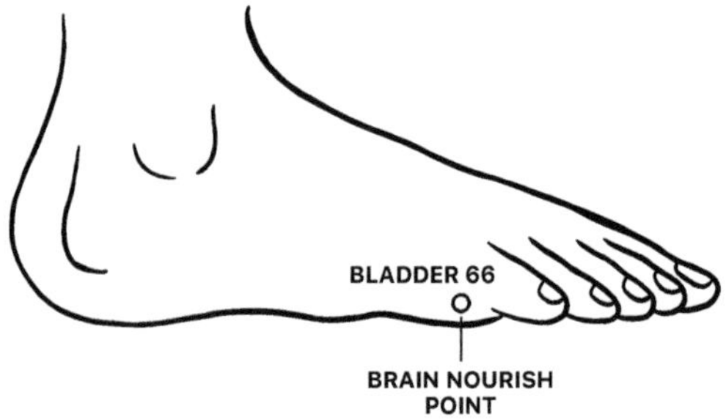

NOURISH THE BRAIN – FLOWER AND GEM ESSENCES

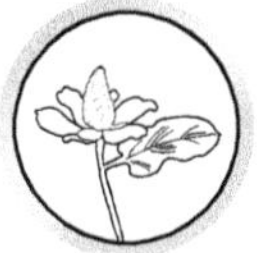

FLOWER ESSENCES

MAJOR ARCHETYPE

YERBA MANSA

Yerba mansa is an essence of tranquility and self-acceptance. It brings the energy of compassion to all the places of judgement within. It is soothing to places of dysfunctional patterning held within the brain and nervous system, supporting these areas to dissolve and fill with the energy of grace. Yerba mansa alleviates anxiety and brings the light of deep healing to the child consciousness. It helps to release deep seated trauma held in the bloodlines where divine love and source connection has been suppressed in the past.

MINOR ARCHETYPES

Mallow

Mallow is an essence of compassion and holds the reminder to love ourselves as we age; it helps to release unhealthy connections to vanity. This essence has a powerful impact on the cellular level, both physically and energetically. It helps to clear toxins and regenerate tissue as well as activating cellular memory to connect, understand, and assimilate past life experiences. Mallow brings healing deep within the DNA and mother and father bloodlines generationally to reach the point of pure energy igniting that in the cells. On another level, this essence is supportive in the dying process for the soul to let go of the earthly realm.

Chaparral

This often-forgotten ancient flower essence increases psychic connection and past life recall, where there are roots in unresolved experience that affect the current life. This essence enhances clarity, memory, focus, and concentration. It is a great aid for new creative projects, problem solving, and out of the box thinking. It is helpful for insomnia and can enhance guidance in dreamtime.

FLOWER ESSENCE ADDITIONS

- ∞ Star of Bethlehem
- ∞ Black eyed Susan

GEM ESSENCE

MAJOR ARCHETYPE

GOLD

Gold essence is akin to bathing the brain and nervous system in liquid light. It enhances cellular communication and connects all meridian points and chakras with the light of divine consciousness. Purifying all physiology, gold is restorative to the nervous system and enhances circulation. It helps to balance extreme emotions from depression to rage. Gold also expands and balances the heart center and supports our ability to bring our heart's desires into actualization.

NOURISH THE BRAIN – INTENTIONS AND AFFIRMATIONS

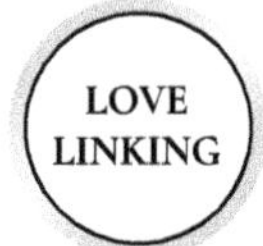

MAJOR ARCHETYPE

LOVE LINKING

MINOR ARCHETYPES

- ∞ My brain easily absorbs water and nutrients into every cell and my DNA is cultivated with life and vitality

- ∞ My brain and nerves are permeated with the light of unconditional love
- ∞ Every point of connectivity in my brain and nervous system is infused with love

MINOR ARCHETYPES

- ∞ I allow myself to feel good and have fun living my life
- ∞ My brain is marinating in the pink light of unconditional love
- ∞ I fill my cells with loving connection

NOURISH THE BRAIN – MEDITATION MUDRA

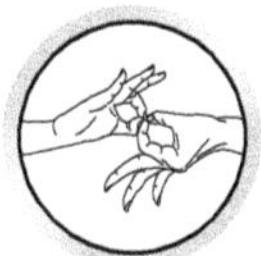

Dharma Chakra Mudra

Feeling the unity and attunement of all my light wheels,
I weave through life renewed and balanced.

The Dharma chakra mudra frees the brain and the heart from suffering and helps link them together with a bond of love and truth. This feeling of truth amplifies in length through all the seven chakras as this mudra integrates the energy of all the chakras as one. It nourishes the spinal column, nervous system, and brain by creating a clear channel of free-flowing energy up through each chakra and into the brain stem. By working daily with this mudra, you will find that by speaking your truth, your brain will be emotionally balanced and neurologically synchronized.

Dharma Chakra Mudra Alignment

1. Touch the tips of the index fingers to the tips of the thumbs of each hand.
2. Place the left palm in front of the belly button, solar plexus, and place the right palm above it, facing outward.

3. Gently extend all the other fingers except the thumb and index fingers.
4. Take a deep breath, let your body relax.
5. You may now either do the meditation below or 10 minutes of Infinity *Ocean Breath.*
6. You may also use this mudra at any time you are feeling anxious or fearful about a current illness or life changing circumstance.

∞ To access the mudra meditation please go to www.zenergymedicinals.com

∞ As you inhale your essential oil for 30–45 seconds, invite a blessing from the divine consciousness to infuse your brain, your nervous system, your mind, all your neural pathways with the remembrance of peace and unity.

∞ Form the Dharma chakra mudra with your hands and take several breaths to open and align the spinal or kundalini power. Feel the connection with each vertebra from the coccyx to the cervical vertebrae and up into the brain. Visualize a rod of chartreuse light extending from the base of your spine up through the crown of your head, nourishing all the nerves extending out of each vertebra and communicating with all the nerves throughout the physical body creating an impression of oneness. This feeling will be subtle but as you practice this mudra more frequently you will become more attuned to this sensation.

∞ Connect in with the core of the Earth and allow yourself to be filled with great abundance, protection, and solidarity, sealing any leaks or tears with light.

∞ Breathe in light of divine consciousness, allowing all the energy centers above the heart to recalibrate from the cosmic perspective. We call for the template of peace and the opalescent ray.

∞ This light ray carries a vibrational template for peace, spiritual illumination, and divine love. This ray holds the breath of higher cosmic energy. Breathe in as this opal light floods your entire being with a wave of peace, calm, and spiritual connection and fills your brain, nervous system, and all pathways with that beautiful and gentle frequency. Healing all the places of shadow of darkness, of forgetting, of separation, and disconnection.

- ∞ Invite this opalescent light to come in through the cellular membrane and ease into the portal of your DNA your mother and father bloodlines drinking in this opalescent light. Bathe your being in the vibration of peace.
- ∞ Opal light, clearing, nourishing, activating the remembrance of peace and unity that exists within us all.
- ∞ With each breath, feel the openness extending through your nervous system with the light of peace, the memory of unity.
- ∞ Repeat the intention three times either silently or aloud: "Feeling the unity and attunement of all my chakras, I weave through life renewed and balanced."
- ∞ May the light of peace spread exponentially within the hearts of all beings on this planet.

NOURISH THE BRAIN – SACRED GEOMETRY

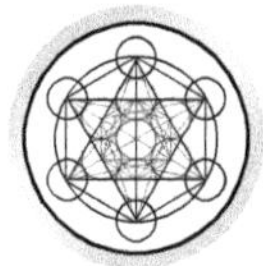

MAJOR ARCHETYPE

NOURISH THE BRAIN SACRED GEOMETRY – METATRON'S CUBE

This sacred geometry, Metatron's cube, is a combination of the flower of life and the five platonic solids hidden in the inside of the outer circles. This intricate pattern symbolizes the brain's intimate connection to life and source. It signifies the flow of energy through the brain and spinal cord connecting our source energy to the cosmic energy above and below. When using it during your meditations and on your FPW it will assist your mind and etheric body from a place of negativity to positivity. Brain Boosting Bliss!

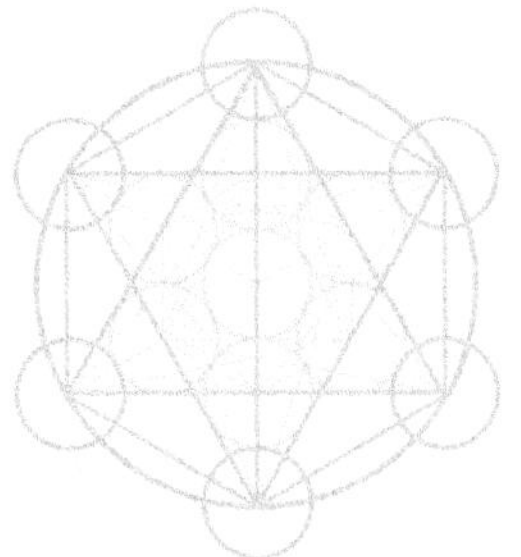

NOURISH THE BRAIN – NUTRITION

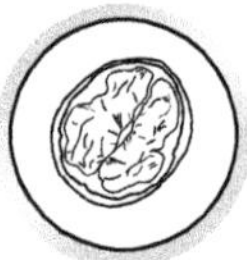

MAJOR ARCHETYPE

WALNUTS

Brain boosting walnuts look like the brain, and you guessed it, they have an affinity for nourishing the brain. They are a marvelous plant source of omega-3 fatty acids called Alpha-linolenic acid (ALA). Omega-3 fats are important for brain nourishment; they build all the cell membranes of the body and the brain. They are the building blocks of the neurons and imperative for brain function (Balk & Lichtenstein, 2017).

Walnuts also support a healthy aging process preventing frontal lobe disease and Alzheimer's; they decrease inflammation in the nervous system and reduce oxidative damage. Studies have shown that consuming a regular serving of walnuts per day (1–1.5 ounces) improves memory, cognitive function, and learning skills.

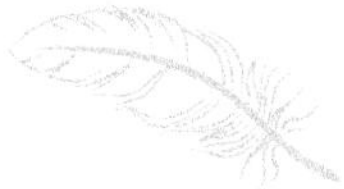

Are you looking for new ways to eat your walnuts? Try roasting them in the oven with a light spray of ghee, tossed with rosemary and sea salt – Yummy!

MINOR ARCHETYPE

Wheat Germ Oil

Wheat germ is a neuroprotective oil rich in vitamin E. It coats the cells of the brain in a thin layer of fat adding protection and reducing inflammation. It is also high in B vitamins and detoxifies the frontal lobe of the brain reducing the risk of Alzheimer's disease.

Wild Caught Salmon

Wild caught salmon is well known for its omega-3 fatty acid content. Fatty acids are essential for brain development and function mainly because the brain is composed of 60 percent fat. Without healthy fats the brain is not able to function fully at optimal level. Docosahexaenoic acid, DHA, is the primary structural component of omega-3 fatty acids and it nourishes the cell membrane, reduces inflammation, and produces more efficient neurotransmitters.

NUTRITIONAL ADDITIONS

∞ Ghee (grass fed)

NOURISH THE BRAIN – DISCOVERY DIVE – MINDFULNESS AND MOOD

Mindfulness offers a simple yet potent aspect to enhance well-being through the mind–body connection. It fosters a sense of empowerment and deliberate intention to create harmony in your life through presence. Being mindful invites you to pay attention to the present moment without judgement or analysis. When we can present our intention, attention, and heart to those places within us that call for enrichment and calm, we create the conditions for consistent betterment in our mood and emotional response.

We are going to play a game of "bridging the gap." Write down five aspects of mood that you would like to experience more of. What state of mind or feeling experience would you like to permeate more of your day-to-day life?

Spend a few minutes of introspection and honestly evaluate your general state of feeling and emotions now.

How can you cultivate a daily mindful practice to bridge this gap and lift your mood, feeling, and emotional response? How can you encourage a sense of lightness, grace, and openness to feeling great?

Consider the notion that you are the captain of your mood and that your energy and cells are swimming within you ready for your empowering command and navigation in the sea of potential. You are powerful beyond measure. By harnessing the presence and power of your breath, your mind through visualization and meditation, you can create new, healthier habit patterns of emotional response and lift your mood, enhancing every way you relate to yourself and the world around you.

FREEDOM PHOTON WHEEL™

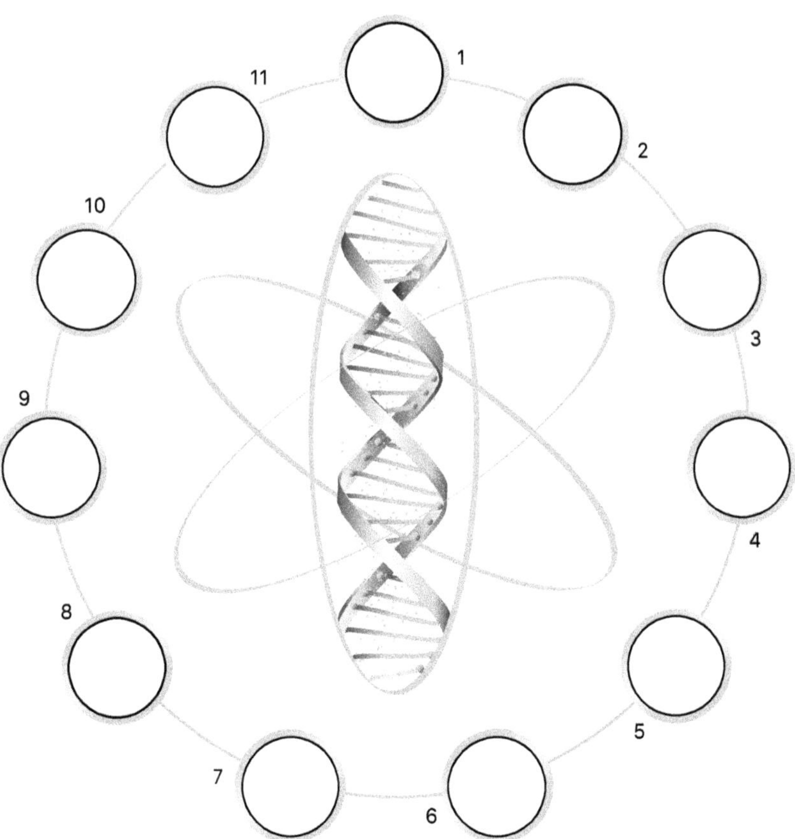

NOURISH THE BRAIN
YOUR PERSONAL FREEDOM PHOTON WHEEL RITUAL

Moon Phase

Perform your ritual during any moon phase.

Intention

"I allow the grace of the Divine to marinate my entire being and my genetic lineage with love, peace, and clarity."

Select, Align, and Activate

Select your interventions according to the instructions in Chapter Five. Inhale and apply your chosen essential oil for 30–45 seconds. Use your botanical tincture or tea as directed. You may also listen to the meditation and use the mudra from this chapter while attuning your FPW.

Affirm

"Divine Consciousness, assist me in allowing full spectrum healing light through my lineage, my mother and father bloodlines so that I have the greatest experience of grace."

ACTIVATE THE BRAIN

Consider the brain from a holographic perspective. Through understanding that our brain is a supercomputer requiring specific chemical balance, and that we consistently are faced with the nature of disruption from internal and external stress, from trauma to nutritional deficiencies and environmental toxins in our air and food and earth; we are in a perpetual state of flux and shift. By creating new healthy habit patterns with our eleven alchemical systems of intervention, we can support the regulation of our brain chemistry. This balance allows feelings of positivity, benevolence, and healthful emotional response to fill our systems cellularly and energetically.

The ability of plant and vibrational medicine to connect, communicate, and restore balance to the nervous system is unparalleled. Brain, body, mind, and nervous system generating a sense of positive feeling, mood, and emotion drive our ability to broaden our consciousness. Through better and more clear decision making, new experience of high sense perception, and an understanding of expanded realities, possibility, and connection to the Divine, we expand.

What is the ultimate quest from the human perspective? We are all seekers on a journey of healing, awakening, transformation, with the goal of self-mastery and the actualization of our soul purpose. Once we are full on our path, we all thirst for enlightenment, a direct connection to divine consciousness that holds all acceptance, understanding, and unification.

AW I have had a few such moments in my life. They lasted only seconds but completely transcended space and time. In these moments, I could hear a tone that sounded like liquid gold; it was deep and almost guttural, like the toning one would hear in a Buddhist temple high in the Himalayas. Through these moments, I could see the complete connection of everything in my life, my family, the planet, and the entire universe connected and unfolding perfectly. Everything is connected. Somewhere everything makes sense. And everything is connected through love. Our prayer for your brain activation is the remembrance of this truth, which is held within you. As much as it may seem like it exists in a galaxy far, far away, it is alive and breathing truth in each of your trillions of cells awaiting your gaze, your intention, and your openness to receive it.

BRAIN ACTIVATE FREEDOM PHOTON WHEEL

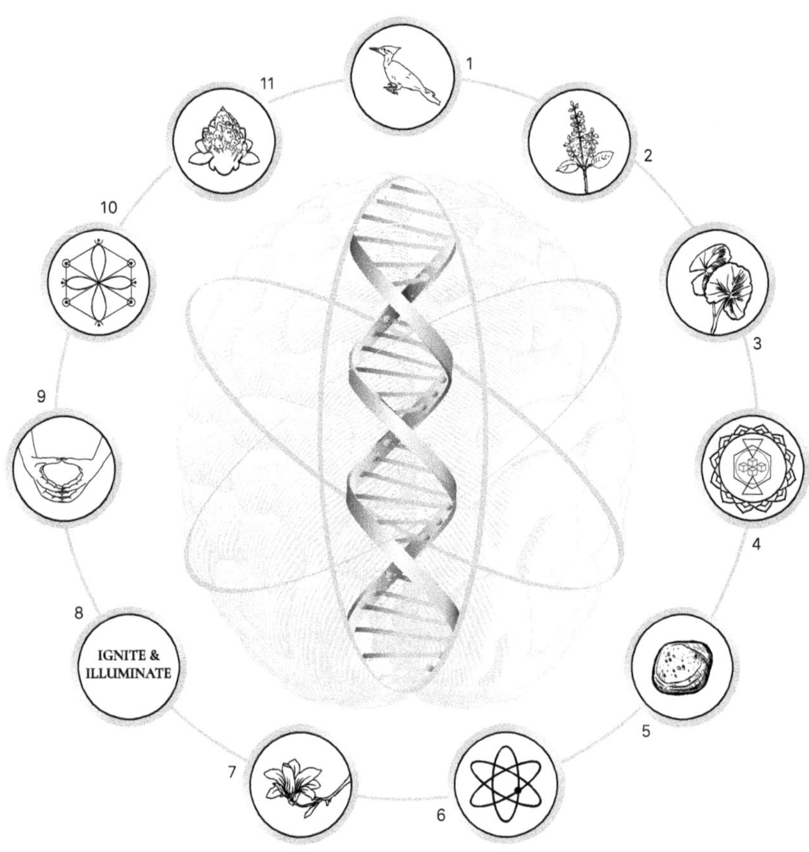

1 Alchemy Animal: Pileated Woodpecker
2 Aromatherapy: Tulsi
3 Botanical: Gotu Kola
4 Light Wheel: Pustakagara
5 Crystal: Fulgurite
6 Photon Vibration
7 Flower or Gem Essence: Japanese Magnolia
8 Intention: Ignite & Illuminate
9 Meditation Mudra: Hakini
10 Sacred Geometry
11 Nutrition: Romanesco Broccoli

BRAIN ACTIVATE
INFINITY INFLUENCERS

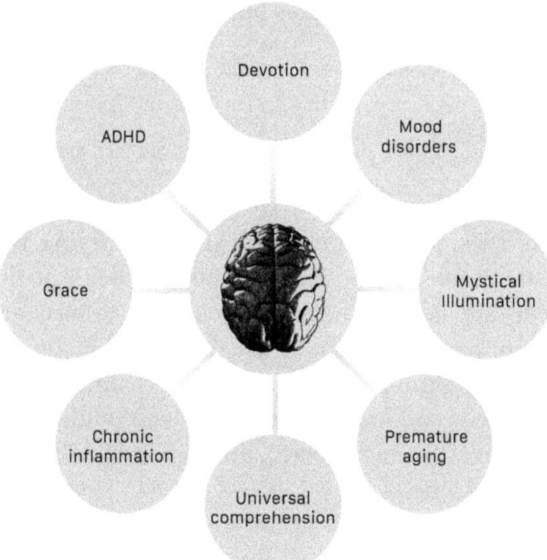

ACTIVATE THE BRAIN – ALCHEMY ANIMALS

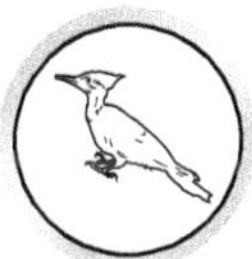

MAJOR ARCHETYPE

PILEATED WOODPECKER

Opportunity is knocking – are you going to let it in? That's the message of this grandiose woodpecker. Time to seize the moment or it's going to pass you by. Are you ready? It could be it's time to finish a project you have in the works or maybe you have been meaning to start a new project you have been dreaming about. Well, the woodpecker says, "What are you waiting for?" The pileated woodpecker also symbolizes it's time to connect to the rhythm of the Earth through your spinal rhythm. Time to shake that booty and move – feel the rhythm and heartbeat flowing within.

Creature Connection: "I call upon you, vibrant bird of flight. I give heed and listen to the opportunities before me. I lovingly embrace them with every cell of my being."

MINOR ARCHETYPES

Dragonfly

The dragonfly flies so fast you might miss her flying by unless you are paying attention. This is the symbolic message of the dragonfly. Wake up, dear one. All the messages you need to hear are all around you and within, just listen. Since the dragonfly is also a creature of air and water, she signifies what lies on the surface is not the true meaning – you need to look deeper or fly deep within yourself for the authentic meaning. It's time to break through an illusion you have been carrying for a long time.

Creature Connection: "I call upon you, alchemy animal of light. As my thoughts create my reality, I envision my dreams into existence. I invite and welcome the messages of the elemental world of air and water."

Coral

The coral signifies that great change is on the horizon and it is time to be stable. Get your roots down! With the guidance of the coral, you will be able to move through all upcoming transitions effortlessly with an embodied sense of patience.

You will need spiritual and emotional support during these next phases of transformation. Reach out to a loved one. Take time to visit healing waters, like the ocean, to be in the flow and let the universe guide you. It's time to love, heal, and nurture your body.

Creature Connection: "Wherever I am, I am grounded. I trust in myself. I welcome and surrender completely to the transformation yet to come."

ACTIVATE THE BRAIN – AROMATHERAPY

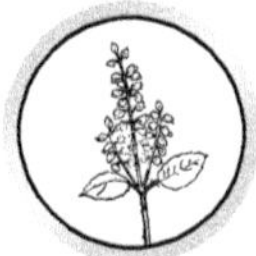

MAJOR ARCHETYPE

TULSI – *Ocimum basilicum*

Part extracted: Flower and Leaves

Core properties: Analgesic, antifungal, anti-infectious, antirheumatic, antiviral, carminative
Safety: nontoxic, nonirritant

Tulsi is a plant medicine of devotion. It allows us ease in accessing our higher self, activating and clearing the higher levels of the auric field before lighting up our cells, igniting and illuminating our consciousness.

AW I came to know tulsi on my first journey to India upon visiting a temple in Mysore. We had the opportunity to purchase sacred plants, including tulsi and davanna for offering inside the temple. It was not until after the temple meditation had concluded that I personally experienced tulsi, as once certain plants are purchased for offering, you cannot inhale the aroma that is given as a devotion to the deity. I did finally experience tulsi, the aroma sweet, herbaceous, connoting holiness as if the spirit of tulsi is neither a priest nor a priestess, yet something intertwining both and elevating those two earthly concepts; activating the remembrance of holiness within our beings as a portal to open the cells, flowing this remembrance deep throughout our DNA.

Tulsi helps to open the crown center or light wheel at the top of our head, along with the higher chakras, inviting the infinite light of divine consciousness while simultaneously opening the heart to the sweetness of life. It aligns the connection to root chakra or Muladhara light wheel to allow for the higher levels of light to move fully down the channel, activating all the cells, meridian points, and energy centers with renewed devotion. Devotion for all the higher universal and cosmic realms above. Devotion to the sacred heart of humanity into the self as a divine representation of light and devotion to the Earth, as a sacred chosen home for the evolution of all consciousness and kingdoms of life on the planet.

Tulsi is purifying, toning, and stimulating. It's an excellent plant for digestion, vitality, and vibrancy. It helps to increase clarity and psychic vision. It's also an excellent adaptogen, supporting the body's resilience to stress.

AW The healing and awakening I found in India is one of the greatest blessings of my life.

After returning from my first visit, I created this blend called Visions of India. It was one of my most popular products for many years until the ingredients became more difficult and costly to procure. I offer it as a transcendent gift for those of you inclined to source the sacred and precious oils held therein. India called me for many years, spoke to me in my dreams, and healed some of the deepest parts of my being. If you feel a call and it has not yet been your time, may this formula nourish a deep part of your soul with its aromatic and vibrational medicine.

Activate the Brain – Visions of India

- ∞ 3 drops Jasmine absolute (*Jasminum sambac*)
- ∞ 5 drops Mitti attar (an attar of the baked earth of southern India)
- ∞ 6 drops Sontaka attar (an attar of the white ginger lily)
- ∞ 3 drops of Cardamom essential oil (*Elettaria cardamomum*)
- ∞ 5 drops of Tulsi essential oil (*Ocimum tenuiflorum*)

Mix into a 60 ml bottle of distilled water and place on your altar for three days before misting with sacred intentions.

MINOR ARCHETYPES

Rosemary – *Rosmarinus officinalis*

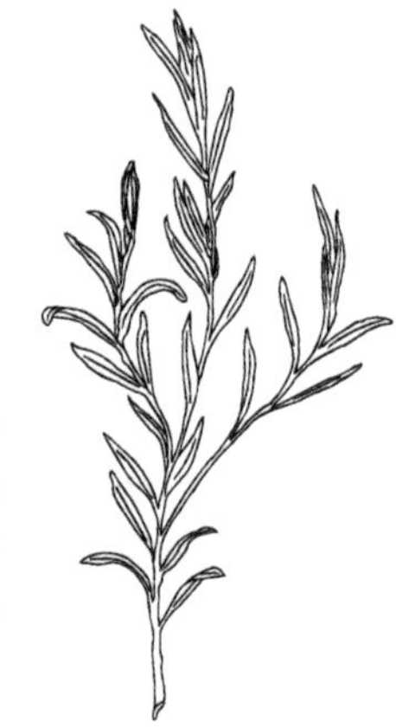

Part extracted: Flower and Leaves

Core properties: analgesic, antidepressive, astringent, carminative, cephalic, cholagogue, cordial, digestive, diuretic, emmenagogue, hepatic, hypertensive, nervine, rubefacient, stimulant, sudorific, and tonic

Safety: nontoxic, nonirritant, avoid in pregnancy and pregnancy and those with epilepsy, use at dilutions under 2.5 percent

A great activator of all mental function and process, rosemary ignites, inspires, and awakens the potential of our mind from focus and concentration to memory and clarity. This oil offers potent brain alchemy. Rosemary has the uncanny ability to clear brain fog, calm the monkey mind, while simultaneously opening and energizing the pathways for both logical and creative thinking. It is helpful for those who overthink to the point of being unable to make decisions.

This oil is indicated for those that tend to have disjointed thoughts as well as mental and physical energy that comes in spurts versus a consistent stream. Flow encapsulates the medicine of rosemary. It facilitates flow of bright, positive energy from the heavens above to the Earth below, cleansing the auric field, strengthening the nervous system, and opening a stream of higher consciousness. This creates a fluid conduit for the higher self to anchor with greater ease and trust. Rosemary ignites the cells with the remembrance of our divine consciousness while supporting physical and mental levels of peak performance.

Historically, rosemary was esteemed for its versatility. From the spiritual perspective it offers protection, purification, and benevolence. Emotionally, it offers courage and the strength to experience new terrain in life and accomplish goals that may seem at first intangible. Rosemary awakens our inner hero or heroine and helps to dissolve victim threads of consciousness. It increases physical vitality and stamina and is beneficial for circulation, digestion, and the muscular system. Rosemary strengthens the heart on all levels and aids our ability to let go of emotions and habitual patterns that no longer serve us. This oil is also helpful for colds, flus, headaches, particularly those related to obsessive thinking.

Rosemary offers three main chemotypes, which indicates a subspecies with similar appearance but different chemical constituents. Rosemary verbenone has a smoother aromatic profile and will be recommended for use in the following blend.

Activate the Brain – Rosemary Bath to Increase Self Confidence

∞ 3 drops of Rosemary essential oil (*Rosmarinus officinalis CT verbenone*)
∞ 2 drops of Juniper essential oil (*Juniperus communis*)

- ∞ 3 drops of Lavender essential oil (*Lavandula angustifolia*)
- ∞ 2 drops Cypress essential oil (*Cupressus sempervirens*)

Blend into 15 ml olive or coconut oil and add to warm water. Luxuriate in the bath for at least 20 minutes with your intention.

Peppermint – *Mentha piperita*

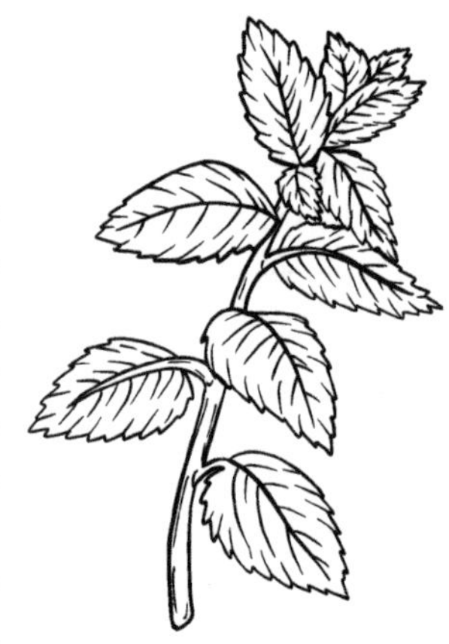

Part extracted: Leaves and Flowers

Core properties: Analgesic, anesthetic, antiseptic, antigalactagogue, antiphlogistic, antispasmodic, astringent, carminative, cephalic, cholagogue, cordial, decongestant, emmenagogue, expectorant, febrifuge, hepatic, nervine, stimulant, stomachic, sudorific, vasoconstrictor, and vermifuge.
Safety: nontoxic, irritant to skin and mucous membranes, use at under 1 percent dilution during pregnancy and breastfeeding, avoid for children under two years of age.

Peppermint's medicine is one of invigoration, bringing strength, fortitude, and clarity to our physiology, emotions, and our will. Always the eternal optimist, mint is none the shy of its mission. Awaken! It encourages us to awaken our youthful vitality, as well as our outlook, clearing away clouded and distorted perception and jadedness towards the wonder and possibility that life has to offer at any age.

The power of mint is felt when used on the skin, diluted of course, and its ability to cool and calm the emotions and mind, while stimulating energy for Qi (chi) flow in the body, and the alignment of the energy bodies. Peppermint fuels energy also at the spirit level to support endurance and the completion of projects, seeing things through for tasks and life lessons, when there is a resistance at the last moment.

Peppermint medicine is potent alchemy for the office and the boardroom to clear heavy energy resulting from confusion and disagreement and brings clarity to the situation at hand. Clearing resistance is a powerful mantra of peppermint. It strengthens the mental body, helps to focus, and breaks up energy blockages around the belief system. Clearing deep layers of mental fog, peppermint is supportive to those who have difficulty making decisions or taking control of their lives, releasing the need for approval, acceptance, and directive from others. Peppermint has an affinity for the throat chakra and encourages us to speak our truth while simultaneously reminding us to keep our cool and that our truth is ours alone, not something to be projected or superimposed on another.

Peppermint is excellent for coughs, colds, enhancing immunity and is, helpful for nausea, and stomach disorders. It is a must for your aromatic arsenal, and we highly recommend the Yakima US variety. This oil is helpful for athletes physically for its analgesic and anti-inflammatory support at the muscular level, and supportive emotionally and energetically for drive and endurance and emotional fortitude as an activator for the mental functions.

The strength and potency of this oil should be used sparingly and respectfully.

Activate the Brain – Peppermint Mist of Empowerment

- 5 drops of Peppermint essential oil (*Mentha piperita*)
- 15 drops of Lavender essential oil (*Lavandula angustifolia*)
- 1 drop of Lemongrass essential oil (*Cymbopogon citratus*)
- 3 drops of Tulsi essential oil (*Ocimum tenuiflorum*)
- 4 drops of Fennel essential oil (*Foeniculum vulgare*)

Blend into a 60 ml bottle of distilled water. Shake well before use. Infuse with the intention to empower your home, personal, and office space and mist freely avoiding contact with eyes.

ADDITIONAL ESSENTIAL OILS

Fennel – *Foeniculum vulgare*

BRAIN ACTIVATE AROMATHERAPY
DNA BLUEPRINT BENEFITS

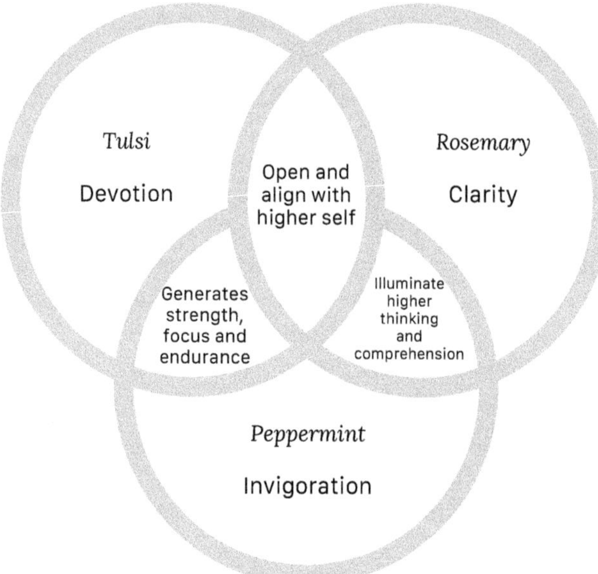

ACTIVATE THE BRAIN – BOTANICAL MEDICINE

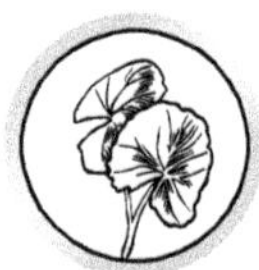

MAJOR ARCHETYPE

GOTU KOLA – *Centella asiatica*

Part Used: Fresh or dried leaf and stem

Gotu kola is a rejuvenating nervous system tonic stimulating the function of the brain. It has a synergistic relationship with the heart and increases cerebral and cardiovascular blood circulation. It also works as a DNA neurotransmitter nervine or relaxant, balancing the two hemispheres of the brain supporting all mood disorders: anxiety, stress, worry, and depression. Gotu kola is an incomparable herb for repairing cellular and connective tissue damage both orally and topically. It accelerates wound healing and repair by collagen formation and increasing antioxidant levels. Gotu kola has also long been used to reinforce the integrity of the hair, skin, and nails.

Gotu kola has been used as a tea by the mystics and yogis to enhance meditation, opening both the sixth and seventh light wheels to the higher light wheels of spiritual connection. If you look at the leaf of Gotu kola, you will notice that it resembles the brain, this is called the doctrine of signatures. Emotionally it harmonizes the left and right hemispheres of the brain, generating a profound spiritual awareness. Gotu kola further connects the nervous system and brain circuitry by lighting up the cells like the lights on a switchboard, enhancing neuron activation.

When using this herb during meditations you will quickly access spiritual states of connection to your higher self.

Activate the Brain – Gotu Kola Physical Uses

Activate: Regenerates cellular membrane and DNA
Nervous System: Brain tonic, antiaging, increases intelligence, memory, panic attacks, and stabilizes mood
Adrenal System: Nervine, rejuvenating, longevity, and alterative and anxiety
Cardiovascular System: Diuretic and blood purifier
Venous System: Varicose veins
Digestive: Bitter, digestive, and laxative
Reproductive: Venereal disease
Immune System: Detoxes the immune system and anti-inflammatory.
Integumentary System: Stimulates hair and nail growth, repairs scar tissue, connective tissue builder and all chronic skin diseases

Activate the Brain – Gotu Kola Emotional Uses

Uplifts mood – depression and anxiety
Connects the brain and the heart (think from the heart)
Gives strength emotionally – clarity and truth

Activate the Brain – Gotu Kola Energetic Uses

Wakens the sixth and seventh light wheels – herb of enlightenment
Deeper meditations
Use in ceremony to boost life force

Activate the Brain – Gotu Kola Dosage

Powder: 1 g 3x/day
Infusion: 1 tablespoon per 236 ml water – infuse 8 min, drink 3 cups/day
Topical: paste or oil for skin conditions

Activate the Brain – Gotu Kola Cautions and Contraindications

Pregnancy

Activate the Brain – Freedom for Alignment

This formula activates the nervous system and all the seven light wheels
Combine equal amounts of the following extracts:

1. Chickweed – *Stellaria media* – Grounding
2. Black cohosh – *Actea racemosa* – Sensuality
3. Licorice – *Glycyrrhiza glabra* – Enthusiasm
4. Hawthorn – *Crataegus monogyna* – Passion
5. Lemon balm – *Melissa officinalis* – Communication
6. Ginkgo – *Ginkgo biloba* – Intuition
7. Gotu kola – *Centella asiatica* – Unity

Directions:
Orally: 1 ml 2x/day in the morning and evening and topically rub 1 drop over each light wheel location 2x/day. See image for application.

BRAIN ACTIVATE TINCTURE PLACEMENT

Apply 1 drop topically over each light wheel 2x/day.

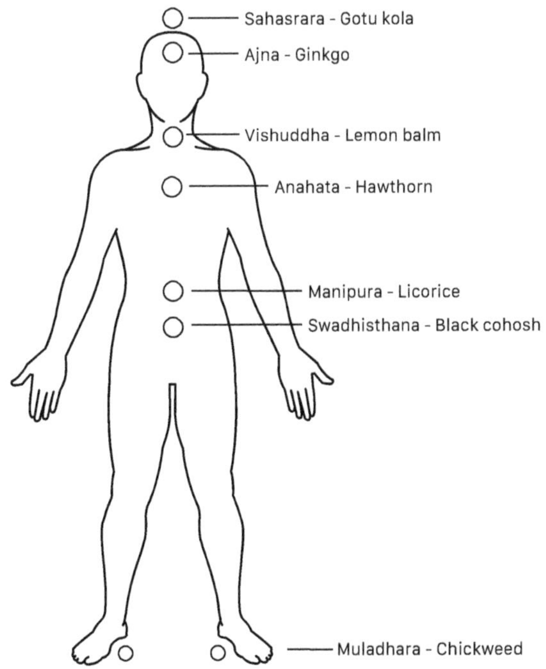

MINOR ARCHETYPES

Lion's Mane – *Hericium Erinaceus*

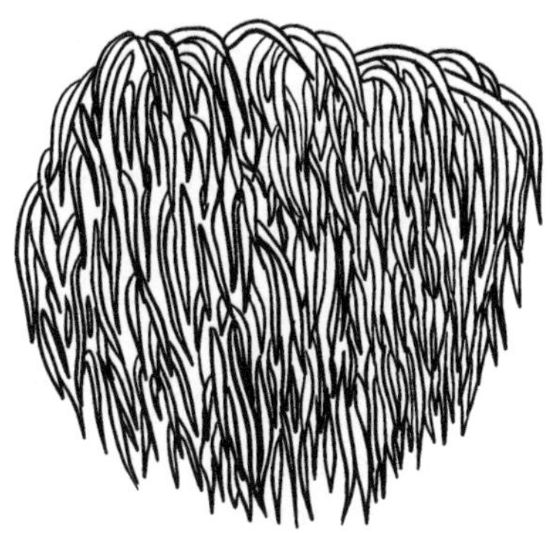

This brain activating mushroom, Lion's mane, is white and hairy resembling a lion's mane as it grows. It has been studied and shown to improve clarity, memory, and cognitive function. A tremendous Alzheimer's and early onset dementia prevention. Lion's mane's antioxidant properties regenerate the neurons and neural pathways of the brain facilitating quick recovery in brain and spinal injuries.

Lion's mane is also an anti-inflammatory for the nervous system and other areas of the body. It expedites the body in recovery from chronic inflammatory conditions by cellular and DNA regeneration.

This soft-hearted fungus additionally, reinforces the functioning of the hippocampus. This is the region of the brain we lovingly call the "switching station for all sensation." It processes emotional responses and memories decreasing high levels of anxiety and depression during nervous system dysfunction.

Activate the Brain – Lion's Mane Physical Uses

Activate: Stimulates brain cell and DNA growth reducing cellular damage
Nervous System: memory, protects against dementia and brain degeneration, recovery from brain and spinal injuries, boosts mental function and mood disorders
Adrenal System: Adrenal fatigue and chronic stress
Cardiovascular System: Antioxidant and reduces risk of heart disease
Immune System: anticancer, anti-inflammation
Endocrine: Balances blood sugar
Digestive System: Protects the gastric mucosa
Liver: Improves fat metabolism and lowers cholesterol levels
Immune System: Enhances immune function against pathogens

Activate the Brain – Lion's Mane Emotional Uses

Brings softness to a hardened heart
Breaks through emotional barriers
Creates lightness in difficult conversations

Activate the Brain – Lion's Mane Energetic Uses

Opens the energetic body connection to the Earth
Initiates communication with the fungi elemental realm
Frees and releases blocked memories of trauma

Activate the Brain – Lion's Mane Dosage

Powder: 2500–3000 mg per day

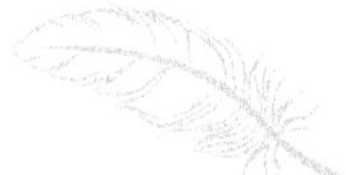

Activate the Brain – Lion's Mane Freedom to Focus

Add 4–8 g Lion's mane to your favorite green smoothie or coffee for daily brain activation.

Ginger – *Zingiber officinalis*

Part Used: Rhizome

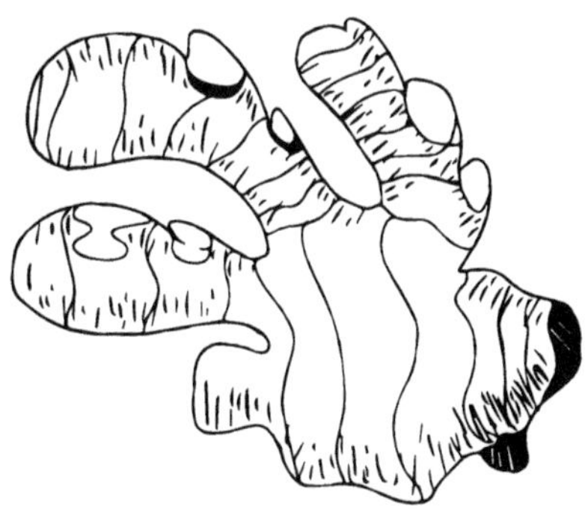

Ginger! Who doesn't love this spicy and fragrant root? It's spicy, sweet, bitter, pungent, and goes with just about every botanical on the planet – a great ally to know and use daily. Ginger is well used around the world for healing and has many different names. We love the Sanskrit name Vishwabhesaj which means "universal medicine." This describes this brain activator ally perfectly. You can use it for a plethora of physical ailments.

Ginger is rich in antioxidants protecting the brain from oxidative damage that can lead to premature cell aging and damage of the DNA. Since the brain functions on oxygen and glucose it is more vulnerable to damage from free radicals. Did you know, one of the reasons smiling is so great for the brain is that it brings in more oxygen. Ginger's constituents, like turmeric, increase the activity of neurotransmitters and blood circulation in the brain, enhancing mood and function. Ginger also assists the brain's connection to the rest of the body by improving vagus nerve function. This nerve runs from the brain and many other important organs – check out the diagram below to see the route.

VAGUS NERVE

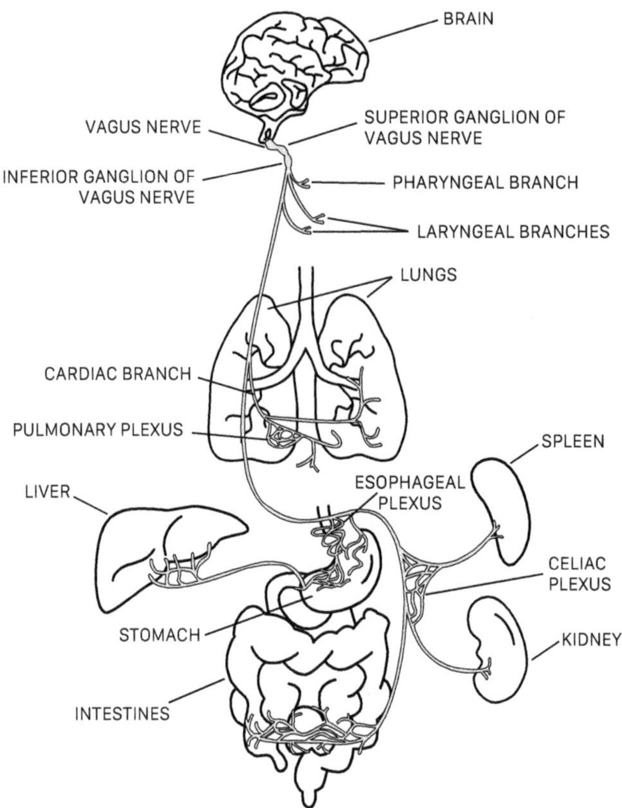

Ginger is the botanical ally of empowerment. It will shift the thought process of the brain from one of victimization to one of confidence and purpose. Ginger soothes yet activates the nervous system reducing the feelings of stress, sadness, anxiety, lethargy, and fatigue. Be creative and add ginger to formulas as an activating synergist as well as adding it to different culinary delights.

Activate the Brain – Ginger Physical Uses

Activate: Turns on gene and DNA regulation
Nervous System: Memory, antioxidant, dementia
Adrenal System: Improves energy
Cardiovascular System: Antioxidant, reduces platelet aggregation, and stimulates circulation
Immune System: Antibiotic
Digestive System: Reduces nausea, stimulates appetite, reduces gas, digestive upset, and motion sickness
Endocrine: Reduces blood sugar
Reproductive: Morning sickness and painful periods
Liver: Reduces cholesterol
Immune System: Acute colds (nasal congestion)
Musculoskeletal: Headaches (topical) and arthritis
Integumentary System: Cold extremities

Activate the Brain – Ginger Emotional Uses

Inspires optimism in times of despair
Liberates the victimization trauma loop
Empowers you to find your life purpose

Activate the Brain – Ginger Energetic Uses

Activates and connects to the dream world
Spices up passion in relationships
Raises earth power (fire) into the second and seventh light wheels

Activate the Brain – Ginger Dosage

Decoction: 4 g root simmered in 236 ml water for 30 minutes. Drink 1–3 cups per day
Powder: 4 g 3x/day
Tincture: 0.5–1 ml 3x/day

Activate the Brain – Ginger Cautions and Contraindications

Caution: Sensitive stomachs and large gallstones
Contraindicated in large amounts in pregnancy

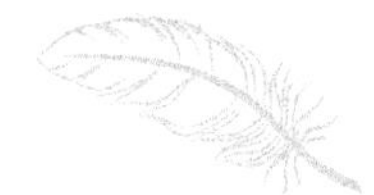

Detox the Brain Freedom to Live Your Highest Potential – Ginger Fizz

Ginger Fizz increases energy to the brain for a real zing!

Ingredients:
226 g peeled and finely chopped fresh
Ginger root – *Zingiber officinalis*
473 ml boiling water
10 ml raw honey or other sweetener of your choice
15 ml fresh lemon or lime juice
118 ml carbonated water

Directions:
Combine ginger and boiling hot water, simmer for 8 minutes and strain. Let cool.
Then, add honey, lemon juice, and carbonated water to 236 ml of your ginger mixture.
Drink right away to get that fizzy rush!
Note – you can substitute ginger for fresh turmeric for a detox fizz.

BOTANICAL ADDITIONS

∞ Bilberry – *Vaccinium myrtillus*
∞ Reishi – *Ganoderma lucidum*
∞ Eleutherococcus – *Eleutherococcus senticosus*
∞ Garlic – *Allium sativum*
∞ Artichoke Leaf – *Cynara scolymus*
∞ Peppermint – *Mentha piperita*

BRAIN ACTIVATE BOTANICAL MEDICINE
DNA BLUEPRINT BENEFITS

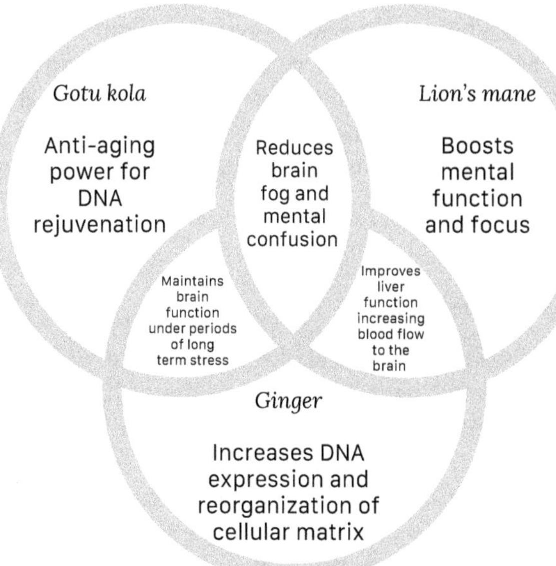

ACTIVATE THE BRAIN – LIGHT WHEELS

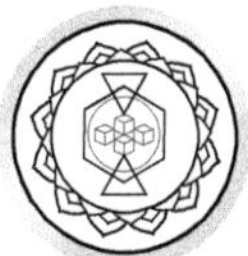

The activate light wheels engage the brain for immediate activation and healing. After using these light wheels in conjunction with the mudra/meditation section you will feel lighter and find a closer connection to your inner joy and original purpose. Be open and feel the light fill every cell of your brain with life.

MAJOR ARCHETYPE

THE 164th LIGHT WHEEL, PUSTAKAGARA

This light wheel, Pustakagara meaning library in Sanskrit, is the portal or doorway to the Akashic Records. With this light wheel the "key" to this dimension has been unlocked for you. This light wheel specifically gives you access to any books or recordings to heal and activate your DNA. When working with this light wheel, you are now able to access any knowledge and tools to help you activate the parts of your brain that have been previously unused or not accessed for healing.

MINOR ARCHETYPE

∞ The 9th light wheel, Seva

The ninth wheel is the light wheel of selfless service, or Seva. The word service here might not have the same meaning that you are familiar with. With this light wheel, service means service to your higher self or the Divine. Seva opens the soul's blueprint. A soul blueprint is a detailed map of the knowledge of your soul. What is in complete alignment with you. Your soul blueprint is unique to you and unlike anyone else's. Access to this blueprint brings your DNA back into alignment of your true purpose and calibration with who you truly are.

LIGHT WHEEL COLORS

MAJOR ARCHETYPE

COPPER

Copper invites in the richness and fullness of life. Surrounding yourself with the copper color will have a calming effect, balancing emotions and stimulating psychic awareness. It deepens the connection to the Earth and symbolizes the need to explore a situation genuinely – don't be afraid to get your hands dirty and dig deep for solutions. When wearing copper around the neck, it enhances the energy flow and helps to smooth disruptions in the auric field.

SOUNDS

∞ TRI-AHH

Toning Tri-Ahh opens to higher universal and cosmic realms, activates the psychic centers, connects to the star seed races and interdimensional beings and accelerates spiritual development. Use this sound frequency and vibration by saying it aloud in repetition for two to eight minutes.

ACTIVATE THE BRAIN – CRYSTALS AND STONES

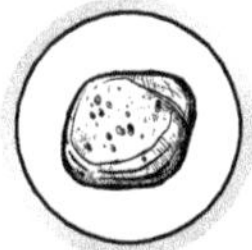

MAJOR ARCHETYPE

FULGURITE

Fulgurite is a powerful activator for awakening the kundalini and spiritual transformation.

It is a stone of acceleration, rapidly clearing stuck emotions from the emotional body and cellular structures. Its potent energy moves through the DNA and mother and father bloodlines to clear belief systems of confusion and misunderstanding of the Divine. This stone is helpful for easing the energetic and emotional dissonance associated with head trauma.

MINOR ARCHETYPES

∞ Black Kyanite

Black kyanite breaks up patterns of negativity from negative self-talk to patterns of self-abuse and self-sabotage. This crystal helps to break up the outer layer of energy calcification of trauma at the cellular level to allow the other alchemical interventions like herbs, essential oils, and nutrition to penetrate their healing energy more deeply.

∞ Sugilite

Sugilite assists in activating the psychic centers and pineal gland. It brings insight in meditation and dreamtime and assists in anchoring of the higher self. It assists in anchoring spiritual teachings in the auric field down to the level of the cellular consciousness and DNA.

CRYSTAL ADDITIONS

- ∞ Amethyst
- ∞ Gold

BRAIN ACTIVATE CRYSTAL GRID

Drink a glass of clean water with 3 drops each of Japanese Magnolia and Heulandite essences. This crystal attunement is best done in the early or mid day for 20-30 minutes. You may choose to listen to music like Solfeggio tones. Cleanse crystals immediately after use. (See Appendix C).

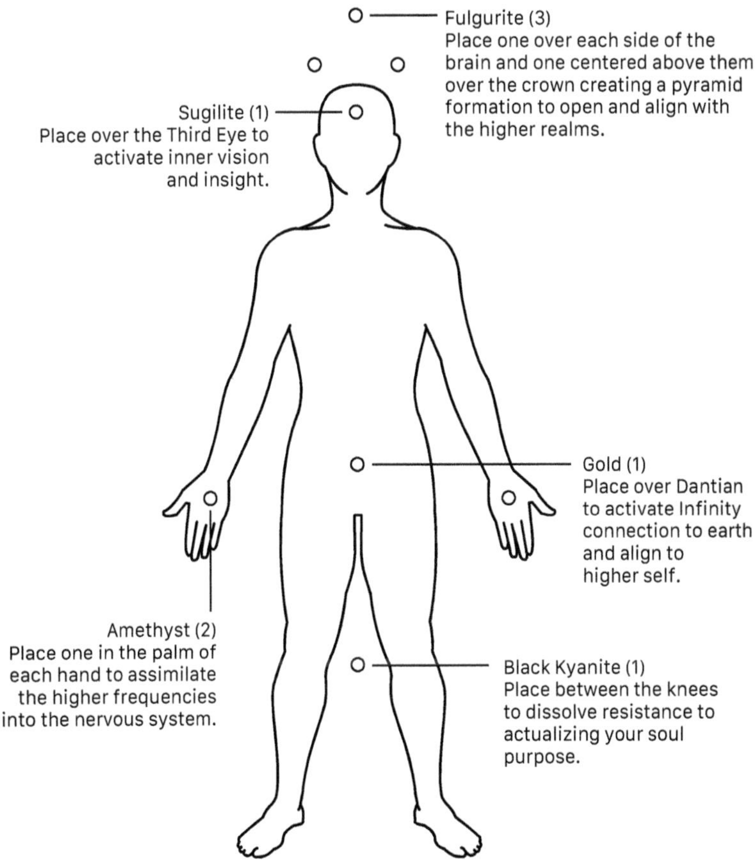

ACTIVATE THE BRAIN – ENERGETIC AND VIBRATIONAL TECHNIQUES

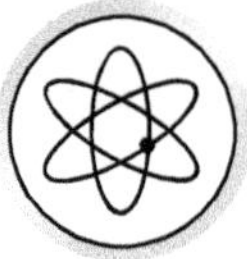

MAJOR ARCHETYPE

ACTIVATE THE BRAIN HYDROTHERAPY

∞ 4 drops of Tulsi essential oil (*Ocimum tenuiflorum*)
∞ 2 drops of Fennel essential oil (*Foeniculum vulgare*)
∞ 2 drops Rosemary essential oil (*Rosmarinus officinalis CT verbenone*)
∞ 3 drops of Lemon essential oil (*Citrus limonum*)
∞ 10 drops of Copper Gem Essence
∞ 10 drops of Gold Gem Essence

Add all ingredients to the bath and soak for at least 20 minutes.

MINOR ARCHETYPES

Activate the Brain Water Ceremony

This form of vibrational alchemy imprints the vibration, life force, and specific healing energy of the crystal into one of the most nourishing and restorative elements, water. Taken on an empty stomach in the morning allows for a rapid cellular response and often a tangible feeling of shift of emotion energy and awareness.

Can be done during any moon phase. Take your cleansed and programmed crystal and add it to a glass or pitcher of fresh clean water. Wrap your hand around the vessel and align your intention to infuse the water molecules with the consciousness of love, gratitude, and the desire to activate your brain with enlightened illumination. To enhance the alchemy of the intervention, infuse with a copper-colored light. After 20 minutes, remove the crystal, thank it for sharing its vibration and drink the water as desired. NOTE: Remember to strain crystal prior to drinking and enjoy with the intention of allowing the spectrum of vibration to permeate and heal at the cellular level.

Needed:
1 piece of Fulgurite
1 vessel of water
Infuse as instructed above and drink throughout the day. Refrigerate unused portions for later use.

Activate the Brain EOBT

Place one drop of tulsi essential oil between the first two fingertips of the right hand, inhale deeply and tap the Yin Tang for 30 seconds with the intention of activating the brain and nervous system with full illumination.

Location: On the forehead midway between the upper border of the eyebrows.

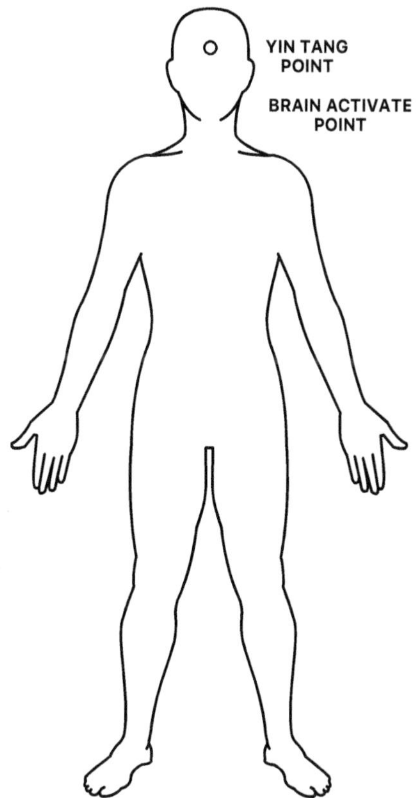

ACTIVATE THE BRAIN – FLOWER AND GEM ESSENCES

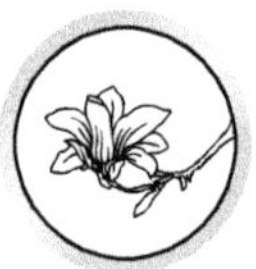

FLOWER ESSENCES

MAJOR ARCHETYPE

JAPANESE MAGNOLIA

Japanese magnolia is an essence of illumination and connection with divine consciousness. At the cellular level, it activates the coding for unity. It lifts and expands the higher levels of the auric field so that the lower levels can decompress, clear, align, and then to expand within this new template.

MINOR ARCHETYPES

Holly

Holly serves as a kick-starter to our vital life force and brings an energy of laser focus, clarity. It strengthens and repairs the structured levels of the energy field, the first, third, fifth, and seventh, the last of which connects with our crown chakra or light wheel.

Manzanita

Manzanita is an essence of joy and connection that activates light and consciousness at the pineal gland and expands that vibration throughout the body and auric field. It brings the energy of sweetness and appreciation of the simple pleasures in life. It reminds us to feel light and free of overwhelm, overthinking, and overdoing.

GEM ESSENCE

MAJOR ARCHETYPE

HEULANDITE

Heulandite essence expands our ability to perceive our multidimensional nature and opens us to extraterrestrial presence. It helps to expand the meridian points to receive higher levels of light quotient and encourages us to open our heart and connection to the divine source within it.

ACTIVATE THE BRAIN – INTENTIONS

MAJOR ARCHETYPE

IGNITE and ILLUMINATE

MINOR ARCHETYPES

∞ My eternal flame within shines brightly for all to see
∞ My neurons are fully energized by the rays of the sun
∞ I am one with the divine light of cosmic consciousness

ADDITIONAL INTENTIONS

∞ I am able switch on all areas of my brain at any moment
∞ I am connected to the cosmic light and collective conscious
∞ My soul path is glowing with true knowledge
∞ I am the light eternal

ACTIVATE THE BRAIN – MEDITATION AND MUDRA

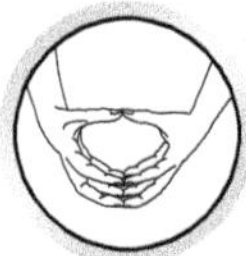

Hakini Mudra

My cells and soul sing in illuminated unison,
I am one with all the wisdom and connectivity of the universe.

The Hakini mudra opens the frontal lobe, and the pineal and pituitary glands of the brain connected to the third eye, ajna chakra. The pineal gland secretes melatonin and serotonin which the brain activates during visualization and meditation exercises. The pituitary gland is the major endocrine hub for hormone production and sends messages to the rest of the glands for adjustments and balance ranging from metabolism to sleep. This area is also the command center for the subtle mind and shines brightly, like the moon, connecting deeply to the innate wisdom of your inner being or soul.

Hakini Mudra Alignment

1. Place the hands facing each other at the level of the third chakra, the solar plexus.
2. Gently touch all fingers and thumbs of both hands together.
3. Hold the hands lightly open in the shape of a circle as if holding a ball of light.
4. Take a deep breath, let your body relax.
5. You may now either do the meditation below or 10 minutes of *Oscillating Brain Breathing* (to access the *Oscillating Brain Breathing* please visit the website www.zenergymedicinals.com). Use this mudra for connecting the right and left sides of the brain when you are experiencing disconnection from your brain and body.
6. The Hakini mudra can be used for distance and global healing by visualizing the globe of light in between your hands to connect with another person needing healing or visualize the globe of light expanding to stretch around the entire planet.

- ∞ To access the mudra meditation please go to www.zenergymedicinals.com

- ∞ Please apply your essential oil and inhale it for 30–45 seconds.
- ∞ Hold the Hakini mudra and take several breaths. Visualize the front and center of your brain being filled with light. Feel your breath moving up from your root chakra or coccyx to the brain. You feel energy moving through the entire body – it might feel tingly and lighter.
- ∞ Connect to the Earth and invite your body to be filled with amber light. Now open to the universal connection of divine consciousness and the great light of Source.
- ∞ As we align with the greater dimensional frequencies available to the Earth during this time of great shift, call forth your spiritual teachers and guides to hold you in the light.
- ∞ Envision a golden merkaba of light and universal divine consciousness filled with light language, and sacred geometric formations. It merges with the higher levels of your auric field; feel a quickening, a tingling as it begins to recalibrate your system holographically from your cellular DNA level to the highest level of the auric field and back down from the aura to the cellular consciousness.
- ∞ Breathe as your entire nonphysical and physical body recalibrates. The higher chakras align themselves, strengthening and elongating the hara line. Breathe as your system fills with light.
- ∞ On the next breath, envision a golden infinity symbol vertically coming down from the presence of divine consciousness, pulsating gold and opalescent light. It encapsulates your entire field.
- ∞ Bathe the brain and nervous system in crystalline light until it begins to shine like a diamond in its highest state of perfection, of light, of clarity, the highest ability to attract and emanate divine light.
- ∞ All pathways begin to reformat and realign with this frequency of diamond light. See, feel, allow, imagine all the synapses in the brain firing, healing with reparation to the myelin sheath, down through the spine and throughout the nervous system. The entire system, holographically reformatting with this crystalline light through the blood, the bone, the bone marrow.
- ∞ Invite in the highest experience of enlightenment in accordance with your "I Am" presence for this lifetime, the unified perspective of understanding for all that exists within the universe and within your place as a child of divine light.

- ∞ Allow the universal wisdom to imprint itself through your cellular structures and DNA.
- ∞ With each breath, feel each cell of the brain filled with light and illuminated with power. Repeat the intention three times either silently or aloud: "My cells and soul sing in illuminated unison. I am one with all the wisdom and connectivity of the universe."
- ∞ Offer a great prayer of gratitude for yourself. All the energies of light that's around you, all that is possible from this moment forward.

ACTIVATE THE BRAIN – SACRED GEOMETRY

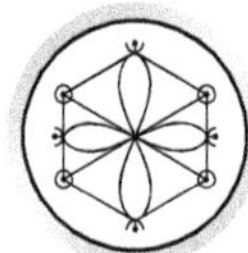

MAJOR ARCHETYPE

ACTIVATE THE BRAIN SACRED GEOMETRY

This intentional and original depiction of sacred geometry converges the pinnacle of divine consciousness with that of the human form. Here the brain is illuminated within the framework of the original genetic blueprint, where full recognition of human potential can be experienced, assimilated, and understood. This activation broadens the potential for accessing higher universal concepts along with the neural pathway comprehension of the schematics needed to actualize them. Incorporate this image into your meditation when beginning new projects, particularly those that benefit the planet from a humanitarian perspective.

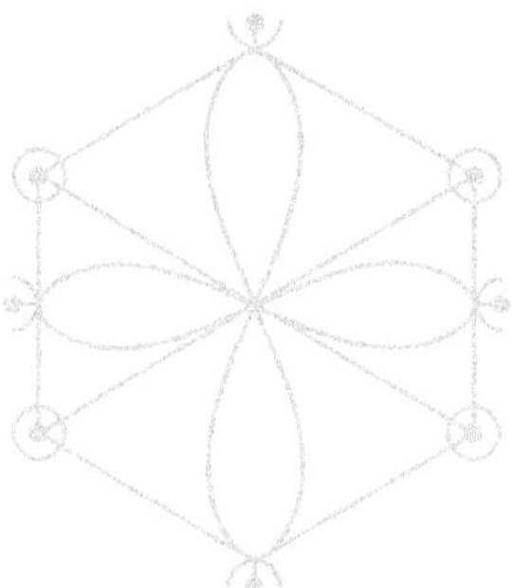

ACTIVATE THE BRAIN – NUTRITION

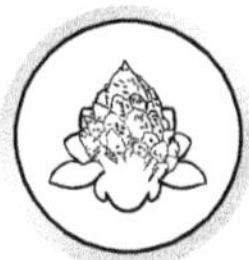

MAJOR ARCHETYPE

ROMANESCO

We love this antioxidant packed vegetable that looks like a plant from outer space resembling the complexity of tubes and fractals making up the brain. This vegetable contains the fat-soluble vitamin K which is essential for forming sphingolipids. Sphingolipids are a type of fat densely packed into the neurons facilitating higher cognitive function and protection against DNA damage.

Romanesco is also a super source of CoQ10 which plays an important part in mitochondrial ATP synthesis. With CoQ10, your brain is given more energy and also more antioxidants, reducing oxidative damage. You can think more clearly, make quicker decisions, and access deeper information and genetic code more quickly with CoQ10.

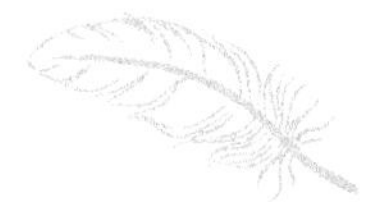

Prepare this vegetable as you would cauliflower or broccoli. We love it lightly steamed in a Greek salad tossed with red onion, feta cheese, parsley, capers, and lemon.

MINOR ARCHETYPES

Liver

Liver is an organ meat that has fallen out of popularity, but it is a super star nutritional profile. It's packed with vitamins A, B2, and B12, iron, copper, and choline. B12 is key for the formation of healthy DNA and red blood cells. Choline has also been shown in studies to improve cognitive function, boost mood, and prevent anxiety.

Pumpkin Seeds

Pumpkin seeds are high in key brain micronutrients copper, zinc, magnesium, and iron, helping with impaired brain function, preventing neurodegenerative disorders, and improving nerve signaling. They are also rich in antioxidants protecting the brain from oxidative damage and DNA malfunction.

NUTRITIONAL ADDITIONS

- ∞ Borage oil
- ∞ Blackcurrant oil
- ∞ Flaxseed oil
- ∞ Vitamin D Foods: organ meats, liver, egg yolks, shrimp
- ∞ Vitamin K Foods: egg yolks, butter, dark leafy greens
- ∞ Avocados

ACTIVATE THE BRAIN – DISCOVERY DIVE – ILLUMINATION

What does it mean to be fully illumined? Once you get on that superhighway, how long can you stay there? Is it indefinite? Illumination is part of the journey. Art of the Renaissance time period often depicted a golden halo over the head of the subject. This halo represents more than the auric field of the individual, it connotes the light of inspiration, of expansion, and yes, illumination. Illumination allows us to integrate our masculine, feminine, and child aspects and healing through our bloodlines. This process allows us to integrate the wisdom of experience both at a soul and cell level and to then allow the infinite energy of the cosmos to enter us fully, expanding our consciousness. When the soul consciousness merges with our cellular consciousness, we have created the conditions for illumination and enlightenment.

As you consider these questions, we would like you to invite in a completely new perception and experience of what it means to be illumined, ignited, and firing at all levels of cognition and clarity. As you are reading this, all the cells of your brain are being activated and connected to the collective consciousness. Feel the Lightning of Your Freedom!

Do I feel connected to the light of the Divine? What is my experience of this connection? Do I want to enhance it? If so, how?

How can I better care for myself from a perspective of nutrition and exercise to support my illumination on a mind–body level?

Do I crave a greater understanding of esoteric or mystical philosophy? In what areas?

Do I feel a sense of grace in my daily experience of self and relationships with others?

A single pathway of practice to activate all these aspects is meditation. Cultivating a meditation practice starting with five minutes of consistency a day and then increasing will benefit illumination on every level. Through these pages, you have many, many options and alchemical interventions to enrich your practice and experience.

FREEDOM PHOTON WHEEL™

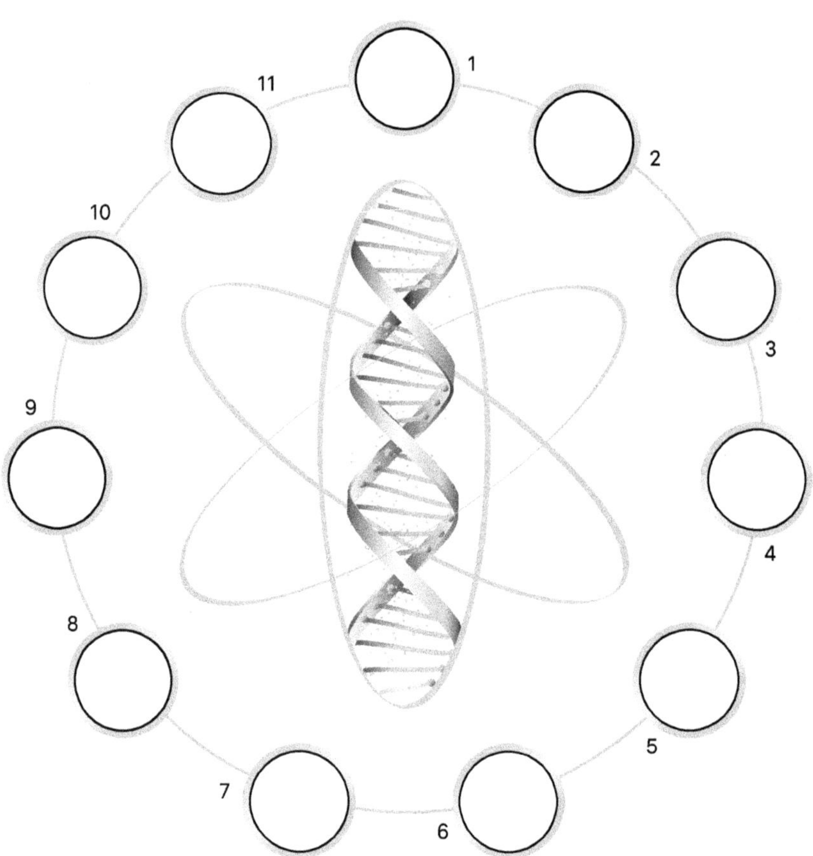

ACTIVATE THE BRAIN
YOUR PERSONAL FREEDOM PHOTON WHEEL RITUAL

Moon Phase

It is best to perform your ritual when the moon is waxing from the new moon to the full moon, to align with the phase. However, the power of your intention and momentum is key so if you are inspired at another time, go for it.

Intention

"I call forth, activate, and allow the highest level of light quotient in accordance with my I Am presence to flood my brain and entire being with the light of unity consciousness."

Select, Align, and Activate

Select your interventions according to the instructions in Chapter Five. Inhale and apply your chosen essential oil for 30–45 seconds. Use your botanical tincture or tea as directed. You may also listen to the meditation and use the mudra from this chapter while attuning your FPW.

Affirm

"Divine Consciousness, please assist me in healing that I have carried through my lineage, my mother and father bloodlines so that I allow the fullest experience of illumination leading to enlightenment. I invite in an enlightened understanding of the universe and my integral place within it."

CHAPTER 9

Conclusion and Integration

∞ To access the meditation please go to www.zenergymedicinals.com

Here we are together at seemingly the end. You may have an inkling, though, it is merely the beginning of another chapter. This is perhaps the most important chapter of all, as it is the very first of your own book, your new story of life, health, well-being, and empowerment. Invite in the intention for deep integration, and to create and experience life from effortless intention.

As the superhero of your own life and the hero or heroine of the story of your past, you have the power of love and light within to guide a brand-new life of freedom, abundance, vibrancy, and joy. Your soul and your cells have been invited into unity and greater understanding of the plight and power of divine consciousness in human form, beyond living a limited perception and experience of reality.

As a multidimensional being ignited and alive with the spark of the Divine in each cell and DNA, you understand you are a powerful cocreator of life experience for the express purpose of your soul's growth, ultimately understanding all perspectives of the human experience to the zenith of self-mastery, enlightenment, and the actualization of your soul purpose.

The beauty of integration is that as we heal, we expand in understanding and compassion. We then integrate, assimilating the wisdom at the soul and cell level to be able to share it with others as an act of transcendence. As each layer surfaces and clears we deepen the journey inward; there is no end while we are within the body. There is always more to learn, experience, grow, and share until each one recognizes their individual freedom, their sovereignty, and interconnectedness.

If we were to speak or to sing one word or idea to you, it would be that of REMEMBER. Remember who you are, remember the light and the grace that dances deep within and all around you. Remember the healing your DNA has experienced throughout this book. You can revisit this book to Detox, Nourish, Activate the DNA over and over again. As you spiritually transform, so do your cells in the never-ending infinity loop of healing. The simplicity of your purpose is remembrance of this truth. It is then that your high path, your soul purpose will surface for the joy of excavation.

Integration is not perfection. Humanity is blessed yet flawed in perfect imperfection. Imperfection is the beauty and the uniqueness of YOU! We offer the perspective that integration offers you to invite in the understanding of everything you have experienced in life and your "treasure map," all the depths of pain, the abuse, betrayal, and all levels of dysfunction that you have risen from. We invite you to stand up straight, tall, and proud, and have an "over the shoulder" moment. Look back through your path and see how far you have come, how strong you are, and how bright you shine.

Choosing life from effortless intention is liberation. It allows us to connect to the heavens above, the Earth below, remember our divine connection and invite in our intentions to form with ease and grace. We let go of the need to create from ego, will, and mind, and open our hearts to miracle consciousness and then allow in the organic nature of evolution to flow through us creating experience far beyond what we could think possible. This is your birthright. This is the gift of your divine light. We stand in glorious recognition of you. All of you. Claim your greatness. Celebrate the New You!

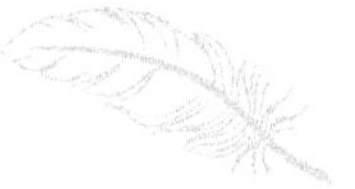

Ceremonial Oil to Remember and Invite Blessing from Your Ancestors

- ∞ 2 drops Rose Otto essential oil (*Rosa damascena*)
- ∞ 1 drop Spikenard essential oil (*Nardostachys jatamansi*)
- ∞ 1 drop Immortelle essential oil (*Helichrysum italicum*)
- ∞ 2 drops Ylang Ylang essential oil (*Cananga odorata superior extra*)
- ∞ 2 drops Geranium essential oil (*Pelargonium graveolens*)
- ∞ 1 drop Jasmine absolute (*Jasminum grandiflorum*)
- ∞ 1 drop Sandalwood essential oil (*Santalum austrocaledonicum*)
- ∞ 5 ml Gardenia monoi

Blend all ingredients and infuse with the intention below. Apply sparingly to the wrists and heart, inhaling deeply. Coming full circle, or perhaps we should say full infinity, the sacred geometric symbol and concept of infinite, holographic healing woven through this journey from the first chapter, we invite you for ceremony. In this sacred, intentional practice we invite you to remember the glory and magnificence of who you truly are. Invoke a blessing from your ancestors, who are encircling you with their love and their light. Your intention can be broad or specific depending on what you long for in this moment. Regardless, know it is heard, held in love, and on its way to actualization.

APPENDIX A

Aromatherapy Formulations

Safety

- Keep out of reach of children.
- Do not use essential oils internally.
- If accidental ingestion occurs, consult a family physician or poison control immediately.
- Some essential oils can cause skin irritation – dilute prior to use (if irritation – redness, swelling, itching) does occur, wash area with unscented soap, place a few drops of vegetable oil or unscented cream on skin, and allow the skin to breathe).
- Sensitization – involving the immune system – may occur with first application yet tends to show signs with prolonged use of same or similar oil. It often occurs in those with general skin sensitivities and/or allergies or when skin is damaged. Shows the same signs as irritation.
- Patch test to determine irritation/sensitization by placing 2 drops of blend (double the planned concentration) on the inside of the elbow, place a band-aid over it, wait 24 hours and remove, checking to see if irritation has occurred. Repeat this process to check for signs of sensitization.

- Some essential oils can be phototoxic – causing increased sensitivity to sunlight; for example, bergamot (Citrus bergamia). Avoid. A UV rays for 12 hours after skin application.
- Always use CAUTION if: pregnant, diabetic, epileptic, have high blood pressure, or in conjunction with homeopathy or prescription drugs.
- Essential oils are not water soluble. If essential oil should accidentally end up in your eye, place one drop of the closest vegetable oil into the eye, then dip a Q-tip in your vegetable oil and trace the outline of your eye.
- Avoid extended use of the same essential oils.
- Sometimes, too little information can be dangerous. If you are interested in working with essential oil please consider many of the educational resources available and at minimum READ, READ, and READ.

Always use dark (blue/brown) glass for storing and mixing oils and remember to shake before each use to maintain the proper balance. Keep essential oils out of heat and direct sunlight. Any blends that are mixed in carrier oil will have a shelf life of up to 6 months.

What to look for when purchasing

- Common name
- Latin name
- Part of plant
- Method of distillation
- Country of origin
- Knowledgeable staff
- The bottles should be amber or blue to deflect UV rays and should contain reducer droppers to prevent evaporation and oxidation.

Massage oils

Use a 2½ percent dilution – 15 drops per ounce of 1 E0, or a combination of 3–5 apricot kernel, almond oil, and jojoba make excellent carrier oils for your bends.

The power of SYNERGY. You will hear this term often in reference to herbs and essential oils. When you combine more than one ingredient, in this case an essential oil, the formula becomes more potent and effective than if you are using the isolate, or single ingredient. Create your formulas to blend 3–5 ingredients for best results. By using no more than 5 ingredients, your blend will contain the clarity needed for healing vs. becoming muddled in its effectiveness by adding too many ingredients.

Bath

Blend the essential oils with (1–2 tablespoons) or without a carrier (add 5–7 drops of blend – synergy) to add to warm bath water, preferably when the person is in the bath, and swish the water to disperse oils in water.

Inhalation

For inhalation try 2–3 drops on a pillowcase or handkerchief inhaling throughout the day or night.

Or try a clay candle, pottery, or nebulizing diffuser, which disperses the essential oil molecules into the air (antimicrobial effect and other biochemical effects).

Spray mist

30 drops of your essential oil synergy to 2 oz distilled water. Remember that essential oils are not water soluble. If you are not adding an emulsifier, shake well prior to use.

APPENDIX B

Botanical Formulations

Tinctures, glycerites, and spirits are concentrated herbal medicinals that are compact and easy to take. They are the alchemy of herbal medicine making and are made by suspending the plant's vital force in an alcohol or glycerin-based menstruum. These healing forms of herbal medicine have been used for centuries to increase immune support, vitality, and longevity, as well as to treat the myriad conditions to which we are subjected throughout our lifetime. Because they are highly concentrated, a little goes a long way. For instance, one could take 20 capsules to equal the potency of 1½ teaspoons of tincture. In addition, tinctures, glycerites, and spirits are immediately absorbed into the bloodstream upon ingestion, resulting in a quickened effect on the body.

Cordial

Prepare ingredients:

- Grind dried herbs (mortar and pestle, coffee grinder, blender, etc.) or chop fresh herbs
- Chop any desired fruit into small pieces

- Choose a jar that allows for a small amount of leftover space not utilized by liquid or solid content
- Place prepared herbs and fruit into a jar
  - Fresh herbs: fill jar ¾ full (fresh herbs take up more space and contain water)
  - Dried herbs and fruit: fill jar ¼ to ½ full
- Pour selected alcohol over herbs. Brandy is traditionally used but tequila, vodka, gin, pure grain alcohol, rum, whiskey, wine, and port are also good options.
  - Make sure the alcohol covers the ingredients by at least 2 inches
- Lid, label, and date jar
- Store in a cool dark place for 2–6 weeks.
  - Shake consistently
  - Check to make sure ingredients are adequately covered with alcohol. Add more alcohol if there is any exposed plant material as mold and fermentation can result
- Decant
  - Place a funnel into the mouth of an additional jar
  - Place muslin or cheesecloth into the funnel
  - Pour the maceration into the funnel
- Sweeten
  - Sugar, honey, molasses, fruit concentrates, simple syrup, stevia, and glycerin are all options
  - Traditionally, cordials are relatively sweet; as much as ½ part of sweetener to 1 part alcohol maceration

Decoctions

A decoction is used for plant constitution that requires more time and heat for extraction, like mineral salts or bitter constituents. Decoctions are also used for hard plant parts, like barks, roots, and seeds.

- Place one cup of water on the stove in a small pan and bring to a boil.
- Add boiling water to 1 tbsp of dried herb in a glass mason jar. Screw lid on the jar.
- Steep covered for 20 minutes.
- Strain the herb using a metal strainer and press out as much liquid from the herb as possible.
- Drink the decoction as directed.

Fluid extracts

A fluid extract or tincture is a 1:1 ratio of dry plant to liquid equivalent.

- Harvest the plant matter.
- Combine the menstruum and herb.
- Make sure that the menstruum covers the herb by at least an inch. This ensures that your preparation spoil due to the herb's exposure to oxidation or microbial growth.
- Label, and store in a cool, dark place.
- Shake daily, pouring your intention and love into your medicine, until ready to press. Typically, fluid extracts need to macerate for 30 days.
- Strain and press the liquid out through cheesecloth or muslin. The remaining liquid is your fluid extract.
- Bottle in dark colored bottles and label. Store in a cool place.

Infusions

An infusion is a process used to extract constituents such as vitamins, enzymes, and volatile oils from plant materials, usually the aerial parts consisting of flowers and leaves.

- Using a clean quart jar, fill about 1/5 of the jar with herb(s).
- Pour boiling water over and fill the jar, loosely cover with a lid.
- Allow to infuse for at least 4 hours.
- Strain out the herbs
- Add more water at this point, if you'd like as the infusion will be quite strong or you can drink as is.

Infused medicinal oil

Medicinal oils can be used as food or medicine depending on the fixed oil used and the herbs chosen for maceration. Ideal oils for infusions include olive, sesame, almond, jojoba and castor oils.

When making infused oils you can choose to use either fresh or dried herbs; however, when using fresh herbs there are some extra steps that need to be followed in order to ensure that your oils do not spoil. It is important to keep your temperature between 100° and 125°F

(38–52°C). Temperatures that go below 100°F (38°C) will require a longer extraction time, and those that exceed 125°F (52°C) risk the loss of medicinal value.

Double Boiler Method

This method is suitable for both fresh and dried herbs.

- Place chopped herbs and oil in a double boiler and bring to a low simmer.
- Slowly heat for 30–60 minutes, checking frequently to be sure the oil is not overheating.
- Then lower the heat, the longer the infusion, the better the oil.
- Strain the oil through cheesecloth or muslin.
- When the oil has been poured off, put the herbs in the cloth and wring thoroughly.
- Store in a dark, sterilized, labeled bottle in a cool, dark area.

Pressing the infused oil

- Place a strainer lined with cheesecloth in a bowl.
- Pour the oil through the strainer.
- Pick up all sides of the cloth and bring them together at the top.
- Twist the cloth, squeezing the remaining oil from the herbs.
- Filter the oil through cheesecloth again if a clear solution is desired.
- Store the oil in a dark-colored bottle with a tight fitting lid, and label your preparation.
- Shelf life: one year if kept in a cool, dark area.

Oxymiel

An oxymiel is a specialized honey mixture combined with vinegar. This medium is useful as a carrier for herbal infusion, decoctions, concentrates, and tinctures.

- Fill a pint jar 1/4 full of your choice of herb.
- Cover with equal parts apple cider vinegar and honey to fill the jar.
- Stir to incorporate.

- Wipe any liquid off the rim and top with a tight-fitting plastic lid. Alternatively, place a piece of parchment paper under a metal canning lid and ring to keep the vinegar from touching the metal.
- Shake jar until thoroughly mixed.
- Store the jar in a cool, dark place to extract for a minimum of two weeks.
- Shake jar at least twice a week to assist in extraction.
- Strain out herbs through a fine mesh strainer.
- Pour strained oxymiel into a glass jar.
- Label and date.
- Store in a cool, dark place until ready to use. When stored properly, shelf life is approximately 6 months.

Herbal compress

- Combine 3 tablespoons of desired herbs with 236 ml of boiling water.
- If using a hot compress, let the mixture cool to the touch as not to burn the skin.
- If using a cool compress, let your tea cool, or place in the refrigerator to cool quickly.
- Soak a clean piece of fabric/cotton material in the tea and squeeze excess herbal liquid out of the cloth.
- Place the soaked cloth on your skin and wrap around the area in need. Let sit and enjoy the healing herbal sensation.

Sitz bath

The sitz bath is an immersion bath with the person seated in a tub with water covering the hips, buttocks, and lower abdomen. It is used to decrease congestion and increase circulation to the pelvic and lower abdominal organs.

Contraindications

Do not use alternating sitz baths in persons with hemorrhages, menorrhagia, prolapses, acute lung congestion, acute inflammation, painful conditions with spasms or colic, and heart problems.

Supplies
1 tub/bathtub/sitz tub
Hot water
6–8 cups decoction of herb tea
Bath thermometer

Directions
Prepare the tub with hot water at 105–110°F (40–43°C), so that it comes ½ inch above your navel. This temperature is slightly higher than the average hot tub. Do not let the water temperature exceed 120°F (49°C) degrees. Prepare the alternate tub with cold water at 45°F (7°C), so that it comes ½ inch below your navel.

- ∞ Sit in a hot tub for 2–5 minutes.
- ∞ After 3–5 minutes, sit in a cold tub for 20–60 seconds.
- ∞ Make three complete cycles between the hot and cold tubs (3x hot/ 3x cold).
- ∞ Always start treatment with the hot bath and finish treatment with the cold bath.
- ∞ Dry off completely and rest in bed for at least 30 minutes.
- ∞ Add hot water to the hot tub if the temperature falls below 105 degrees.

The greater the contrast between the hot and cold water, to a resonable degree, the stronger the treatment.

APPENDIX C

Cleansing and Care of Crystals

Clearing and Charging Crystals

After receiving your crystal, it is important to clear and charge it to establish pure energy as well as clarity of intention for its use. You can then clear on a monthly basis or as you feel is needed.

Clearing a Crystal

1. Clearing any past programming or energy from your crystal, envision a laser of white light emanating from your third eye light wheel. See this white light permeating the crystal with the intention for it to be cleared and cleansed.
2. Place in the sun, particularly at midday for an hour after rinsing it in cool water.
3. Bury in the ground for three nights.
4. Charging a Crystal. Hold in your right hand and command that it be activated with the energy consciousness of divine will. Now your crystal is ready for sacred practices, meditation, healing, and creative manifestation.

GLOSSARY OF TERMS

Adaptogen: Adaptogens or adaptogenic substances are used in herbal medicine for the claimed stabilization of physiological processes and promotion of homeostasis.

Akashic records: An etheric collection of each human souls' lifetime (past and present) containing karmic information and soul level contracts.

Alterative: An agent used to improve elimination of metabolic waste.

Analgesic: An analgesic or painkiller is any member of the group of herbs or pharmaceuticals used to achieve analgesia, relief from pain.

Anhidrotic: An agent that reduces sweating.

Antiallergic: An herb that counters an allergy.

Antiarrhythmic: Herbs used for regulating heart rhythms.

Antibacterial: An agent that fights against bacteria and bacterial infections.

Anticatarrhal: An herb that reduces the production or rate of mucus.

Antifungal: An agent that fights against a fungus or mold.

Antigalactagogue: An herb that decreases the secretion of milk from nursing mothers.

Anti-inflammatory: The property of a substance or treatment that reduces inflammation or swelling.

Antimicrobial: An agent that kills microorganisms or stops their growth.

Antioxidant: An agent that prevents oxidation, a process believed to be the initiating factor in the development of many disease conditions.

Antirheumatic: Herbs that act to treat rheumatic conditions by decreasing inflammation, swelling, and pain.

Antisclerotic: An herb that decreases or prevents hardening of the tissues.

Antiseptic: An agent used to prevent, resist, and counteract infection.

Antispasmodic: Herbs which relieve spasm of involuntary muscle in organs and muscles.

Antiphlogistic: An herb that reduces inflammation and fever.

Antitussive: Herbs which are used to suppress or relieve cough.

Antiviral: Herbs that inhibit the development of viruses.

Aphrodisiac: An agent that arouses or is held to arouse sexual desire.

Astringent: An astringent acts to contract and tighten, or constrict body tissues, usually locally after topical medicinal application, like a styptic.

Aquaretic: An aquaretic is used to promote aquaresis, the excretion of water without electrolyte loss.

Bitter: An agent that has a bitter taste but also promotes digestive function and improves appetite.

Blueprint: The etheric map of an individual's soul purpose infused with the highest potentials of creation.

Cardiotonic: An agent which has a beneficial action on the heart.

Carminative: An agent which improves digestion and relieves the discomfort of flatulence and/or colic.

Cephalic: Herbs used to clear mind and brain disorders such as memory loss.

Cholagogue: An herb that promotes the discharge of bile from the digestive system.

Cicatrisant: An herb that is used to heal a wound by increasing the formation of scar tissue.

Choleretic: An herb that increases secretion of bile from the liver.

Cytophylactic: An herb that protects an organ by creating new cells.

Demulcent: Herbs which contain mucilage.

Depurative: An agent capable of removing toxins and waste from the body system.

Diaphoretic: An agent that increases perspiration and elimination through the skin, often used to reduce temperature in fevers.

Diuretic: An agent that increases the production and flow of urine.

Emetic: An agent that induces vomiting.

Emmenagogue: An agent that promotes menstruation.

Expectorant: An agent which promotes the removal of excess mucus from the lungs and air passages.

Febrifuge: An herb that reduces fever.

Genetic Blueprint: The sequence of the human genome represents our genetic blueprint.

Great Central Sun: Cosmic source of Divine light and omniscience.

Hepatic: An agent used to strengthen, tone, and stimulate bile secretion improving liver function.

Hepatoprotectant: Those herbs which are used to cure or prevent liver damage.

Hypoglycemic: An agent used to lower raised blood sugar levels in the body.

Hypotensive: An agent that lowers blood pressure.

Laxative: Laxatives, purgatives, or aperients are substances that loosen stools and increase bowel movements. They are used to treat and/or prevent constipation.

Lymphatic: These herbs are "blood purifiers" as lymphatic herbs have an ability to move lymph and can increase lymphatic flow, moving fluid and protein away from areas of inflammation so that fresh lymph (rich in oxygen and nutrients needed for tissue repair) can replace them.

Immunomodulator: A substance which stimulates or suppresses the components of the immune system including both innate and adaptive immune responses.

Immunostimulatory: A substance that increases the ability of the immune system to fight infection and disease.

Merkaba: Etheric light body comprised of two pyramid sacred geometric forms that surround the body and connect to higher levels of consciousness.

Meridian: In traditional Chinese medicine (TCM), a form of alternative medicine that originated in China, meridians are invisible energy pathways, or channels, that run through the body.

Nervine: An agent that tones and strengthens the nervous system.

Organoleptic: Involving the use of sense organs.

Organophosphates: Any organic compound whose molecule contains one or more phosphate ester groups, especially a pesticide.

Oxytocic: Herbs that induce labor by stimulating contractions of the muscles of the uterus. These are also considered as uterotonics.

Polyphenols: Any of a group of naturally occurring compounds found significantly in fruits, vegetables, cereals, coffee, tea, and wine, and widely studied for properties believed to promote health and fight disease.

Purgative: Herbs that produce very strong laxative effects and watery evacuations. These herbs increase bowel movements.

Rubefacient: A substance for topical application that produces redness of the skin, e.g., by causing dilation of the capillaries and an increase in blood circulation.

Sedative: Herbs used to relieve irritability and promote calm and tranquil feelings.

Sudorific: An herb that induces extreme sweating.

Telomere: A region of repetitive nucleotide sequences associated with specialized proteins at the ends of linear chromosomes.

Tonic: An herb that tones the tissues.

Trophorestorative: The "trophic" state is representative of the vital capacity of a system or tissue in the body. Often these herbs have tissue specificity within the body, such as endocrine, skin, lungs, heart, stomach, and female reproductive organs.

Vasoconstrictor: An agent that causes constriction of the blood vessels.

Vermifuge: An herb that destroys and expels intestinal worms.

Vulnerary: An agent that promotes healing of external wounds and cuts.

REFERENCES

Andersson, U., Berger, K., Högberg, A., Landin-Olsson, M., & Holm, C. (2012). Effects of rose hip intake on risk markers of type 2 diabetes and cardiovascular disease: a randomized, double-blind, cross-over investigation in obese persons. *European Journal of Clinical Nutrition, 66*(5): 585–590. doi: 10.1038/ejcn.2011.203.

Balk, E. M., & Lichtenstein, A. H. (2017). Omega-3 fatty acids and cardiovascular disease: Summary of the 2016 Agency of Healthcare Research and Quality evidence review. *Nutrients, 9*(8): 865. doi: 10.3390/nu9080865.

Basu, A., Rhone, M., & Lyons, T. J. (2010). Berries: emerging impact on cardiovascular health. *Nutrition Review, 68*(3): 168–177. doi: 10.1111/j.1753-4887.

Clare, B. A., Conroy, R. S., & Spelman, K. (2009). The diuretic effect in human subjects of an extract of Taraxacum officinale folium over a single day. *Journal of Alternative & Complementary Medicine, 15*(8): 929–934. doi: 10.1089/acm.2008.0152.

De Araujo, Q. R., Gattward, J. N., Almoosawi, S., Silva, M. D., Dantas, P. A., & De Araujo Júnior, Q. R. (2016). Cocoa and human health: From head to foot – a review. *Critical Reviews in Food Science and Nutrition, 56*(1): 1–12. doi: 10.1080/10408398.2012.657921.

Emoto, M. (2005). *The Hidden Messages in Water*. London: Pocket.

Fallon, S., Enig, M. G., Murray, K., & Dearth, M. (2005). *Nourishing Traditions: The Cookbook that Challenges Politically Correct Nutrition and the Diet Dictocrats*. Washington, DC: New Trends.

Farooq, S. M., Boppana, N. B., Devarajan, A., Sekaran, S. D., Shankar, E. M., Li, C., Gopal, K., Bakar, S. A., & Gerber, R. (2000). *Vibrational Medicine for the 21st Century: The Complete Guide to Energy Healing and Spiritual Transformation* (p. 377). New York: Eagle Brook.

Herz, C., Tran, H. T., Márton, M. R., Maul, R., Baldermann, S., Schreiner, M., & Lamy, E. (2017). Evaluation of an aqueous extract from horseradish root (*Armoracia rusticana radix*) against lipopolysaccharide-induced cellular inflammation reaction. *Evidence-Based Complementary and Alternative Medicine*: 1950692. doi: 10.1155/2017/1950692.

Hewlings, S. J., & Kalman, D. S. (2017). Curcumin: A review of its effects on human health. *Foods (Basel, Switzerland)*, *6*(10): 92. doi: 10.3390/foods6100092.

Karthik, H. S., & Ebrahim, A. S. (2014). C-phycocyanin confers protection against oxalate-mediated oxidative stress and mitochondrial dysfunctions in MDCK cells. *PLoS One*, *9*(4): e93056. doi: 10.1371/journal.pone.0093056. Erratum in: PLoS One. *9*(7): e103361. Asokan, Devarajan [corrected to Devarajan, Asokan].

Kössler, S., Nofziger, C., Jakab, M., Dossena, S., & Paulmichi, M. (2012). Curcumin affects cell survival and cell volume regulation in human renal and intestinal cells. *Toxicology*, *292*(2–3): 123–135. doi: 10.1016/j.tox.2011.12.002.

Massa, N. M. L., Silva, A. S., Toscano, L. T., Silva, J. D. G. R., Persuhn, D. C., & Gonçalves, M. da C. R. (2016). Watermelon extract reduces blood pressure but does not change sympathovagal balance in prehypertensive and hypertensive subjects. *Blood Pressure*, *25*(4): 244–248. doi: 10.3109/08037051.2016.1150561.

Pourmasoumi, M., Hadi, A., Najafgholizadeh, A., Joukar, F., & Mansour-Ghanaei, F. (2020). The effects of cranberry on cardiovascular metabolic risk factors: A systematic review and meta-analysis. *Clinical Nutrition*, *39*(3): 774–788. doi: 10.1016/j.clnu.2019.04.003.

Rull, G., Mohd-Zain, Z. N., Shiel, J., Lundberg, M. H., Collier, D. J., Johnston, A., Warner, T. D., & Corder, R. (2015). Effects of high flavanol dark chocolate on cardiovascular function and platelet aggregation. *Vascular Pharmacology*, *71*: 70–78. doi: 10.1016/j.vph.2015.02.010.

Tahri, A., Yamani, S., Legssyer, A., Aziz, M., Mekhfi, H., Bnouham, M., & Ziyyat, A. (2000). Acute diuretic, natriuretic and hypotensive effects of a continuous perfusion of aqueous extract of Urtica dioica in the rat. *Journal of Ethnopharmacology*, *73*(1–2): 95–100. doi: 10.1016/s0378-8741(00)00270-1.

Xiong, X. J., Wang, P. Q., Li, S. J., Li, X. K., Zhang, Y. Q., & Wang, J. (2015). Garlic for hypertension: A systematic review and meta-analysis of randomized controlled trials. *Phytomedicine*, *22*(3): 352–361. doi: 10.1016/j.phymed.2014.12.013.

BIBLIOGRAPHY

Andrews, E. (2006). *Animal Speak: The Spiritual & Magical Powers of Creatures Great & Small*. Woodbury, MN: Llewellyn.

Barnes, J., Anderson, L. A., & Phillipson, J. D. (2002). *Herbal Medicines: A Guide for Health-Care Professionals*. 2nd revised edition. London: Pharmaceutical.

Battaglia, S. (1995). *The Complete Guide to Aromatherapy*. Brisbane, Australia: Perfect Potion.

Bender, S. S., & Sise, M. T. (2008). *The Energy of Belief: Psychology's Power Tools to Focus Intention and Release Blocking Beliefs*. Santa Rosa, CA: Energy Psychology Press.

Brennan, B. A. (1988). *Hands of Light: A Guide to Healing Through the Human Energy Field*. New York: Bantam.

Brennan, B. A. (2017). *Core Light Healing: My Personal Journey and Advanced Concepts for Creating the Life You Long to Live*. Carlsbad, CA: Hay House.

Chevallier, A. (2016). *The Encyclopedia of Herbal Medicine*. London: Dorling Kindersley.

Craydon, D., & Bellows, W. (2005). *Floral Acupuncture: Applying the Flower Essences of Dr. Bach to Acupuncture Sites*. Berkeley, CA: Crossing.

Cunningham, D. (1992). *Flower Remedies Handbook: Emotional Healing & Growth with Bach & Other Flower Essences*. New York: Sterling.

Cunningham, S. (1995). *Cunningham's Encyclopedia of Crystal, Gem and Metal Magic*. St. Paul, MN: Newellyn.

Dava Michelson Five Element Acupuncture. https://davamichelson.com (accessed June 16, 2020).

Gladstar, R. (2008). *Rosemary Gladstar's Herbal Recipes for Vibrant Health: 175 Teas, Tonics, Oils, Salves, Tinctures, and Other Natural Remedies for the Entire Family*. North Adams, MA: Storey.

Gladstar, R. (2012). *Medicinal Herbs. A Beginner's Guide. 33 Healing Herbs to Know, Grow, and Use*. North Adams, MA: Storey.

Godfrey, A., & Saunders, P. R. (2010). *Principles & Practices of Naturopathic Botanical Medicine*. Toronto, Canada: Canadian College of Naturopathic Medicine Press.

Gonzalez, G. (2012). *Holographic Healing: 5 Keys to Nervous System Consciousness*. Kingston, WA: Quantum Neurology Registered Publications.

Green, J. (1940). *The Herbal Medicine-Maker's Handbook: A Home Manual*. 4th revised edition. Forestville, CA: Simplers Botanical.

Gueniot, G., & Ledoux, F. (2012). *Phytembryotherapy: The Embryo of Gemmotherapy*. Brussels: Éditions Amyris.

"Gurudas". (1985). *Gem Elixirs and Vibrational Healing. Vol. 1*. Boulder, CO: Cassandra.

"Gurudas". (1986). *Flower Essences and Vibrational Healing*. Albuquerque, NM: Brotherhood of Life.

Hoffmann, D. (2003). *Medical Herbalism: The Science and Practice of Herbal Medicine*. Rochester, VT: Inner Traditions/Bear.

Inner Search Foundation (1990). *Life Plan: Finding Your Real Self. The Journey Through Life*. Mumbai, India: Inner Search Foundation.

Kaminski, P., & Katz, R. (2004). *Flower Essence Repertory: A Comprehensive Guide to North American and English Flower Essences for Emotional and Spiritual Well-being*. Nevada City, CA: Flower Essence Society.

Katz, M. (2004). *Gemstone Energy Medicine: Healing Body, Mind and Spirit*. Portland, OR: Natural Healing Press.

Katz, M. (2005). *Wisdom of the Gemstone Guardians*. Portland, OR: Natural Healing Press.

Le Page, J., & Le Page, L. (2014). *Mudras: For Healing and Transformation*. 2nd edition. Sebastopol, CA: Integrative Yoga Therapy.

Le Page, J., Le Page, L., Rezek, S., & Barbosa, C. E. (2013). *Mudras: for Healing and Transformation*. Sebastopol, CA: Integrative Yoga Therapy.

Lipton, B. H. (2015). *The Biology of Belief: Unleashing the Power of Consciousness, Matter & Miracles*. Carlsbad, CA: Hay House.

Mackenna, B. R., & Callander, R. (1997). *Illustrated Physiology*. New York: Churchill Livingstone.

Melody. Love Is in the Earth: A Kaleidoscope of Crystals (1995). Wheat Ridge, CO: Earth-Love Publishing House.

Mercier, P. (2007). *The Chakra Bible*. New York: Sterling.

Mojay, G. (1997). *Aromatherapy for Healing the Spirit: Restoring Emotional and Mental Balance with Essential Oils*. Rochester, VT: Healing Arts, 2003.

Mojay, G. (2005). *Aromatherapy for Healing the Spirit: a Guide to Restoring Emotional and Mental Balance through Essential Oils*. London: Gaia.

Nemerov, H. (1977). "The Consent". In: *The Collected Poems of Howard Nemerov*. Chicago, IL: University of Chicago Press.

Pizzorno, J. E., Murray, M. T., & Joiner-Bey, H. (2016). *The Clinician's Handbook of Natural Medicine*. St. Louis, MO: Elsevier.

Price, L. (1999). *Aromatherapy for Health Professionals*. 2nd edition. London: Harcourt.

Prophet, M. L., & Prophet, E. C. (2003). *The Masters and Their Retreats*. Corwin Springs, MT: Summit University Press.

Ross, J. (2004). *The Mood Cure: The 4-Step Program to Take Charge of Your Emotions – Today*. New York: Penguin.

Rudd, R. (2013). *Gene Keys: Embracing Your Higher Purpose*. London: Watkins.

Rudd, R. (2018). *The Seven Sacred Seals: Portals to Grace*. Poole, UK: Gene Keys Publishing.

Scheffer, M. (2001). *Encyclopedia of Bach Flower Therapy*. Rochester, VT: Healing Arts.

Schneider, M. S. (2015). *A Beginner's Guide to Constructing the Universe: The Mathematical Archetypes of Nature, Art, and Science*. New York: Harper.

Shamballa, R. (2019). *100 Chakra System: An Introduction to Negative Energy Release Work*. Bloomington, IN: Balboa.

Simmons, R., Ahsian, N., & Raven, H. (2015). *The Book of Stones: Who They Are & What They Teach*. East Montpelier, VT: Heaven & Earth.

Tilgner, S. M. (1999). *Herbal Medicine from the Heart of the Earth*. Creswell, OR: Wise Acres, 2009.

Wright, M. S. (1988). *Flower Essences: Reordering Our Understanding and Approach to Illness and Health*. Warrenton, VA: Perelandra.

GENERAL INDEX

www.ingramcontent.com/pod-product-compliance
Ingram Content Group UK Ltd.
Pitfield, Milton Keynes, MK11 3LW, UK
UKHW020615180726
13836UKWH00010B/2486